Guidelines for the
Blood Transfusion Services in the United Kingdom

8th edition 2013

London: TSO

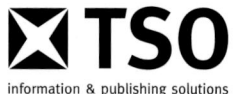
information & publishing solutions

Published by TSO (The Stationery Office) and available from:

Online
www.tsoshop.co.uk

Mail, Telephone, Fax & E-mail
TSO
PO Box 29, Norwich, NR3 1GN
Telephone orders/General enquiries: 0870 600 5522
Fax orders: 0870 600 5533
E-mail: customer.services@tso.co.uk
Textphone 0870 240 3701

TSO@Blackwell and other Accredited Agents

Published with the permission of the 4 UK Blood Services on behalf of the Controller of Her Majesty's Stationery Office.

© Crown Copyright 2013

You may re-use this document/publication (not including logos) free of charge in any format or medium, under the terms of the Open Government Licence. To view this licence, visit http://www.nationalarchives.gov.uk/doc/open-government-licence or write to the Information Policy Team, The National Archives, Kew, Richmond, Surrey TW9 4DU; or email: psi@nationalarchives.gsi.gov.uk.

First published 2013
Eighth edition 2013
First impression 2013

ISBN 9780117081673

J002703291   c10   2/13

Contents

Preface to eighth edition		xv
Chapter 1	**Introduction**	**1**
	1.1 Development of the Red Book	1
	1.2 Organisation of the UK Blood Services	2
	1.3 Other institutions involved in developing guidelines and regulations relevant to the UK	2
	1.4 References	5
Chapter 2	**Quality in Blood and Tissue Establishments and hospital blood banks**	**6**
	2.1 Introduction	6
	2.2 Key European initiatives	7
	2.3 Other standards	9
	2.4 Systems	12
	2.5 Application of a quality management system	13
	2.6 Quality management system	14
	2.7 Reporting of incidents to external bodies	21
	2.8 References	23
Chapter 3	**Care and selection of whole blood and component donors (including donors of pre-deposit autologous blood)**	**25**
	3.1 Introduction	25
	3.2 General principles	26
	3.3 Assessment of fitness to donate	26
	3.4 Informed consent	27
	3.5 Donor age	28
	3.6 Frequency of donation	29
	3.7 Volume of donation	29
	3.8 Medical history of donors	30
	3.9 Genetically determined conditions	31
	3.10 Donors on treatment with medications (drugs)	31
	3.11 Transfusion-transmissible infectious diseases	32
	3.12 Travel history	32
	3.13 Prion-associated diseases including sporadic Creutzfeldt-Jakob Disease (CJD) and variant CJD (vCJD)	32
	3.14 Physical examination of donors	33
	3.15 Blood tests	33
	3.16 Donors of pre-deposit autologous donations	35
	3.17 Donors of immune plasma	35
	3.18 References	35

	Appendix I	Extra-corporeal volume tables	36
	Appendix II	Citrate anticoagulants and the avoidance of citrate toxicity	37
	Appendix III	Volume of blood processed per pass	38

Chapter 4 Premises and quality assurance at blood donor sessions   39

4.1	Premises	39
4.2	Staffing and training principles for donation sessions	41
4.3	Collection of the donation	41
4.4	Donor identification	42
4.5	Labelling	42
4.6	Records	42
4.7	Control of purchased material and services	43
4.8	Protection and preservation of product quality	44
4.9	References	45

Chapter 5 Collection of a blood or component donation   46

5.1	Information to be provided to prospective donors of blood or blood components	46
5.2	Information to be obtained from donors by Blood Establishments at every donation	47
5.3	Haemoglobin screening	47
5.4	Preparation of the venepuncture site	48
5.5	Preparation of the blood pack	48
5.6	Performance of the venepuncture	49
5.7	Whole blood donation	49
5.8	Component donation by apheresis	50
5.9	Information to be provided to the donor post-donation	51
5.10	Adverse reactions in donors	51
5.11	Adverse events	52
5.12	Donor compensation	52
5.13	References	
	Appendix I Points of care	52
	Appendix II International Haemovigilance Network categories for donor adverse events	54
	Appendix III International Haemovigilance Network definition of severe donor adverse events	56

Chapter 6 Evaluation and manufacture of blood components   57

6.1	Scope of the guidelines	57
6.2	Setting and maintaining specifications	57
6.3	Component and process monitoring tests	58
6.4	Component processing	61
6.5	Component shelf life	63
6.6	Labelling	64
6.7	Component storage	64
6.8	Non-conforming components and biohazards	66
6.9	Component release	66
6.10	Release of components which do not conform to specified requirements	67
6.11	Transportation of blood components	67

	6.12	Component recall and traceability	69
	6.13	References	69

Chapter 7 Specifications for blood components — 70

7.1	Leucocyte depletion	70
7.2	Other component specifications	71
7.3	Production advice	72
7.4	Whole Blood, Leucocyte Depleted	73
7.5	Red Cells, Leucocyte Depleted	75
7.6	Red Cells in Additive Solution, Leucocyte Depleted	77
7.7	Red Cells, Washed, Leucocyte Depleted	79
7.8	Red Cells, Thawed and Washed, Leucocyte Depleted	81
7.9	Platelets, Pooled, Buffy Coat Derived, Leucocyte Depleted	83
7.10	Platelets, Apheresis, Leucocyte Depleted	86
7.11	Platelets in Additive Solution and Plasma, Leucocyte Depleted	88
7.12	Platelets in Additive Solution, Leucocyte Depleted	90
7.13	Granulocytes, Apheresis	92
7.14	Granulocytes, Pooled, Buffy Coat Derived, in Platelet Additive Solution and Plasma	93
7.15	Fresh Frozen Plasma, Leucocyte Depleted	95
7.16	Fresh Frozen Plasma, Methylene Blue Treated and Removed, Leucocyte Depleted	97
7.17	Cryoprecipitate, Leucocyte Depleted	100
7.18	Cryoprecipitate Pooled, Leucocyte Depleted	102
7.19	Cryoprecipitate, Methylene Blue Treated and Removed, Leucocyte Depleted	104
7.20	Plasma, Cryoprecipitate Depleted, Leucocyte Depleted	105
7.21	Components suitable for use in intrauterine transfusion, neonates and infants under 1 year	107
7.22	Red Cells for Intrauterine Transfusion (IUT), Leucocyte Depleted	107
7.23	Whole Blood for Exchange Transfusion, Leucocyte Depleted	109
7.24	Red Cells for Exchange Transfusion, Leucocyte Depleted	112
7.25	Red Cells for Neonates and Infants, Leucocyte Depleted	114
7.26	Red Cells in Additive Solution for Neonates and Infants, Leucocyte Depleted	117
7.27	Fresh Frozen Plasma, Neonatal Use, Methylene Blue Treated and Removed, Leucocyte Depleted	119
7.28	Cryoprecipitate, Methylene Blue Treated and Removed, Leucocyte Depleted	122
7.29	Platelets for Intrauterine Transfusion, Leucocyte Depleted	124
7.30	Platelets for Neonatal Use, Leucocyte Depleted	126
7.31	Irradiated components	128
7.32	References	130

Chapter 8 Evaluation of novel blood components, production processes and blood packs: generic protocols — 131

8.1	Aims and introduction	131
8.2	Evaluation of new red cell components for transfusion	134
8.3	Evaluation of new platelet components for transfusion	137
8.4	Evaluation of new fresh frozen plasma/cryoprecipitate components for transfusion	141
8.5	Generic protocol for the evaluation of apheresis equipment	144

	8.6	Generic protocol for the evaluation of blood packs for whole blood donations and apheresis collections	145
	8.7	References	153

Chapter 9 Microbiology tests for donors and donations: general specifications for laboratory test procedures — 154

	9.1	General requirements	154
	9.2	Microbiology screening	156
	9.3	Specific assays	162
	9.4	Reinstatement of blood donors	167
	9.5	Recommended standards for the reduction of bacterial contamination of blood components	168
	9.6	Recommended standards for microbiological screening	172
	9.7	Recommended standards for environmental monitoring of processing facilities	174
	9.8	Investigation of suspected bacterial contamination of blood components	176
	9.9	References	177

Chapter 10 Investigation of suspected transfusion-transmitted infection — 178

	10.1	General considerations	178
	10.2	Assessment of validity of the possible diagnosis of TTI	178
	10.3	Non-bacterial TTI: identification of possible infectious donations	179
	10.4	Investigation of possible bacterial TTI	179
	10.5	Closing TTI investigations	179
	10.6	Look-back investigations	180

Chapter 11 Reagent manufacture — 182

	11.1	Guidelines for reagent manufacture	182
	11.2	Specifications, performance evaluation and quality control of blood grouping reagents	188
	11.3	Reference preparations	203
	11.4	Recommended serological techniques for reagent testing	205
	11.5	References	212

Chapter 12 Donation testing (red cell immunohaematology) — 213

	12.1	Scope	213
	12.2	General requirements	213
	12.3	Samples	213
	12.4	Reagents and test kits	214
	12.5	Equipment	214
	12.6	Test procedure	214
	12.7	Reporting of results	215
	12.8	Release of tested components	215
	12.9	Laboratory test categories	215
	12.10	Mandatory testing of blood donations	215
	12.11	Additional testing	218
	12.12	Donations found to have a positive direct antiglobulin test	220
	12.13	Automated testing	220
	12.14	Manual testing	220

Chapter 13	**Patient testing (red cell immunohaematology)**	**221**
13.1	Scope	221
13.2	Sample acceptance and labelling	221
13.3	Pre-transfusion testing	222
13.4	Antibody quantification and titration	225
13.5	Post-examination	226
13.6	References	226

Chapter 14	**Guidelines for the use of DNA/PCR techniques in Blood Establishments**	**228**
14.1	Safety precautions	228
14.2	Avoidance of contamination	228
14.3	Working practices	229

Chapter 15	**Molecular typing for red cell antigens**	**230**
15.1	Introduction	230
15.2	Clinical applications of blood group molecular typing	230
15.3	ABO typing by molecular genetics	231
15.4	Methods available for molecular blood grouping	231
15.5	External quality assurance	232
15.6	References	233

Chapter 16	**HLA typing and HLA serology**	**234**
16.1	Preamble	234
16.2	Introduction	234
16.3	Terminology and nomenclature	235
16.4	Reagents	235
16.5	Testing of HLA genes and gene products	239
16.6	Testing for HLA-specific antibodies	239
16.7	Leucocyte crossmatching in blood transfusion	244
16.8	Application of HLA/HPA testing to patients and donors	245
16.9	References	249

Chapter 17	**Granulocyte immunology**	**250**
17.1	Reagent manufacture/reference preparations/cell panels	250
17.2	Nomenclature	251
17.3	HNA typing methods	252
17.4	HNA antibody detection methods	252
17.5	Donor testing	253
17.6	Patient testing	253
17.7	References	254

Chapter 18	**Platelet immunology**	**255**
18.1	Reagent manufacture/reference preparations	255
18.2	Methods	257
18.3	Donor testing	258
18.4	Patient testing	258
18.5	References	259

Chapter 19 Tissue banking: general principles — 260
- 19.1 Regulatory environment in the UK — 260
- 19.2 Reference documents for tissue banking — 260
- 19.3 Data protection and confidentiality — 261
- 19.4 References — 261

Chapter 20 Tissue banking: selection of donors — 263
- 20.1 General considerations — 263
- 20.2 Consent — 263
- 20.3 Medical and behavioural history — 264
- 20.4 Tissue-specific donor considerations — 266
- 20.5 Donor testing — 266
- 20.6 Living donor samples — 266
- 20.7 Deceased donor samples — 267
- 20.8 Follow-up — 267
- 20.9 Autologous tissue donation — 268
- 20.10 Archiving of donor samples — 268
- 20.11 Release criteria — 269
- 20.12 References — 269

Chapter 21 Tissue banking: tissue retrieval and processing — 270
- 21.1 General considerations — 270
- 21.2 Retrieval — 271
- 21.3 Transportation conditions from retrieval site to Tissue Establishment — 272
- 21.4 Bacteriostasis and disinfection — 272
- 21.5 General guidelines for tissue processing — 274
- 21.6 Tissue storage — 277
- 21.7 Tracking of tissues — 280
- 21.8 Notification of serious adverse events and reactions — 281
- 21.9 Additional guidelines for skeletal tissue retrieval and processing — 281
- 21.10 Cardiovascular tissue retrieval and processing — 282
- 21.11 Skin retrieval and processing — 283
- 21.12 Ocular tissue retrieval and storage — 284
- 21.13 References — 285

Chapter 22 Haemopoietic progenitor cells — 286
- 22.1 Introduction — 286
- 22.2 Terminology — 288
- 22.3 Policy and procedure requirements — 289
- 22.4 Safety requirements — 289
- 22.5 Adverse events and reactions — 289
- 22.6 Donor selection, consent and testing — 290
- 22.7 Collection facilities for HPC-A, HPC-M, HPC-C and TC — 291
- 22.8 Component definitions — 293
- 22.9 Haemopoietic progenitor cell processing standards — 294
- 22.10 Storage of cellular therapy products — 295

22.11 Testing of haemopoietic progenitor cell donors and components including therapeutic cells 297
22.12 Labelling, packaging, transportation and temperature controls 299
22.13 Release 301
22.14 Transportation 303
22.15 Thawing and infusion 303
22.16 Disposal of haemopoietic progenitor cells 304
22.17 Records 304

Chapter 23 Specification for the uniform labelling of blood, blood components and blood donor samples 306

23.1 Introduction 306
23.2 The labelling system 307
23.3 Barcode reading and interpretation 308
23.4 Donation identification numbers (DIN) 313
23.5 Blood group labels 316
23.6 Component labels 322

Chapter 24 Specification for the uniform labelling of human tissue products using ISBT 128 325

24.1 Introduction 325
24.2 The labelling system 326
24.3 General requirements 327
24.4 Tissue product labels 330

Chapter 25 Standards for electronic data interchange within the UK Blood Transfusion Services 341

25.1 Introduction 341
25.2 Control of message structures 341
25.3 General protocol 342
25.4 Envelope definition 342
25.5 Message protocols 342
25.6 Protocol 000001 – blood component dispatch information 343
25.7 Protocol 000002 – blood derivative dispatch information 346
25.8 Protocol 000003 – reagent dispatch information 346
25.9 Protocol 000004 – blood component dispatch acknowledgement 348
25.10 Protocol 000005 – blood component fate information 349

Chapter 26 Specification for blood pack base labels 352

26.1 Introduction 352
26.2 Specification 352
26.3 Manufacturers' blood pack catalogue and lot numbers 355

Chapter 27 Specification for labelling consumables used in therapeutic product production **357**

    27.1 Introduction 357
    27.2 Specification 357
    27.3 Manufacturers' catalogue and lot numbers 359
    27.4 References 359

Annex 1 Standards available from the National Institute for Biological Standards and Control **360**

Annex 2 ISBT 128 check character calculation **366**

Annex 3 Trial components **368**

Definitions **369**

Abbreviations **374**

Index **378**

Figures and tables

Figures

Figure 1.1	Standing Advisory Committees of the Joint UKBTS/HPA Professional Advisory Committee	2
Figure 3.1	Volume of blood processed per cycle vs donor haematocrit.	38
Figure 6.1	Algorithm for the selection of quality monitoring methods	59
Figure 8.1	Generic flowchart of apheresis equipment acceptance	146
Figure 9.1	Serology screening: blood donations	158
Figure 9.2	Serology screening and stem cell donations	159
Figure 9.3	Molecular screening: blood donations	160
Figure 9.4	Molecular screening for tissue and cell donors	160
Figure 9.5	Action chart – blood donor reinstatement following confirmation of screen reactivity as non-specific	167
Figure 9.6	Action chart – tissue and cell donor reinstatement following confirmation that screen reactivity is not indicative of current or past infection	169
Figure 9.7	Platelet components testing algorithm	171
Figure 9.8	Red blood cell algorithm	172
Figure 16.1	Algorithm for laboratory investigation of platelet refractoriness	247
Figure 16.2	Algorithm for laboratory investigation and reporting of TRALI case	248
Figure 21.1	An example of increasing inactivation of bacteria related to increasing the dose of the sterilant	275
Figure 23.1	Layout of labels on the manufacturer's base label	308
Figure 23.2	Two concatenation processes	310
Figure 23.3	ISBT 128 donation number sets (with and without Blood Establishment text)	313
Figure 23.4	Labels showing the use of flag characters	316
Figure 23.5	ABO/Rh blood group label layouts showing 'Do not use after' with and without time	317
Figure 23.6	Label for unit with use limitations	320
Figure 23.7	Example of a component label layout	323
Figure 24.1	Label positioning: option 1 (example; see cautionary note in text)	328
Figure 24.2	Label positioning: option 2 (example; not to scale)	328
Figure 24.3	Base label design: square format	331
Figure 24.4	Base label design: horizontal format (not to scale)	331
Figure 24.5	Donation identification number label set	332
Figure 24.6	Donation number label dimensions	333
Figure 24.7	Donation number showing process control/flags characters	333
Figure 24.8	Form boxes designed to enable accurate recording	333
Figure 24.9	Tissue product label template	334
Figure 24.10	Product label (example)	335
Figure 24.11	Tissue release status label	335
Figure 24.12	Status label (example)	335
Figure 24.13	Expiry date label (example)	340
Figure 26.1	Base label layout: dimensions in millimetres for 400 mL to 600 mL pack	352
Figure 26.2	Symbols used on blood packs and on critical consumables (ISO 3826-2, ISO 15223-1 and EN 980)	354

Tables

Table 2.1	List of some key inspection/licensing/accreditation/certification standards	10
Table 3.1	Extra-corporeal volume tables	36
Table 3.2	Citrate anticoagulants	37
Table 6.1	Discard limits	58
Table 7.1	Whole Blood, Leucocyte Depleted – additional tests	74
Table 7.2	Red Cells, Leucocyte Depleted – additional tests	76
Table 7.3	Red Cells in Additive Solution, Leucocyte Depleted – additional tests	78
Table 7.4	Red Cells, Washed, Leucocyte Depleted – additional tests	81
Table 7.5	Red Cells, Thawed and Washed, Leucocyte Depleted – additional tests	83
Table 7.6	Platelets, Pooled, Buffy Coat Derived, Leucocyte Depleted – additional tests	85
Table 7.7	Platelets, Apheresis, Leucocyte Depleted – additional tests	87
Table 7.8	Platelets in Additive Solution and Plasma – additional tests	89
Table 7.9	Platelets in Additive Solution, Leucocyte Depleted – additional tests	91
Table 7.10	Granulocytes, Apheresis – additional tests	93
Table 7.11	Granulocytes, Pooled, Buffy Coat Derived, in Additive Solution and Plasma – additional tests	95
Table 7.12	Fresh Frozen Plasma, Leucocyte Depleted – additional tests	97
Table 7.13	Fresh Frozen Plasma, Methylene Blue Treated and Removed, Leucocyte Depleted – additional tests	100
Table 7.14	Cryoprecipitate, Leucocyte Depleted – additional tests	102
Table 7.15	Cryoprecipitate Pooled, Leucocyte Depleted – additional tests	104
Table 7.16	Plasma, Cryoprecipitate Depleted, Leucocyte Depleted – additional tests	106
Table 7.17	Red Cells for Intrauterine Transfusion (IUT), Leucocyte Depleted – additional tests	109
Table 7.18	Whole Blood for Exchange Transfusion, Leucocyte Depleted – additional tests	111
Table 7.19	Red Cells for Exchange Transfusion, Leucocyte Depleted – additional tests	114
Table 7.20	Red Cells for Neonates and Infants, Leucocyte Depleted – additional tests	116
Table 7.21	Red Cells in Additive Solution for Neonates and Infants, Leucocyte Depleted – additional tests	118
Table 7.22	Fresh Frozen Plasma, Neonatal Use, Methylene Blue Treated and Removed, Leucocyte Depleted – additional tests	121
Table 7.23	Cryoprecipitate, Methylene Blue Treated and Removed, Leucocyte Depleted – additional tests	124
Table 7.24	Platelets for Intrauterine Transfusion, Leucocyte Depleted – additional tests	126
Table 7.25	Platelets for Neonatal Use, Leucocyte Depleted – additional tests	128
Table 8.1	Steps for evaluation of novel components	132
Table 8.2	Evaluation of new red cell components for transfusion: recommended tests	136
Table 8.3	*In vitro* assessment	139
Table 8.4	Evaluation of new platelet components for transfusion	140
Table 8.5	Evaluation of novel plasma components	143
Table 8.6	Summary of testing numbers required for evaluations and validations	147
Table 9.1	Screening required for blood donations	156
Table 9.2	Screening required for tissue and stem cell donations	157
Table 11.1	Label colour coding	188
Table 11.2	Grading system for serological tests	189
Table 11.3	Requirements for conventional blood typing reagents	191

Table 11.4	Chequerboard test format	210
Table 11.5	Complement C3 and C4 activation	212
Table 12.1	Minimum release criteria for blood products with antibodies of probable clinical significance	217
Table 12.2	Test monitor red cell samples	219
Table 15.1	Some blood group polymorphisms and associated gene sequence changes	232
Table 16.1	HLA antigens that are defined by serological typing (with broad specificities shown in brackets)	240
Table 16.2	Characterisation of HLA-specific antibodies	242
Table 17.1	Current nomenclature for HNA and corresponding antibodies	251
Table 18.1	Current HPA nomenclature	256
Table 21.1	Temperature/time relationships for banked tissues	273
Table 21.2	Minimum donor/recipient data set to be kept	280
Table 22.1	Requirements for the timing of testing	298
Table 22.2	Label content adapted from FACT-JACIE	300
Table 22.3	Label content for HPC-C adapted from NetCord-FACT	302
Table 23.1	Standard blood group classifications	318
Table 23.2	Usage limitation	318
Table 23.3	Blood group and donation use label text	318
Table 24.1	Statements of product status	337
Table 25.1	Envelope definition	343
Table 25.2	Message protocol numbers	343
Table 25.3	Message protocol 000001: blood component dispatch information: administration line	344
Table 25.4	Message protocol 000001: blood component dispatch information: dispatch line	344
Table 25.5	Message protocol 000001: blood component dispatch information. Field 10: red cell phenotype field – antigen codes	345
Table 25.6	Message protocol 000001: blood component dispatch information. Field 14: platelet-specific phenotype	346
Table 25.7	Message protocol 000002: blood derivative dispatch information: administration line	346
Table 25.8	Message protocol 000002: blood derivative dispatch information: dispatch line	347
Table 25.9	Message protocol 000003: reagent dispatch information: administration line	347
Table 25.10	Message protocol 000003: reagent dispatch information: dispatch line	348
Table 25.11	Message protocol 000004: blood component dispatch acknowledgement: administration line	348
Table 25.12	Message protocol 000004: blood component dispatch acknowledgement: dispatch line	349
Table 25.13	Message protocol 000005: blood component fate information: data line	350
Table 25.14	Message protocol 000005: blood component fate information. Field 8: wasted classification code	351
Table 26.1	Blood bag base label dimensions (width × depth)	355
Table 26.2	Manufacturers' Codabar codes	356
Table A1.1	Serological, virological and other preparations	360
Table A1.2	Coagulation preparations – WHO International Standards	364
Table A1.3	Coagulation preparations – British Standards	364
Table A2.1	Mapping from characters to ISO 7064 check values	366
Table A2.2	Example of displayed numbers	367

Preface to eighth edition

An in-depth service review of the Joint UKBTS/HPA Professional Advisory Committee (JPAC) conducted in 2009/10 concluded that the work of JPAC was perceived as being of high value, and that the outputs were valid and based on sound professional advice and expertise. One of the most important of these outputs is this publication. Due to undertaking the review, it has been several years since the publication of the seventh edition of the *Guidelines for the Blood Transfusion Services in the United Kingdom* (known as the Red Book). During this time numerous updates have been made to the website version and issued as change notifications. All chapters have been reviewed in preparation for this edition, revised where appropriate, and in addition some chapters have been removed and one added. It is not therefore feasible to indicate where changes have been introduced in the text, although any major changes will have been approved by JPAC prior to their inclusion.

At the time of publication of the seventh edition, the European Directives on blood and tissues and their translation into UK law had just come into force. The legal requirements of these are now well embedded into the practice of blood transfusion and tissue transplantation in the UK and continue to be reflected in these Red Book guidelines.

The most up-to-date version of the Red Book can always be found on the JPAC website, www.transfusionguidelines.org.uk. In this increasingly electronic age, we conducted a website survey among users of the Red Book in 2010 to determine whether a hard copy version was still required. Out of 223 respondents, 173 (78%) confirmed that they would prefer to have the Red Book available in both electronic and hard copy format. Working practices continue to change rapidly, however, and we will continue to monitor users' requirements in this area, particularly when deciding how future editions should be presented.

The JPAC website, in addition to hosting these guidelines, is the home of the *Donor Selection Guidelines* for blood, tissues, stem cells and cord blood, the *Handbook of Transfusion Medicine* and other transfusion-related areas. In addition, position statements and background documents written by the JPAC Standing Advisory Committees providing evidence for changes in the guidelines are posted, together with the minutes of JPAC meetings. The website is now 10 years old, and a redevelopment is being planned.

We wish to thank the Chairs and Members of the JPAC Standing Advisory Committees for their efforts and enthusiasm in reviewing the chapters for this edition, and for their continuing work in ensuring that these guidelines remain up to date and representative of best practice in transfusion and transplantation medicine. In particular I would like to thank Caroline Smith, JPAC Manager, for her unstinting work in preparing the material and organising the publication of this edition.

We are very happy to receive comments on this edition from users of the Red Book. These should be addressed to me.

Dr Sheila MacLennan (Editor)
Professional Director, Joint UKBTS/HPA Professional Advisory Committee
NHS Blood and Transplant
Bridle Path
LEEDS
LS15 7TW

sheila.maclennan@nhsbt.nhs.uk

Chapter 1
Introduction

1.1 Development of the Red Book

Guidelines for the Blood Transfusion Services in the United Kingdom was first published in 1990 by HMSO. It was compiled by experts from the then Regional Transfusion Centres and the National Institute for Biological Standards and Control (NIBSC), and aimed to define guidelines for all materials produced by the United Kingdom Blood Transfusion Services (UKBTS) for both therapeutic and diagnostic use. The driving force for this joint initiative, which started in 1987, was the imminent European Union (EU) Directive which would bind member states to introduce product liability by July 1988. It was understood that human blood and substances derived from it would be defined as 'products' in terms of this Directive, and guidelines against which manufacturers could be inspected would be required.

Since then seven editions of the Red Book (as the guidelines became known) have been published. They are compiled by a group of experts both from within the Blood Transfusion Services and from the wider NHS and universities, now called the Joint UKBTS/HPA Professional Advisory Committee (JPAC).

The Red Book contains guidelines reflecting best practice, sets standards to be met by the products, describes technical details of the processes involved and states the legally binding requirements introduced in 2005 under the Blood Safety and Quality Regulations, Statutory Instrument 2005 No. 50.[1] More detailed information about the regulatory environment relating to blood and tissues in the UK can be found in Chapter 2.

Guidelines reflect best practice and are developed by professionals in the field. JPAC consists of such professionals in blood transfusion and tissue transplantation, appointed for their expertise from throughout the UK. The Red Book reflects their work as it is implemented in the UK. The book concentrates on the products rather than their use. Clinical use of blood and blood components is outlined in the *Handbook of Transfusion Medicine*,[2] produced by collaboration between JPAC and the British Committee for Standards in Haematology (BCSH).

Professional guidelines are not legally binding but, as they reflect consensus best practice, may be taken into account by the UK judiciary. Such national guidelines have to take into account EU Directives, which have to be transposed into UK law, and these are legally binding.

JPAC, with its Standing Advisory Committees (SACs), undertakes regular review of the guidelines in the light of developments in the field, both scientific and regulatory. The overall aim is to ensure as far as possible the safety of blood transfusion in the UK, for both the donor and the patient. Changes in the guidelines are therefore likely to occur, and these will be notified on the JPAC website, www.transfusionguidelines.org.uk, where an up-to-date version of the guidelines can always be found.

The work of JPAC is conducted through expert SACs. The current SACs of JPAC are shown in Figure 1.1.

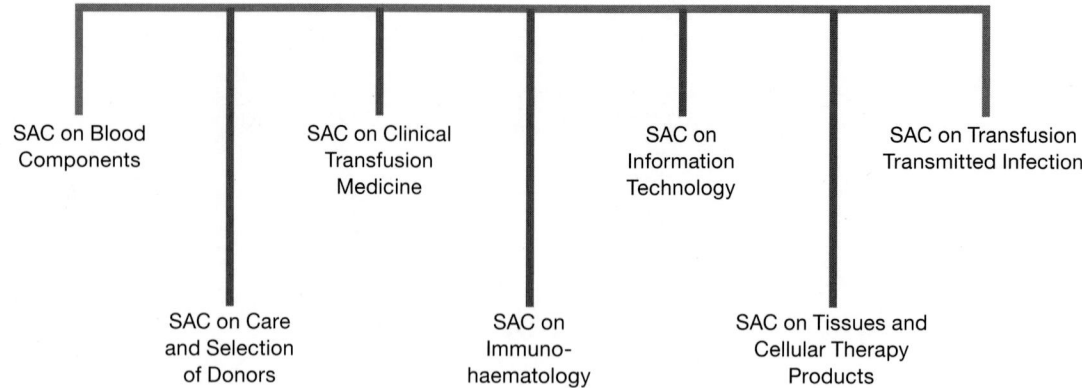

Figure 1.1 Standing Advisory Committees of the Joint UKBTS/HPA Professional Advisory Committee

1.2 Organisation of the UK Blood Services

There are four national Blood Services/Blood Transfusion Services in the UK:

- NHS Blood and Transplant (NHSBT), a Special Health Authority within the NHS, which provides Blood Services and tissues in England and North Wales, and organs for the whole of the UK.

- The Scottish National Blood Transfusion Service (SNBTS), which is managed by NHS National Services Scotland.

- The Northern Ireland Blood Transfusion Service (NIBTS), which is managed by the Northern Ireland Blood Transfusion Special Agency.

- The Welsh Blood Service (WBS), which is provided and managed by Velindre NHS Trust.

These are Blood Establishments.

Following devolution of governments in the UK, the UK Blood Services Forum was established in 1999 comprising the chief executives and medical directors of the four services, and JPAC became accountable to the medical directors, who themselves are accountable to their chief executives. The close working relationship with NIBSC (subsequently part of the Medicines and Healthcare products Regulatory Authority (MHRA) from April 2013) has been maintained through the Director of NIBSC.

1.3 Other institutions involved in developing guidelines and regulations relevant to the UK

A brief description of some international organisations and their interrelationships is required for an understanding of the regulatory environment in the UK.

1.3.1 World Health Organization

www.who.int

Established in 1948 as the United Nations' specialised agency for health, the World Health Organization (WHO) is governed by 194 member states through the World Health Assembly. Its aim is the attainment of the highest possible levels of health by all people, and clearly the availability of safe blood contributes to this aim.

The WHO produces recommendations, programmes and educational materials. The Global Collaboration in Blood Safety programme started in 1995. It was recognised that with the increased movement of populations and plasma and plasma-derived medicinal products, blood safety could only be improved through global collaboration. Consensus proposals and recommendations are addressed to the participant countries.

WHO guidelines and recommendations are not legally binding in any of the 194 countries; however, EU legislation in this field states that the advice emanating from the WHO has to be taken into account by the member states when formulating their own legislation.

1.3.2 The Council of Europe and the European Union

The Council of Europe (CoE) and the EU are two totally distinct organisations. They are easily and often confused as much of the same terminology is used. In 2012 the CoE had 47 member states with approximately 800 million inhabitants and the EU had 27, with a population of 502 million. All member states of the EU are member states of the CoE.

1.3.2.1 Council of Europe

www.coe.int

Founded in 1949, one of the Council of Europe's founding principles was the promotion of increased cooperation between member states to improve the quality of life for the population of Europe. In the field of health the CoE has consistently addressed ethical issues; the most important of these is the non-commercialisation of human substances: blood, tissues and organs. In the 1950s member states started to cooperate in blood transfusion activities. Through its committees and working parties composed of national experts, including representation from JPAC, the CoE has produced recommendations to ensure the quality of blood components and tissues and publishes guidelines as annexes to the recommendations – *Guide to the Preparation, Use and Quality Assurance of Blood Components*[3] and *Guide to Safety and Quality Assurance for the Transplantation of Organs, Tissues and Cells.*[4] These annexes are updated regularly to take account of advances in worldwide knowledge and technology.

Neither the recommendations nor the guidelines are legally binding but they are generally regarded as constituting basic best practice and many form the basis of EU Directives, which are legally binding in EU member states.

1.3.2.2 European Union

www.europa.eu

The EU was first proposed by the French Foreign Minister Robert Schuman in 1950, following the devastation of the Second World War. It was conceived to prevent further such wars. Initially it consisted of six countries. The European Coal and Steel Community (ECSC) was created in 1951: coal and steel had played a major role in the Second World War and cooperation over these assets was seen as a means of preventing further such cataclysms. The European Atomic Energy Community (EAEC or Euratom) came into force in 1958, as did the European Economic Community (EEC) created by the Treaty of Rome in 1957. The Treaty of Maastricht 1992 (the Treaty on the European Union) amended the three existing treaties giving the three Communities (ECSC, EAEC and EEC) increased powers. The EEC was renamed the European Community (EC). A 'competence' in EU terminology is a subject over which it has legislative powers. These competences are agreed by the treaties and outlined in the *acquis communautaire*. Competence in the field of blood and blood components was conferred on the EU by the Treaty of Amsterdam 1999 Article 152. It is important to note that this Article stipulates that 'member states cannot be prevented from maintaining or introducing more stringent protective measures as regards standards of quality and safety of blood and blood components'.

In 2012 the EU does not have competence over member states' healthcare services or clinical practice. This means that the laws governing blood, blood components and tissues extend only to cover the safety of the products and not their clinical use.

The five key EU institutions are:

- Parliament: elected by the peoples of the member states.
- Council of the European Union: representing the governments of the member states.
- European Commission: the driving force and executive body.
- European Court of Justice: ensuring compliance with EU law.
- European Court of Auditors: controlling sound and lawful management of the European budget.

The European Commission is the only body that can initiate legislation; the processes whereby legislation is proposed and finally adopted are complex.

Issues regarding health come under a Co-decision Procedure, which means that both the European Parliament and Council (European Council not Council of Europe) have to agree the Commission proposals.

There is open consultation on any proposed legislation. The texts of the Directives and stages in the consultation process can be found online at www.europarl.eu

Directives come into force on the day they are published in the *Official Journal of the European Union* (*OJ*) but defined time for transposition and implementation is allowed.

EU member states in 2012 were: Austria, Belgium, Bulgaria, Cyprus, Czech Republic, Denmark, Estonia, Finland, France, Germany, Greece, Hungary, Ireland, Italy, Latvia, Lithuania, Luxembourg, Malta, The Netherlands, Poland, Portugal, Romania, Slovakia, Slovenia, Spain, Sweden and the United Kingdom.

Candidate countries in 2012 were: Croatia, FYR Macedonia and Turkey.

1.3.3 European Pharmacopoeia

www.pheur.org

This CoE initiative was ratified by the EU and 30 participating member states. Pharmacopoeias are collections of standardised specifications that define the quality of pharmaceutical preparations, their constituents and even their containers. The European Pharmacopoeia (Ph Eur) monographs are binding on the EU and the participating member states.

The success of the Biological Standardisation Programme for medicines for human use of the European Pharmacopoeia Secretariat led to further collaboration between the Commission of the EU and the CoE. The European Pharmacopoeia Secretariat changed its name to the European Directorate for the Quality of Medicines & HealthCare (EDQM).

Blood transfusion activities in the EDQM are managed by the Department of Biological Standardisation, Network of Official Medicines Control Laboratories (OMCL) and Healthcare Department.

The European Medicines Agency (EMEA, www.ema.europa.eu) is a decentralised body of the EU based in London. Its main responsibility is the protection and promotion of public health through the evaluation and supervision of medicines for human and veterinary use. The EMEA coordinates the evaluation and supervision of medicinal products throughout the EU.

The Committee for Medicinal Products for Human Use (CHMP, part of the EMEA) is involved in evaluating industrially prepared plasma derivatives.

The CoE and EU work together in this field. Industrially prepared, fractionated plasma products are medicinal products and the Ph Eur monographs are mandatory.

Blood components are not 'medicinal products' and are now regulated by the EU Blood Safety and Quality Directives (see Chapter 2).

1.3.4 United Kingdom

www.cabinetoffice.gov.uk

The UK is one member state in the EU, although since 1997 there has been devolved government in Wales and Scotland and sporadically in Northern Ireland. EU legislation must be transposed into member states' own legislation within a defined time frame.

An account of European decision-making and transposition is given in the *Transposition Guide: How to Implement European Directives Effectively*.[5] This is available at www.bis.gov.uk.

The EU Directives regarding blood and blood components are transposed into The Blood Safety and Quality Regulations 2005[1] under Section 2(5) of the European Community Act (Maastricht 1992) and are binding across the UK.

1.4 References

1. Statutory Instrument 2005 No. 50. The Blood Safety and Quality Regulations 2005. Available at www.legislation.gov.uk.

2. *Handbook of Transfusion Medicine*, third edition. Available at www.transfusionguidelines.org.uk.

3. Council of Europe (2010). *Guide to the Preparation, Use and Quality Assurance of Blood Components*, 16th edition. Council of Europe Publishing.

4. Council of Europe (2010). *Guide to Safety and Quality Assurance for the Transplantation of Organs, Tissues and Cells*, fourth edition. Council of Europe Publishing.

5. *Transposition Guide: How to Implement European Directives Effectively*. Available at www.gov.uk/government/publications/implementing-eu-directives-into-uk-law

Chapter 2
Quality in Blood and Tissue Establishments and hospital blood banks

2.1 Introduction

2.1.1 The quality environment

Until fairly recently, there was no formal regulation to cover blood tissues or cells. Indeed, they were all formally excluded when the Good Manufacturing Practice (GMP) Directive[1] was updated in 2003.

This omission was deliberate, in the knowledge that separate legislation was planned for blood (the 'Blood Directives') and tissues and cells (the 'Tissues and Cells Directives'). All of this legislation is described in more detail below. This legislation has changed the regulatory landscape for the Blood Services (now known as Blood Establishments), hospital blood banks (which are now subject to regulatory scrutiny for the first time) and for tissue and cell banks (which are now under formal regulation for the first time and known as Tissue Establishments).

In this chapter, the impact of these new regulatory requirements is discussed and the management of a quality management system which meets these new regulations is described based on the requirements for the Blood Safety and Quality Directives. The requirements for Tissues and Cells Directives are similar.

The key requirements for Blood Establishments and for hospital blood banks are defined in the Blood Safety and Quality Regulations (Statutory Instrument 2005 No. 50),[2] and are enforced by the Medicines and Healthcare products Regulatory Agency (MHRA). Those for tissues and cells are defined in the Human Tissue (Quality and Safety for Human Application) Regulations, 2007 (Statutory Instrument 2007 No. 1523),[3] and are enforced by the Human Tissue Authority (HTA).

These regulations require that Blood and Tissue Establishments are licensed and subject to regular inspection for compliance. Hospital blood banks are not formally licensed, but must submit annual compliance reports to the MHRA. Based on these compliance reports, the MHRA select a number of hospital blood banks for inspection every year and can also decide to do 'for cause' inspections when there is evidence of non-compliance.

The MHRA and HTA have powers to remove licences from Blood and Tissue Establishments, respectively, and the MHRA can issue cease and desist orders to prevent blood banks from continuing in operation. These powers derive from the relevant UK legislation, which is designed to ensure that appropriate standards of performance are achieved and maintained. This inspection process is designed to generate a climate of continual quality improvement, and this chapter will look at the key issues which have to be addressed in achieving an effective quality management system.

2.2 Key European initiatives

2.2.1 European Union Blood Safety and Quality Directives

- Commission Directive 2002/98/EC of the European Parliament and of the Council of 27 January 2003 setting standards of quality and safety for the collection, testing, processing, storage and distribution of human blood and blood components and amending Directive 2001/83/EC.[4]

- Commission Directive 2004/33/EC of the European Parliament and the Council of 22 March 2004 implementing Directive 2002/98/EC of the European Parliament and of the Council as regards certain technical requirements for blood and blood components.[5]

- Commission Directive 2005/61/EC of 30 September 2005 implementing Directive 2002/98/EC of the European Parliament and of the Council as regards traceability requirements and notification of serious adverse reactions and events.[6]

- Commission Directive 2005/62/EC of 30 September 2005 implementing Directive 2002/98/EC of the European Parliament and of the Council as regards Community standards and specifications relating to a quality system for Blood Establishments.[7]

The first two Directives came into force in UK law on 8 February 2005 as the Blood Safety and Quality Regulations 2005 (BSQR),[2] with their requirements becoming effective in November 2005. They set standards of quality and safety for the collection and testing of human blood and blood components, whatever their intended purpose, and their processing, storage and distribution when intended for transfusion. The regulations also cover the collection and testing of blood and blood components for autologous use. In effect, therefore, they cover the whole process from donor to patient – from 'vein to vein'.

The latter two Directives came into force in August 2006 and relate specifically to traceability requirements and notification of adverse reactions and events, and introduce EC standards and specifications relating to a quality system for Blood Establishments. They also added provisions relating to record keeping and traceability of blood and blood components to a new category of facility, defined as a hospital, another facility or service owned or managed by a health service body, a care home, an independent clinic, a manufacturer or a biomedical research institute.

The Directives define certain activities which can only be undertaken by Blood Establishments, namely:

- the collection and testing of blood or blood components, whatever their intended purpose

- the processing, storage and distribution of blood and blood components when they are intended to be used for transfusion.

Hospital blood banks are not permitted to undertake these activities unless licensed as Blood Establishments, but are able to store, distribute and perform compatibility tests on blood and blood components for use within hospital facilities.

2.2.2 *In Vitro* Diagnostic Medical Devices Directive – 98/79/EC[8]

Following implementation of this Directive into UK law, users of *in vitro* devices must ensure that any stock produced and introduced into the supply chain is CE marked, and that only CE-marked stock can be purchased and used. There are a number of other obligations placed upon users; for example, they can be held criminally liable if they knowingly encourage the supply of non-CE-marked *in vitro* devices. The main implication for the Blood Services surrounds the provision of reagents to third parties for their use, where CE marking is required, even if there is no payment for the reagent supplied. This is a complicated piece of legislation. Blood and Tissue Establishments and hospital blood banks are significant users and producers of *in vitro* devices, and they should ensure they are compliant with the legislation and should take appropriate advice to ensure they work within the legislation.

2.2.3 Medical Devices Directive (MDD) – 93/42/EEC[9]

This Directive has been brought into UK law. It was, however, amended by Directive 98/79/EC to recognise the definition of an *in vitro* diagnostic device, which was not originally defined, and to ensure there were common definitions between the two Directives, such as the precise meaning of 'putting into service'. It is anticipated that, while Blood and Tissue Establishments and hospital blood banks may not manufacture medical devices, they are key users of such devices, from blood bags to donation beds, so knowledge of the legislation may be beneficial.

At the time of writing (late 2012) a European Consultation is in progress to review the effectiveness of the European Devices legislation.

2.2.4 Human Tissue Act 2004[10]

The Human Tissue Act 2004 replaced the Human Tissue Act 1961, the Anatomy Act 1984 and the Human Organ Transplants Act 1989 as they relate to England and Wales, and the corresponding Orders in Northern Ireland.

The Human Tissue Act 2004 covers England, Wales and Northern Ireland. It established the Human Tissue Authority (HTA) to regulate activities concerning the removal, storage, use and disposal of human tissue. Consent is the fundamental principle of the legislation and underpins the lawful removal, storage and use of body parts, organs and tissue. Different consent requirements apply when dealing with tissue from the deceased and the living. The Human Tissue Act 2004 lists the purposes for which consent is required (these are called Scheduled Purposes).

There is separate legislation in Scotland – the Human Tissue (Scotland) Act 2006.

While provisions of the Human Tissue (Scotland) Act 2006 are based on authorisation rather than consent, these are essentially both expressions of the same principle.

2.2.5 The European Union Tissues and Cells Directives

- Directive 2004/23/EC of the European Parliament and of the Council of 31 March 2004 on setting standards of quality and safety for the donation, procurement, testing, processing, preservation, storage and distribution of human tissues and cells.[11]

- Commission Directive 2006/17/EC of 8 February 2006 implementing Directive 2004/23/EC of the European Parliament and of the Council as regards certain technical requirements for the donation, procurement and testing of human tissues and cells.[12]

- Commission Directive 2006/86/EC of 24 October 2006 implementing Directive 2004/23/EC of the European Parliament and of the Council as regards traceability requirements, notification of serious adverse reactions and events, and certain technical requirements for the coding, processing, preservation, storage and distribution of human tissues and cells.[13]

These Directives establish a harmonised approach to the regulation of tissues and cells across Europe. They set a benchmark for the standards that must be met when carrying out any activity involving tissues and cells for human application (patient treatment). The Directives also require that systems are put in place to ensure that all tissues and cells used in human application are traceable from donor to recipient.

The HTA, as one of the Competent Authorities in the UK under the EU Tissues and Cells Directives, has responsibility for regulating tissues and cells (other than gametes and embryos) for human application.

2.2.6 Human Tissue (Quality and Safety for Human Application) Regulations 2007[3]

The Directives were fully implemented into UK law on 5 July 2007, via the Human Tissue (Quality and Safety for Human Application) Regulations 2007. The HTA's remit includes the regulation of:

- procurement
- testing
- processing
- storage
- distribution
- import/export

of tissues and cells for human application.

Establishments where these activities are carried out will normally need a licence. To obtain this, establishments carrying out the above activities are required to meet the standards which are detailed in the Guide to Quality and Safety Assurance for Human Tissues and Cells for Patient Treatment[14] as implemented by HTA Directions 003/2010.

The HTA also publishes Codes of Practice, which provide guidance and lay down expected standards for each of the sectors it regulates (see www.hta.gov.uk).

2.3 Other standards

There are a number of other standards that help define how a quality management system should be designed to meet the needs of a particular aspect of a Service's work. Table 2.1 provides information on some key inspection/licensing/accreditation/certification standards.

They are all applicable within England. Some apply directly to the whole of the UK (e.g. the International Standards), others to England and Wales (e.g. the NHS Litigation Authority Risk management assessment programme). Where there is not a direct cross-reference the reader should investigate further to determine how the standards might apply.

All the primary sources cited here are places where sound advice on management systems to address the various requirements of a modern Blood Service can be found. These will support the design and establishment of a system that can be confidently subjected to an external inspection process. The list is not intended to be exhaustive and by the nature of change is only current at the time of publication. It is for this reason version numbering has not been applied to the available standards; they will be constantly updated.

Table 2.1 List of some key inspection/licensing/accreditation/certification standards

Key standards	Applicable to	Responsible body	Website
BS 15000 IT Service Management Standard	Service management	BSI British Standards HQ, 389 Chiswick High Road, London W4 4AL, UK +44 208 996 9000 BSI Online, Technical Indexes Limited, Willoughby Road, Bracknell RG12 8DW, UK +44 1344 404429	www.bsigroup.com
Caldicott Report 1997, implementation 1998	Confidentiality of patient data	Department of Health, Richmond House, 79 Whitehall, London SW1A 2NL, UK +44 207 210 4850	www.dh.gov.uk
Care Quality Commission	To regulate and inspect health and social care services in England	Care Quality Commission National Correspondence, Citygate, Gallowgate, Newcastle upon Tyne NE1 4PA, UK +44 3000 616161	www.cqc.org.uk
or Healthcare Inspectorate Wales	Healthcare Inspectorate Wales is the independent inspectorate and regulator of all healthcare in Wales	Healthcare Inspectorate Wales, Bevan House, Caerphilly Business Park, Van Road, Caerphilly CF83 3ED, UK +44 29 2092 8850	
or NHS Quality Improvement Scotland	Improving the quality of care and treatment delivered by NHS Scotland	NHS Quality Improvement Scotland, Edinburgh Office, Elliott House, 8–10 Hillside Crescent, Edinburgh EH7 5EA, UK +44 131 623 4300	
or The Regulation and Quality Improvement Authority Northern Ireland Department of Health, Social Services and Public Safety	Responsible for monitoring and inspecting the availability and quality of health and social care services in Northern Ireland, and encouraging improvements in the quality of those services Controls assurance standards	The Regulation and Quality Improvement Authority, 9th Floor, Riverside Tower, 5 Lanyon Place, Belfast BT1 3BT, UK +44 28 9051 7500 Central ALB Governance Unit, Department of Health, Social Services and Public Safety, Castle Buildings, Stormont Estate, Belfast BT4 3SQ, UK +44 28 9052 2792	
European Foundation for Quality Management (EFQM) Self-Assessment	Measurement of the effectiveness and, over time, the improvement in a Blood Service's management system. Helping understand where they are on the path to excellence	British Quality Foundation, 32–34 Great Peter Street, London SW1P 2QX, UK +44 207 654 5000	www.bqf.org.uk www.efqm.org

Key standards	Applicable to	Responsible body	Website
European Blood Inspection System (EuBIS)	European project addressing the safety of blood transfusion	Institut für Transfusionsmedizin und Immunhämatologie, DRK-Blutspendedienst, Klinikum der Johann Wolfgang Goethe Universität, Sandhofstrasse 1, D-60528 Frankfurt am Main, Germany	www.eubis-europe.eu
European Federation for Immunogenetics (EFI)	Histocompatibility and Immunology (H&I) – reference and tissue typing	European Federation for Immunogenetics (EFI), EFI Central Office, c/o Department of Immunohematology and Blood Transfusion, Leiden University Medical Centre, Building 1 E3-Q, PO Box 9600, 2300 RC Leiden, The Netherlands	www.efiweb.eu
Good Automated Manufacturing Practice (GAMP) Guide for Validation of Automated Systems in Pharmaceutical Manufacture	Validation of computer system	International Society for Pharmaceutical Engineering, European Office, 7 Ave des Gaulois, B-1040, Brussels, Belgium +32 2 743 44 22	www.ispe.org
Good Manufacturing Practice (GMP) guidelines	Pharmaceutical environments	The European Commission publishes this online as EudraLex Volume 4	http://ec.europa.eu/health/documents/eudralex/vol-4/index_en.htm
HTA Directions 003/2010 – the standards required under the Human Tissue (Quality and Safety of Tissues and Cells for Human Application) Regulations 2007 HTA Codes of Practice	Tissue banking activity	Human Tissue Authority, 151 Buckingham Palace Road, Victoria, London SW1W 9SZ, UK	www.hta.gov.uk
International standards for unrelated haematopoietic stem cell donor registries WMDA Accreditation Programme	Stem cell and donor registries	World Marrow Donor Association, WMDA Office, Europdonor Foundation, Plesmanlaan 1b, 2333 BZ Leiden, The Netherlands Fax: +31 71 5210457	www.worldmarrow.org/
ISO 17799 Information Security Management	Information security	BSI British Standards HQ, 389 Chiswick High Road, London W4 4AL, UK +44 208 996 9000 BSI Online, Technical Indexes Limited, Willoughby Road, Bracknell RG12 8DW, UK +44 1344 404429	www.bsigroup.com

Table continues

Table 2.1 continued

Key standards	Applicable to	Responsible body	Website
ISO 9000 2000 and ISO 9001 2008 Quality management system requirements	Quality management system	BSI British Standards HQ, 389 Chiswick High Road, London W4 4AL, UK +44 208 996 9000 BSI Online, Technical Indexes Limited, Willoughby Road, Bracknell RG12 8DW, UK +44 1344 404429	www.bsigroup.com
Joint Accreditation ICT Europe and EBMT (JACIE) assessment standard	Stem Cell Immunology – Human Progenitor Cells (SCI – HPC) collection, processing and storage	The Joint Accreditation Committee EBMT-EuroISHAGE (JACIE) Alvaro Urbano-Ispizua, JACIE Office, Hospital Clinic, Villarroel 170, 08036 Barcelona, Spain Tel: +34 93 454 9543 Fax: +34 93 453 1263	www.jacie.org/standards/interim-standards
NHSLA risk management assessment programme for NHS Trusts	Management of claims and litigation	National Health Service Litigation Authority, Napier House, 24 High Holborn, London WC1V 6AZ, UK +44 207 430 8700	www.nhsla.com
PRINCE2	Project control	Cabinet Office, Service Desk, Rosebery Court, St Andrew's Business Park, Norwich NR7 0HS, UK +44 845 000 4999	www.best-management-practice.com
Standards for the Medical Laboratory	Medical laboratories	Clinical Pathology Accreditation (UK) Limited, 21–47 High Street, Feltham TW13 4UN, UK Tel: +44 20 8917 8400 Fax: +44 20 8917 8500	www.cpa-uk.co.uk

2.4 Systems

2.4.1 Quality management system

Within a Blood/Tissue Establishment an effective quality management system (QMS) is a well-designed, structured and organised method of quality assuring the provision of consistent, safe and efficacious products. It also covers all diagnostic activities, reagent production, clinical trials and R&D. It provides both a means to confirm to regulatory bodies, management and customers that the establishment's service is in compliance with relevant standards, and also a basis whereby improvement in quality may be demonstrated.

The European Blood and Safety Quality Directives require that a quality system is to be applied for any blood and blood components circulating in the EC and that member states therefore should ensure that for all blood and blood components including those coming from third countries there is a quality system in place for Blood Establishments equivalent to the quality system provided under these Directives.

The EU Tissues and Cells Directives have equivalent requirements for the provision of a quality management system. These are defined as follows: 'an efficient QMS comprises a series of inter-related elements and a quality system for Blood/Tissue Establishments should embrace the principles of quality management, quality assurance, and continuous quality improvement, and should include personnel, premises and equipment, documentation, collection, testing and processing, storage and distribution, contract management, non-conformance and self-inspection, quality control, blood component recall, and external and internal auditing'.

2.4.2 Good manufacturing practice

The application of GMP is the cornerstone of an effective QMS and provides the structure upon which the elements of the quality system can be built. The objective of GMP is formally stated as being 'to assure the quality of the medicinal product for the safety, well-being and protection of the patient'.[15] The BSQR requires that Blood Establishments and hospital blood banks meet the requirements of good practice. This is taken by the MHRA to mean that Blood Establishments and hospital blood banks should comply with all relevant sections of the EC Guidelines to GMP.[16] This applies to hospital blood banks, even though they are not manufacturing anything, but are part of the distribution chain which is defined as part of the overall manufacturing process.

The EC Guidelines to GMP are described more fully in section 2.6 using the quality system format provided by Directive 2005/62/EC.[7] Elements are presented under separate headings, and in practical terms all of these must be considered for each and every procedure or process to conform to the principles of good manufacturing practice.

2.5 Application of a quality management system

2.5.1 Blood Establishments

Blood Establishments are required under Directive 2005/62/EC[7] to implement EC standards and specifications relating to a quality system for Blood Establishments, taking fully into account the principles of GMP. Article 2 of the Directive identifies the need for Good Practice Guidelines. These are in the process of preparation and the first iteration appears in the Council of Europe's *Guide to the Preparation, Use and Quality Assurance of Blood Components*, Annex 1.[17] Over the next few editions of the guide the contents of the annex will be expanded and elaborated to fully incorporate all relevant aspects of GMP. When complete, it will become the Good Practice Guidelines referred to in Article 2 of Directive 2005/62/EC.[7]

In the absence of a complete guide, the approach we have taken in this chapter is to outline in this section the requirements of a quality management system in the context of the collection, processing, testing, storage and distribution of blood and blood components and tissues.

In addition, Blood Establishments should ensure they are compliant with the specific standards identified within the Blood Safety and Quality Regulations 2005[2] and other relevant standards and guidelines. These elements of the quality management system can be adapted to support other activities that a Blood Establishment may undertake, such as diagnostic testing and reagent production.

Blood Establishments are required to obtain a Blood Establishment Authorisation from MHRA before operating and to ensure that it is maintained through inspections scheduled every 2 years.

2.5.2 Hospital blood banks

Hospital blood banks are required to comply with the elements of the quality system outlined below relevant to their activities (see section 2.6). In addition, they must:

- Maintain donor to recipient traceability. Specifically BSQR (SI 2005 No.50) Regulation 9 (1)(e) requires hospital transfusion laboratories to 'maintain, for not less than 30 years, the data needed to ensure full traceability of blood and blood components, from the point of receipt of the blood or blood component by the hospital blood bank'.

- Undertake mandatory reporting of serious adverse events and serious adverse reactions related to transfusion to the Competent Authority. Specifically BSQR (SI 2005 No. 50) Regulation (1)(f) and Regulation 12B, Directive 2005/62 Annex, section 9.2 requires that 'there are procedures in place for quality assurance within the transfusion laboratory – Reporting Serious Adverse Events (SAE) and Serious Adverse Reactions (SAR)'.

- Complete an annual form, the Blood Compliance Report, developed by the MHRA, in which the laboratory indicates its compliance with the regulations. The form is reviewed by the Inspectorate division of the MHRA and those laboratories where there is deemed non-compliance are inspected as 'for cause' inspections. There may also be some control inspections undertaken to verify the use of the Blood Compliance Report and its completion.

- Establish their bona fides with the supplying Blood Establishment and sign a service level agreement between both parties to outline how compliance will be achieved. This must be done before a hospital blood bank can operate.

2.5.3 Tissue and cell establishments

These establishments should also operate a quality system that reflects the requirements below (section 2.6). The Tissues and Cells Directives are not as explicit on the requirements of a quality management system as the Blood Safety and Quality Directives and a quality system in the context of the Tissues and Cells Directives consists of the following elements: the organisational structure, defined responsibilities, procedures, processes, and resources for implementing quality management, and includes all activities which contribute to quality, directly or indirectly. Experience has shown that the elements below are effective in maintaining quality and safety in the procurement and supply of tissues and cells.

2.6 Quality management system

Note that where key advice is given elsewhere in the guidelines, the relevant sections have been cross-referenced. Where there is not a direct cross-reference, the reader should investigate further the relevant chapters of these guidelines and the standards in Table 2.1.

2.6.1 Personnel and organisation

The Blood Service must ensure that adequate resources are provided to implement and operate the quality management system, to continually improve its effectiveness and to satisfy customer requirements. The physical resources to undertake the work must be suitable to attain the required standards; this will include equipment, consumables, work areas, utilities etc. (see section 4.2 on staffing and training principles for donation sessions).

All personnel shall have up-to-date job descriptions that clearly set out their tasks and responsibilities. Organisations shall assign the responsibility for processing management and quality assurance to different individuals who function independently.

All personnel shall receive initial and continued training appropriate to their specific tasks. Training records shall be maintained. Training programmes shall be in place and shall include good practice.

The contents of training programmes shall be periodically assessed and the competence of personnel evaluated regularly.

There shall be written safety and hygiene instructions in place adapted to the activities to be carried out and in compliance with requirements.

2.6.2 Premises

2.6.2.1 General

Premises including mobile sites shall be adapted and maintained to suit the activities to be carried out. They shall enable the work to proceed in a logical sequence so as to minimise the risk of errors, and shall allow for effective cleaning and maintenance in order to minimise the risk of contamination (see section 6.4 on component processing).

2.6.2.2 Donation area

There shall be an area for confidential personal interviews and assessment of individuals to determine their eligibility to donate. This area shall be separated from all processing areas (see section 4.1 on premises at blood donor sessions).

2.6.2.3 Collection area

Collection shall be carried out in an area intended for safe donation, appropriately equipped for the initial treatment of donors experiencing adverse reactions or injuries from events associated with donation, and organised in such a way as to ensure the safety of both donors and personnel as well as to avoid errors in the collection procedure (see section 4.1 on premises at blood donor sessions).

2.6.2.4 Testing and processing areas

There shall be a dedicated laboratory area for testing that is separate from the processing area with access restricted to authorised personnel.

2.6.2.5 Storage areas

Storage areas shall provide for properly secure and segregated storage of different categories of blood, blood components, tissues and materials including quarantine and released materials and donations collected under special criteria (e.g. autologous donation).

Provisions shall be in place in the event of equipment or power failure in the main storage facility (see section 6.7.1 on the specifications for component storage areas).

2.6.2.6 Waste disposal area

An area shall be designated for the safe disposal of waste, disposable items used during the collection, testing and processing, and for rejected blood or blood components.

2.6.3 Equipment and materials

2.6.3.1 Equipment checks and record keeping

All equipment shall be validated, calibrated and maintained to suit its intended purpose. Operating instructions shall be available and appropriate records kept.

2.6.3.2 Selection of equipment

Equipment shall be selected to minimise any hazard to donors, personnel or blood components.

2.6.3.3 Selection of materials

Only reagents and materials from approved suppliers that meet the documented requirements and specifications shall be used. Critical materials shall be released by a person qualified to perform this task. Where relevant, materials, reagents and equipment shall meet the requirements of Directive 93/42/EEC[9] for medical devices and Directive 98/79/EC[8] for *in vitro* diagnostic medical devices or comply with equivalent standards in the case of collection in third countries (see section 4.7 on the control of purchased material and services).

2.6.3.4 Inventory records

Inventory records shall be retained for a period acceptable to and agreed with the Competent Authority.

2.6.3.5 Computerised systems

When computerised systems are used, software, hardware and back-up procedures must be checked regularly to ensure reliability, be validated before use, and be maintained in a validated state. Hardware and software shall be protected against unauthorised use or unauthorised changes. The back-up procedure shall prevent loss of or damage to data at expected and unexpected downtimes or function failures.

2.6.4 Change control

There shall be a system of change control in process. The system's aims shall be to ensure that changes are evaluated and made only if they provide tangible benefits to the organisation as judged by, for example, benefit to patients through risk reduction. It may also be driven by efficiency savings to ensure that maximum resources are devoted to patient care.

The system shall then ensure that the change is planned and implemented in a controlled way, incorporating training for staff in new procedures, and demonstration that the expected outcome has been delivered. Supporting documentation, including for example standard operating procedures (SOPs), shall ensure there is a record of the processes operated before and after the change, that the date of the change is known, and that material processes through the changed system can be identified.

There shall also be a system to ensure that the effectiveness of the newly implemented process is monitored and opportunities for further improvement are investigated and, where relevant, implemented. It shall support the organisation in trying to learn from incidents, complaints and other event information, as analysis of this will help identify potential beneficial changes.

2.6.5 Validation

Validation is a pre-defined exercise to ensure that equipment or a procedure (either current or proposed) is fit for its intended purpose and meets its pre-defined specification. The benefits of validation include assurance that critical aspects of a process are in control, increased probability of uniform product quality, reduced product waste and reduced customer complaints. New equipment, blood packs and manufacturing processes are examples where validation is essential before they are introduced into routine application.

2.6.6 Documentation

Effective documentation, whether in written or electronic format, must be accurate, authorised, controlled at issue and reviewed on a regular basis to ensure that it remains relevant. It provides clear instructions on what to do and prevents errors that may result from spoken communication. Records must be legible and made at the time actions are completed using indelible ink; corrections shall be signed and dated and made so that the original entry can be seen. This ensures consistency of manufacture and service provision, provides objective evidence that tasks have been correctly performed, permits investigation if problems arise and facilitates traceability from donor to patient and vice versa.

Records can be transferred to other media following procedures which meet applicable British or international standards.

Comprehensive documentation includes a hierarchy of documentation starting with:

- a quality manual
- policies
- specifications
- SOPs
- forms and worksheets, batch processing records, labels, equipment logbooks and investigation/validation records.

Effective document control must be practised to ensure that documents being used are current and an archive of superseded documents shall be established to provide an historical record.

2.6.7 Collection

2.6.7.1 Donor eligibility

- Procedures for safe donor identification, suitability interview and eligibility assessment shall be implemented and maintained. They shall take place before each donation and comply with legislative requirements (see section 3.2 on blood donation, and section 20.1 on tissue donation).
- The interview shall be conducted in such a way as to ensure confidentiality (see section 3.4 on informed consent for blood donation, and section 20.2 for tissue donation).
- The donor suitability records and final assessment shall be signed by a qualified health professional (see section 3.4 on informed consent for blood donation, and section 20.2 for tissue donation).

2.6.7.2 Collection of donated blood, blood components and tissues

- The collection procedure shall be designed to ensure that the identity of the donor is verified and securely recorded and that the link between the donor and the blood, blood components and blood samples is clearly established (see Chapter 5 on the collection of a blood component).

- The sterile systems used for the collection of donations and their processing shall be CE marked or comply with equivalent standards if the donations are collected in developing countries. The batch number of the key consumables shall be traceable for each blood component (see section 4.7 on the control of purchased material and services).

- Collection procedures shall minimise the risk of microbial contamination.

- Laboratory samples shall be taken at the time of donation and appropriately stored prior to testing.

- The procedure used for the labelling of records, donations and laboratory samples with donation numbers shall be designed to avoid any risk of identification error and mix-up.

- After collection, the donations shall be handled in a way that maintains their quality at a storage and transport temperature appropriate to further processing requirements.

- There shall be a system in place to ensure that each donation can be linked to the collection and processing system into which it was collected and/or processed.

2.6.8 Manufacture

2.6.8.1 Procedures and controls

Manufacturing processes must follow clearly defined procedures in order to obtain products or services of the requisite quality. The inputs to any process must be controlled: for example the use of approved suppliers to agreed specifications. Goods requiring incoming inspection must be held in quarantine until the inspection has been performed. During manufacture any in-process controls shall be carried out and recorded (see Chapter 7 on specifications for blood components). Statistical techniques may be used to provide confidence that processes remain in control.

2.6.8.2 Calibration

Calibration is a procedure that confirms, under defined conditions, the relationship between values obtained from an instrument or system and those obtained using an appropriate certified standard. Examples include any equipment from which physical measurements are obtained, for example weights, scales, temperature loggers, thermometers, light sources etc.

2.6.8.3 Quality control and quality monitoring

These provide confirmation either during or at completion of a process that manufacturing materials, processes and products meet their pre-defined specification. They may be release requirements (quality control tests), such as a non-reactive microbiological test results or demonstration of the effectiveness of a new batch of reagents (see Chapter 9 on microbiology tests for donors and donations, and section 20.5 on tissue donor testing). They may provide evidence that systems are operating as expected (quality monitoring), such as meeting a stated leucodepletion requirement by random sampling of finished product, or testing white cell content and then subjecting the result to statistical analysis perhaps by the use of control charts (see section 6.3 on component and process monitoring tests). These latter tests would not normally prevent the issue of material.

2.6.8.4 Proficiency testing

Proficiency testing monitors the capability to perform procedures within defined limits of accuracy by analysis of unknown samples. Successful outcomes are dependent on the combined outputs of operators, equipment and process. Proficiency testing exercises are applied to a wide spectrum of laboratory procedures and may be managed on a local or national basis. National External Quality Assurance Schemes (NEQAS) are widely used in the UK.

2.6.8.5 Contract manufacture

When contract manufacture/testing are undertaken the company supplying the goods or service shall have been employed following a formal contracting process. This shall include supplier audit, if the goods or service had been deemed critical, on the basis of a GMP risk assessment, by the organisation letting the contract. The goods and services provided shall be subject to regular monitoring to ensure they comply with the service specified in the original contract and may be subject to ongoing audit depending on the quality of the service/goods provided and their criticality to the organisation letting the contract.

2.6.9 Labelling

At all stages, all containers shall be labelled with relevant information of their identity. In the absence of a validated computerised system for status control, the labelling shall clearly distinguish released from non-released units of blood and blood components (see section 6.6 for labelling of blood components).

The labelling system for the collected donations, intermediate and finished blood components, tissues and samples must unmistakably identify the type of content, and comply with the labelling and traceability requirements.

For autologous blood and blood components, the label also shall comply with requirements.

2.6.10 Release of blood and tissue components

There shall be a safe and secure system to prevent release until all mandatory requirements have been fulfilled (see Chapter 9 on microbiology tests for donors and donations for blood, and section 20.11 on release criteria for tissues). Each establishment shall be able to demonstrate that each blood, blood component, tissue, reagent or diagnostic test result has been formally released by an authorised person. Records shall demonstrate that before a blood component or tissue is released, all current declaration forms, relevant medical records and test results meet all acceptance criteria.

Before release, blood and blood components, tissues and reagents shall be kept administratively and physically segregated from released items. In the absence of a validated computerised system for status control a labelling system shall identify the release status.

In the event that an item fails release due to a confirmed positive infection test result, a check shall be made to ensure that other components from the same donation and components prepared from previous donations given by the donor are identified. There shall be an immediate update of the donor record.

2.6.11 Storage and distribution

Procedures for storage and distribution shall be validated to ensure blood and blood component quality during the entire storage period and to exclude mix-ups of blood components (see section 6.7 on component storage).

Autologous blood, blood components and tissues as well as blood components and tissues collected and prepared for specific purposes shall be stored separately.

Appropriate records of inventory and distribution shall be kept.

Packaging shall maintain the integrity and storage temperature of blood or blood components during distribution and transportation (see section 6.11 on transportation of blood components).

Return of blood, blood components and tissues into inventory for subsequent reissue shall only be accepted when all quality requirements and procedures laid down by the Blood Establishment to ensure tissue and blood component integrity are fulfilled.

2.6.12 Traceability

There must be a system to ensure that material can be traced through the procurement, testing, and production and issue systems to a patient (for blood, see sections 5.2.1 on donor identification, and 5.5.3 on labels). If the material is donated then traceability must be maintained from the donor to the patient. Any products must be uniquely identified to help support traceability. For example, for reagents this can be to batch level. Where appropriate this should be to individual units, for example apheresis donations split into multiple doses. Any material obtained from outside the EU must maintain a standard of traceability to its origin equivalent to that expected within a Blood Establishment. Under the terms of the BSQR, traceability records of blood components must be maintained for a minimum of 30 years. A similar requirement is in place for tissues and cells under the terms of the Tissues and Cells Directive.[11]

2.6.13 Continuous improvement

It is important to take a holistic view using all available information, including information derived from analysis of incidents, errors, near misses and complaints as well as from audit processes, litigation and peer organisations. This approach will help prioritise those improvements that will be most beneficial to patients, donors and staff. As root cause analysis places a significant drain on expert resources it should be targeted on activities that on the balance of risk are most critical to the organisation. This process should be linked to the Blood Establishment's planning process so that improvements that require significant resources can be given sufficient consideration and support in their implementation.

2.6.14 Non-conformance

2.6.14.1 Deviations

Blood components or tissues deviating from required standards shall be released for transfusion only in exceptional circumstances and with the recorded agreement of the prescribing physician and the Blood Establishment physician.

2.6.14.2 Complaints

All complaints and other information, including serious adverse reactions and serious adverse events, which may suggest that defective blood components or tissues have been issued, shall be documented, carefully investigated for causative factors of the defect and, where necessary, followed by recall and the implementation of corrective actions to prevent recurrence. Procedures shall be in place to ensure that the Competent Authorities are notified as appropriate of serious adverse reactions or serious adverse events in accordance with regulatory requirements.

2.6.14.3 Recall

A system (usually, but not necessarily, computer software) shall be in place to allow full traceability of products. This will ensure that efficient recall of products can be effected and that look-back studies can be undertaken. The recall operation shall be capable of being initiated promptly and at any time. It is essential that all recalled products are stored separately and securely until a decision is made on the fate of the product. Records of recall must be maintained. A review of the recall procedures for effectiveness needs to be carried out periodically (for blood, see section 6.12 on component recall and traceability).

2.6.14.4 Serious adverse events and reactions

Serious adverse events (SAEs) and serious adverse reactions (SARs) (as defined in the EU Directives) must be reported to the relevant Competent Authority through the relevant website reporting tool:

- For blood and blood components, these are reported to the MHRA as serious adverse blood reactions and events
- For tissues, these are reported to the HTA as serious adverse events and reactions.

2.6.15 Audit (self-inspection)

Quality audit is a planned process of inspection conducted in an independent and detailed way by competent, trained individuals to ensure that procedures and associated quality assurance comply with the principles of GMP. The results of such inspections shall be recorded and non-compliances reported in writing to a designated individual whose responsibility it is to ensure corrective and preventive actions are applied in an effective and timely manner.

There will also be an opportunity to learn from the problems identified through audit, to identify underlying root cause and possibly to support conclusions on areas to improve, identified through incidents and error reporting. As noted above this process should also be linked to the Blood Service's planning process so that improvements that require significant resources can be given sufficient consideration and support in their implementation.

For Blood and Tissue Establishments, audits shall extend to suppliers of goods and services. The frequency or appropriateness of audit shall be decided on the basis of risk. This can be incorporated into the procurement system.

2.7 Reporting of incidents to external bodies

2.7.1 Serious Hazards of Transfusion (www.shotuk.org)

For blood components, serious adverse reactions and events must be reported to the MHRA (see section 2.6.14.4). However, in addition, blood banks and Blood Establishments are encouraged to report to the Serious Hazards of Transfusion (SHOT) scheme. SHOT collects data on serious sequelae of transfusion of blood components. Through the participating bodies, the information obtained contributes to improving the safety of the transfusion process, informing policy within the transfusion services, improving standards of hospital transfusion practice and aiding production of clinical guidelines for the use of blood components.

Participation in the scheme is voluntary, and covers both NHS and private hospitals in the UK and Ireland. Reports are made via SABRE (see www.mhra.gov.uk/Safetyinformation/Reportingsafetyproblems/Blood/index.htm).

Near misses should also be reported to SHOT. These are incidents where an action has placed a patient at risk. This could include, for example, the placing in stock of incorrectly labelled blood components where the discrepancy in blood group, genotype or test status would have placed a patient at risk of an adverse outcome if the component had been transfused.

It is assumed that if transfusion of products in this 'near miss' category occurs resulting in adverse outcome the incident would be reported back to the supplying service, so that they can investigate, identify root cause and prevent further occurrence. In this case it is important that it is understood that in these situations capturing data about events is not about assigning blame or liability but is about improving systems and reducing risk. Such incidents should also be reported to SHOT.

2.7.2 Devices (www.mhra.gov.uk)

The remit of the Medicines and Healthcare products Regulatory Agency (MHRA) is to enhance and safeguard the health of the public by ensuring that medicines work and are acceptably safe.

Blood Services, blood and tissue banks shall have a mechanism to report problems with medicines, medical devices or *in vitro* diagnostic devices to the MHRA. This will provide an opportunity for problems with medicines and devices to be viewed on a UK or European-wide level.

There may be additional local requirements which also must be met. For example, in Northern Ireland there has been a recent Directive that all critical adverse incidents be reported directly to the Northern Ireland Department of Health, Social Services and Public Safety.

2.7.3 Serious untoward incidents

Serious untoward incidents can be defined as 'something out of the ordinary, or unexpected, with the potential to cause serious harm, and/or likely to attract public and media interest that occurs on NHS premises or in the provision of an NHS or a commissioned service' (NHS London, 2007).[18] Blood Services may choose to refine this definition further.

Many of these incidents will be captured and investigated using a Blood Service's quality management system processes. Investigations shall be undertaken promptly, be coordinated by a board director and shall be considered for reporting externally.

Reports may be referred to:

- Department of Health or equivalent

- National Patient Safety Agency (NPSA), although the lead report should be from the Trust or facility where the patient involvement occurred. If this is not a Blood Service then the final report should contain the blood service's contribution

- National Health Service Litigation Authority (NHSLA) if litigation may result

- NHS Information Authority (NHSIA) for IT-related events

- Police in the case of criminal activity

- Health and Safety Executive (HSE) – RIDDOR

- Department of Health Estates and Facilities for fires

- Local Counter-Fraud Specialist (LCFS) for fraud

- Department of Health Estates and Facilities for defect and failure reporting in plant or facility or associated services

- Other stakeholders identified as relevant during the investigation of the serious untoward incident.

2.8 References

1. Commission Directive 2003/94/EC laying down the principles and guidelines of good manufacturing practice in respect of medicinal products for human use and investigational medicinal products for human use. *OJ*, L 262/22, 14.10.2003.

2. Statutory Instrument 2005 No. 50. The Blood Safety and Quality Regulations 2005. Available at www.legislation.gov.uk.

3. Statutory Instrument 2007 No. 1523. The Human Tissue (Quality and Safety for Human Application) Regulations 2007. Available at www.legislation.gov.uk.

4. Commission Directive 2002/98/EC setting standards of quality and safety for the collection, testing, processing, storage and distribution of human blood and blood components and amending Directive 2001/83/EC. *OJ*, L 33, 08.02.2003, p30.

5. Commission Directive 2004/33/EC implementing Directive 2002/98/EC of the European Parliament and of the Council as regards certain technical requirements for blood and blood components. *OJ*, L 91, 30.03.2004, p25.

6. Commission Directive 2005/61/EC implementing Directive 2002/98/EC of the European Parliament and of the Council as regards traceability requirements and notification of serious adverse reactions and events. *OJ*, L 256, 01.10.05, p32.

7. Commission Directive 2005/62/EC implementing Directive 2002/98/EC of the European Parliament and of the Council as regards Community standards and specifications relating to a quality system for blood establishments. *OJ*, L 256, 01.10.05, p41.

8. Directive 98/79/EC of the European Parliament and of the Council of 27 October 1998 on *in vitro* diagnostic medical devices'. *OJ*, L 331, 07.12.1998, p1.

9. Council Directive 93/42/EEC of 14 June 1993 concerning medical devices. *OJ*, L 169, 12.7.1993, pp1–43.

10. Human Tissue Act 2004. Available at www.legislation.gov.uk/ukpga/2004/30/pdfs/ukpga_20040030_en.pdf.

11. Directive 2004/23/EC of the European Parliament and of the Council of 31 March 2004 on setting standards of quality and safety for the donation, procurement, testing, processing, preservation, storage and distribution of human tissues and cells. *OJ*, L 102, 07.04.2004, p48.

12. Commission Directive 2006/17/EC of 8 February 2006 implementing Directive 2004/23/EC of the European Parliament and of the Council as regards certain technical requirements for the donation, procurement and testing of human tissues and cells. *OJ*, L 038, 09.02.2006, p40.

13. Commission Directive 2006/86/EC of 24 October 2006 implementing Directive 2004/23/EC of the European Parliament and of the Council as regards traceability requirements, notification of serious adverse reactions and events and certain technical requirements for the coding, processing, preservation, storage and distribution of human tissues and cells. *OJ*, L 294, 25.10.2006, p32.

14. Human Tissue Authority, Guide to Quality and Safety Assurance for Human Tissues and Cells for Patient Treatment. Available at www.hta.gov.uk.

15. Medicines and Healthcare products Regulatory Agency (2007). *Rules and Guidance for Pharmaceutical Manufacturers and Distributors 2007.* London: Pharmaceutical Press.

16. EC Guidelines to Good Manufacturing Practice. Available at http://ec.europa.eu/health/documents/eudralex/vol-4/index_en.htm.

17. Council of Europe (2013). Guide to the Preparation, Use and Quality Assurance of Blood Components, 17th edition, Appendix 1.

18. NHS London (2007). Serious Untoward Incident Guidance. www.london.nhs.uk/webfiles/tools%20and%20resources/NHSL_SUI_Guidance.pdf

Chapter 3
Care and selection of whole blood and component donors (including donors of pre-deposit autologous blood)

3.1 Introduction

All blood donors in the UK are non-remunerated volunteer donors. These guidelines relate to the collection of (a) whole blood and (b) components by automated apheresis. Their purpose is to:

- Ensure the safety of volunteer donors and the quality of collected components

- Protect recipients of blood transfusions from adverse effects, such as transmission of infectious diseases or other medical conditions and unwanted effects caused by any medications taken by the donor.

They relate only to whole blood collection and the apheresis of healthy volunteer donors and not to the clinical use of cell separators for plasma exchange and other therapeutic procedures.

A medically qualified consultant must be ultimately responsible for the selection, health and welfare of the donors. He or she should ensure that all staff are appropriately trained and that clinical standards are maintained. Extreme care should be taken to ensure that undue pressure is not put on persons to donate.

The criteria for selecting blood donors are laid down in the current Joint UKBTS/HPA Professional Advisory Committee's (JPAC) *Donor Selection Guidelines*.[1] These apply to donors of (a) whole blood and of (b) components (cells and/or plasma) collected by apheresis. Other than in exceptional circumstances (to be decided by a designated medical officer), donors for apheresis procedures shall meet the usual criteria for ordinary whole blood donations. First-time donors may give components by apheresis. Donors who will be giving platelets should have given at least one sample for mandatory infection screening within the last 2 years and at least 8 weeks prior to their platelet donation. In addition, the following criteria should be observed for apheresis donors:

- For donors between 50 kg and 60 kg in weight, the extra-corporeal volume (ECV) must be calculated and never exceed 15% (see Appendix I to this chapter).

- The minimum pre-donation platelet count must be 150×10^9/L.

- The predicted post-procedure platelet count must not be less than 100×10^9/L.

- Deferral periods for platelet donors following ingestion of drugs affecting platelet function (e.g. aspirin or non-steroidal anti-inflammatory drugs) should be in accordance with the JPAC *Donor Selection Guidelines*.[1]

- For the collection of double units of red cells by apheresis, special considerations apply. Male and female donors must be greater than 70 kg in weight.

- The haemoglobin level to donate double units of red cells must be 140 g/L for both males and females.

Guidelines for donors of pre-deposit autologous donations are outlined in section 3.16. The criteria for donors of tissues and stem cells are found in Chapters 20 and 22.

More detailed and frequently updated criteria are found in the JPAC *Donor Selection Guidelines*.[1] These form a constituent part of this chapter and must be consulted.

3.2 General principles

Only persons in good health shall be accepted as donors of blood or components for therapeutic use.

A prospective donor's medical history must be evaluated on the day of donation by a suitably qualified person who has been trained to use the JPAC *Donor Selection Guidelines*.[1]

If there is any doubt about the suitability of a prospective donor, a donation should not be taken and the details should be referred to the designated clinical support staff.

Each Blood Establishment responsible for the collection of blood should include a medical consultant who will take professional responsibility for the care and selection of donors. The immediate responsibility is that of the healthcare professional in attendance at the session. Patients referred for therapeutic venesection shall not be accepted at donation sessions (but see section 3.9.1 on donors with genetic haemochromatosis).

3.2.1 Donors with hazardous occupations or hobbies

Occupations where a delayed faint may present a hazard either to the donor or to others can be accepted only when the individual is going off duty. This would apply, for example, to train, HGV or bus drivers; heavy machine or crane operators; work involving climbing ladders or scaffolding; and miners working underground.

'Hazardous' hobbies (e.g. gliding, powered flying, car or motor cycle racing, climbing, diving etc.) should not be undertaken on the day of donation.

3.3 Assessment of fitness to donate

The combination of assessing each donor clinically (at every attendance) and testing each donation for markers of infection is essential to maximise donor and recipient safety.

Each donor must undergo an assessment based on the JPAC *Donor Selection Guidelines*[1] to determine his/her eligibility to donate. This requires each donor to complete a questionnaire and answer a series of standard questions relating to their general health, lifestyle, travel history, past medical history and medication.

In addition, as a minimum requirement for all donors on entry to the apheresis programme, their pulse and weight must be assessed and recorded.

If necessary, with the donor's consent, his/her general practitioner may be contacted for further information.

3.4 Informed consent

For consent to a procedure to be legally valid the donor must as a matter of good principle have been told the nature and purpose of the procedure as well as being warned of any substantial or unusual adverse event risk. Therefore, informed consent must be obtained by a trained person, fully conversant with the procedure. A consent form must be signed by each donor before donation.

Leaflets about donation appropriate to the procedure should be available at the session and should be studied by prospective donors to assist in the process of obtaining fully informed consent. In obtaining donor consent, the consenter must satisfy themselves that the donor has read the leaflet and has understood the following information:

- The purpose of the donation and the use of the product (clinical, research or other).
- A description of the procedure and its likely duration.
- An explanation that a voluntary donor can withdraw consent at any stage of the procedure or of an apheresis programme.
- A description of the common risks and discomfort involved in the procedures. These include:
  - for all donors:
    - dizziness and fainting
    - haematoma formation
  - for donors of components by apheresis:
    - citrate toxicity
    - red cell loss if the procedure has to be aborted and it is considered unsafe to return the red cells
    - chilling on reinfusion.

If the donor asks further questions relating to more remote hazards, they must be answered, however unlikely these hazards may be.

It is the responsibility of session staff to ensure that donors clearly understand the nature of the donation process and the associated risks involved as explained in the available literature. The donors must also understand the health check and other medical information presented to them. Donors are asked about confidential and sensitive aspects of their medical history and lifestyle. It is therefore important that blood collection sessions have facilities that offer privacy for donor interviews and that donors are assured of the confidentiality of any information they provide. For the donor's consent to be valid the donor must have capacity to consent. Capacity is defined in the Mental Capacity Act 2005.[2] The five principles of this act state that:

- The person must be assumed to have capacity unless you can establish that they have not.
- No-one should be treated as being unable to make a decision unless the Blood Service has made all practical steps to ensure that they are able to make that decision without success.
- The person may not be deemed unable to make a decision just because they appear to make an unwise decision.

- Any act done or decision made under the Act on behalf of a person who lacks capacity must be done in the best interests of that person.

- One must always consider whether you can do the same thing in a way that is less likely to infringe that person's rights and freedom of action.

We must therefore presume that every donor that we deal with has capacity to make decisions. To have capacity the person must, with the appropriate help and support, be able to understand, retain, use and/ or weigh up the information they are given to make the decision or to communicate their wishes. Just because a person is of a certain age, or has a disability, communication difficulty or medical condition we cannot assume that they lack capacity. Thus staff who consent donors must understand and apply these principles. All donors, be they 17 or 70, should have capacity when they sign their consent and it is the duty of the attending carers and healthcare professionals at the session to ensure that they do have that. Since the Family and Law Reform Act 1969 children have capacity to give consent in medical matters from the age of 16.

Third-party interpreters should not be used except as laid down in the current JPAC *Donor Selection Guidelines*[1] as there is no guarantee of understanding or the accuracy of information provided to or given by the interpreter, particularly if they are a friend, family member or are otherwise known to the donor. Blood Service staff gain sensitive medical and personally identifiable information about donors. They must not disclose information about a donor without their consent to a third party. This includes members of their family and includes the fact that they have attended for donation. Should a family member ring up to make an appointment or to ask a specific question, that specific factual question may be answered but further information about the donor should not be disclosed, e.g. 'My husband has started on treatment for high blood pressure, can he donate?' Answer – 'Yes, once he has been on the treatment for 4 weeks and as long as he has no other problems.'

Should third-party information be given to members of the Blood Service staff it must be handled as per an approved procedure to ensure that the information is acted on in an appropriate fashion and verified if at all possible regardless of the source of that third-party information (i.e. even if it is from an internal UK Blood Service source). All members of staff should be very clear that they have a duty to protect a donor's personal information and they should only disclose this information to people who have a legitimate right to know and should avoid disclosing information unnecessarily within the organisation.

Potential donors who are unable to read the literature should be informed of its contents by a suitably trained member of staff.

3.5 Donor age

Donors shall be between the ages of 17 and 65 years; i.e. from their 17th to 66th birthday inclusive. Regular and returning donors (as defined in the JPAC *Donor Selection Guidelines*[1]) may be allowed to donate beyond their 66th birthday with permission of a physician in the Blood Establishment, given annually.

It is normal practice to set an upper age limit of 60 years (up to 61st birthday inclusive) for first-time donors. However, older donors may be accepted at the discretion of the physician in the Blood Establishment.

3.6 Frequency of donation

3.6.1 Whole blood

An interval of 16 weeks between donations of whole blood is reasonable. The minimum interval is 12 weeks. Normally, no more than three donations should be collected from a female donor and four from a male donor during any 12-month period.

3.6.2 Plasma and plateletpheresis

A donor should not undergo a total of more than 24 plasma/plateletpheresis procedures per annum including not more than 12 leucapheresis procedures per annum. There should normally be a minimum of 2 weeks between plateletpheresis procedures. There should normally be a minimum of 48 hours between leucapheresis procedures and a donor should not normally undergo more than two procedures within a 7-day period.

Not more than 15 litres of plasma should be donated by one donor in a year.

Not more than 2.4 litres of plasma should be donated by one donor in any 1-month period.

After a whole blood donation, or the loss of an equivalent number of red cells during an apheresis procedure, a donor should not normally donate plasma, platelets or leucocytes for a period of 4 weeks.

3.6.3 Double red cell donations

The interdonation interval for donation of double red cells by apheresis should not be less than 26 weeks (6 months) in the absence of iron supplementation. A shorter interval may be acceptable only if confirmation of iron-replete body stores can be accurately demonstrated and monitored.

3.7 Volume of donation

For whole blood a donation of 450 mL±10% is required to ensure the final red cell component meets specification. No more than 15% of the estimated blood volume should be taken during any one donation. In general 470–475 mL of blood, excluding samples, is collected into the main pack.

Attention must be paid during apheresis to the ECV in order to avoid rendering the donor significantly hypovolaemic. Consideration must be given to the following factors:

- donor weight and estimated blood volume
- type of apheresis procedure: intermittent flow or continuous flow
- donor's haematocrit: this influences volume of plasma collected during any one cycle of an intermittent flow procedure (see Appendix III).

For any single apheresis procedure, the final collection volume should not exceed 15% of the total blood volume (TBV) excluding anticoagulant (see Appendix I).

During apheresis procedures the ECV should not exceed 15% TBV (excluding anticoagulant). Some procedures may result in a total ECV of as much as 1 litre. The procedure may need to be adjusted to suit each individual donor's safety tolerance limits. Special considerations should be given during intermittent flow apheresis procedures (see Appendices I, II and III). TBV can be estimated using the Nadler formula (see Appendix I).[3]

ECV is the total volume of blood and plasma removed from the donor at any time. It includes all blood and plasma in collection packs and contained within the machine harness (volumes contained within the collection harness can be obtained by reference to manufacturers' manuals).

Anticoagulant ratio during collection influences the volume of anticoagulant in collected plasma, e.g. anticoagulant in 1:12 ratio forms 14% of the final volume collected in a donor with a haematocrit of 45% (see Appendix II).

3.8 Medical history of donors

3.8.1 General considerations

All donors should clearly understand any information and questionnaire presented to them and must sign an appropriate document which also attests to their consent for the blood to be taken, tested and used for the benefit of patients. Any condition declared shall be discussed with the clinician in attendance at the blood collection session unless clear, unequivocal instructions regarding the responses are available to the member of staff conducting the questioning.

For details of information to be supplied to and obtained from donors see Chapter 5.

Donors whose serum or plasma or cells are to be used for laboratory, as opposed to therapeutic, purposes shall be submitted to the same routine as other donors, but some decisions regarding their suitability to donate may be different (e.g. treatment with certain medications, or on the basis of their medical history). When this is the case, secure mechanisms must be in place to ensure that the donation cannot be released for clinical purposes.

Individuals currently undergoing medical investigations or who have been referred for a specialist opinion or are on a hospital waiting list should normally be deferred. If, however, the condition or potential condition concerned would not of itself be a contraindication to donation they may be able to donate.

Donors taking part in clinical trials cannot be accepted until their involvement in the trial has finished, or the designated clinical support team member has examined the trial protocol and agreed that donors participating in that trial can be accepted. A 'clinical trial' normally implies that the donor is participating in an intervention programme – usually taking a drug or a potential drug which may be either active or a placebo. Participating in questionnaires does not constitute a clinical trial.

All donors should be made aware that recipients are at risk from transfusion, and shall be asked to report any illness that develops within 14 days of donation.

Information about either the donor or the donation which becomes available after the blood or any derivative has been issued or transfused, and which is, or may be, relevant to the safety of that blood for transfusion, should be reported to the appropriate individual, e.g. the consultant in charge of the hospital blood transfusion laboratory. Donor confidentiality must be respected.

The member of staff carrying out the donor assessment must confirm they have done so by signing the donation record. Any reason for deferral, whether temporary or permanent, must be explained to the donor and recorded.

3.9 Genetically determined conditions

An increasing number of genetically determined conditions that potentially affect donor health are being identified, and some donors have had specific tests which confirm that they possess variant genes. These include not only the haemoglobinopathies and thalassaemias, but also more recently discovered conditions such as the thrombophilias (e.g. factor V Leiden). Mere possession of such genetic variants does not debar from donation if the donor is otherwise healthy and fulfils all other selection criteria.

3.9.1 Genetic haemochromatosis

This is a special case. Blood from individuals with genetic haemochromatosis (GH) who have no symptoms arising from their GH is intrinsically safe for transfusion. However, before patients with GH who require continued venesection for the maintenance of their health are accepted as blood donors, the consultant with responsibility for donors must ensure that the following criteria are met:

- The selection criteria/methods for all donors with GH preserve the principles of altruism.

- Blood donated for therapeutic use by any donor known to have GH meets all other criteria (except donation frequency) in the JPAC *Donor Selection Guidelines*.[1] If it is clinically necessary for individuals to donate more frequently than the minimum donation interval, specific permission must be obtained from the designated clinical support officer.

- The donor is under the continuing care of a physician who is able to offer alternative venesection facilities whenever, for any reason, the donor does not meet all other criteria in the JPAC *Donor Selection Guidelines*.[1]

3.10 Donors on treatment with medications (drugs)

Donor deferral for most drugs is based on the underlying illness suffered by the donor (e.g. cardiovascular disease, diabetes, anaemia and malignancies) rather than on the properties of the drug itself. Since, in general, traces of drugs in blood and blood components are believed to be harmless to patients, many people taking medications – even when prescribed – are acceptable as blood donors as long as the reason for which the medication is taken is acceptable.

A pragmatic view should be taken of treatment of infections with antimicrobials. Provided that the donor is in good health, deferral is limited to 2 weeks from full recovery and 1 week after cessation of antimicrobial therapy, whichever is the longer. This is based on what may be regarded as a reasonable recovery period for the infection and is not related to the antimicrobial therapy itself.

Donors taking drugs which are proven or potential teratogens (e.g. vitamin A derivatives) or who are taking drugs that accumulate in tissues over long periods, should not be accepted for blood donation. Some such drugs may be taken to prevent diseases to which the donor – though currently healthy – is prone. A decision to accept should be taken after considering the pharmacodynamics of the specific drug, and its mode of action. The period of deferral after finishing a course of treatment is set out in the JPAC *Donor Selection Guidelines*.[1]

The current JPAC *Donor Selection Guidelines*[1] must be referred to for all donors who have had immunisations recently.

Sporadic self-medication with some drugs (e.g. vitamins, aspirin, sleeping tablets) need not prevent a donation being accepted, as long as the donor is in good health.

If the donor has taken drugs affecting platelet function (e.g. aspirin) within either the last 2 or 5 days (depending on the drug) the donation shall not be used for preparing platelets. A list of such drugs is in the JPAC *Donor Selection Guidelines*.[1] Other drugs or tablets may be acceptable. However, the taking of some drugs may indicate a disease that would automatically make a donor ineligible.

3.11 Transfusion-transmissible infectious diseases

Every effort is made to prevent transmission of disease by careful and appropriate selection of donors. This includes ensuring that the donor is provided with clear, understandable and up-to-date information and also ensuring that the donor has understood this information (see Chapter 5).

Donors must be assessed for their exposure to any risk of acquiring a transfusion-transmissible infection. The latest JPAC *Donor Selection Guidelines*[1] should be consulted for any donor with a relevant exposure history.

3.12 Travel history

Increased and rapid travel of the population may lead to asymptomatic people donating infectious blood. A clear and detailed travel history must be obtained from all donors to minimise the risk of transmission of malaria, *Trypanosoma cruzi* and emerging diseases such as West Nile Virus and Chikungunya virus.

The latest JPAC *Donor Selection Guidelines*[1] should be consulted for any donor with a relevant travel history.

The Blood Services and JPAC maintain close links with the World Health Organization (WHO), the European Centre for Disease Prevention and Control (ECDC) and the UK Health Protection Agency (HPA) and base the donor deferral criteria on the advice obtained. Any changes to current selection guidelines need to be rapidly communicated and this will happen through change notifications and the website www.transfusionguidelines.org.uk

3.13 Prion-associated diseases including sporadic Creutzfeldt-Jakob Disease (CJD) and variant CJD (vCJD)

Individuals who are identified as having an increased risk of developing a prion-associated disease must be permanently excluded from donation. This includes:

- individuals who have received human pituitary-derived hormones
- patients who have received grafts of human dura mater or cornea, sclera or other ocular tissue
- persons identified as being members of a family at risk of inherited prion diseases
- persons who are known to have received an allogeneic tissue or blood transfusion since 1980 (for these purposes, a transfusion is defined as any product containing red cells, platelets, granulocytes, fresh frozen plasma, cryoprecipitate-depleted plasma, buffy coat preparations and intravenous or subcutaneous human normal immunoglobulin and includes mothers whose babies have required intrauterine transfusion)

- persons who have been told that they have been put at increased risk from surgery, transfusion or transplant of tissues or organs
- persons who have been told that they may be at increased risk because a recipient of their blood or tissues has developed a prion-related disorder.

The current edition of the JPAC *Donor Selection Guidelines*[1] provides detailed advice and should be consulted.

3.14 Physical examination of donors

3.14.1 General considerations

A detailed medical assessment procedure must be conducted on all donors, as referred to above, i.e. based on the JPAC *Donor Selection Guidelines*.[1] Particular attention is required for the assessment of first-time or 'returning' donors. Returning donors are defined as those who – although formerly registered as a blood donor with one of the four national Blood Transfusion Services – have not been assessed for donation for 2 years or more.

Assessment of blood pressure is not recommended because the circumstances at blood collection sessions are not conducive to obtaining meaningful measurements. Routine measurement of blood pressure could also give the impression that Blood Establishments offer a general health screening service which might be construed as an inducement to donate.

Inspection of the donor: The donor should be in good health. Note should be taken of poor physique, debilitation, under-nutrition, plethora, jaundice, cyanosis, dyspnoea, intoxication and mental instability. When in doubt the donor should be deferred until further advice has been obtained from a designated clinical support officer.

Weight: The minimum weight for donation is 50 kg (7 stone 12 lb) or 70 kg for donors of double red cells by apheresis. Those who weigh less than 50 kg are more likely to suffer adverse reactions, in particular dizziness and fainting, after a standard donation. This is because the volume taken represents a greater proportion of their blood volume. It should be noted that donors who are obese but are towards the lower weight limit may not have a sufficient blood volume to ensure a safe donation. The estimated blood volume of women weighing less than 65 kg should be calculated and consideration given to ensuring that no more than 15% of this volume is donated by the donor at any one time.

3.15 Blood tests

3.15.1 Estimation of the concentration of haemoglobin in donor blood

The haemoglobin (Hb) concentration should be determined each time a potential donor presents. The acceptable lower limits for venous blood are 125 g/L for female donors and 135 g/L for male donors (140 g/L for all donors of double red cells by apheresis).

Several methods of screening donors for their blood Hb concentration are available (or in development). These include:

- gravimetric method using solutions of copper sulphate on blood samples obtained by fingerprick
- spectrophotometric devices using capillary or venous samples

- non-invasive technology
- full blood count using venous or capillary samples.

The final method chosen must be validated, and validation should include comparison to a full blood count measured on a venous sample.

A donor whose fingerprick sample fails the Hb screening should be offered a test on a sample of venous blood for accurate determination of their Hb concentration. This is to enable the donor to receive appropriate advice either from the donor clinical support officer or the donor's general practitioner. The Hb concentration in the venous sample may be determined immediately at the session if a suitably validated haemoglobinometric device capable of rapid and accurate analysis is available. If the concentration so determined is at or exceeds those quoted above the donor may be invited to give a full donation.

Donors whose Hb concentration is below the minimum values should not be bled. The reason for deferral should be explained and the donors advised to see their own general practitioner if this is considered to be appropriate as defined by Blood Service procedures.

If a quantitative method of Hb determination is employed, before or after the donation, individuals found to have a concentration of Hb above the normal upper limit as indicated in the JPAC *Donor Selection Guidelines*[1] should be referred for further investigations.

3.15.2 Copper sulphate haemoglobin screen

If used, aqueous copper sulphate, coloured blue, with a specific gravity of 1.053, equivalent to 125 g/L haemoglobin, is required to test female donors. If used, aqueous copper sulphate, coloured green, with a specific gravity of 1.055, equivalent to 135 g/L, is required to test male donors. These stock solutions should be colour-coded and labelled accordingly.

Stock solutions shall be stored at room temperature in tightly capped, dark glass containers to prevent evaporation and contamination. Copper sulphate solutions are temperature sensitive and must be stored and used within the temperature ranges specified in the Blood Service's procedures.

3.15.3 Additional tests for component donors

In addition, component donors should have the following blood tests performed at the initial visit:

- full blood count for all donors
- serum albumin and total serum protein levels for plasma donors (total serum protein has no relevance to platelet donors).

The lower limit of acceptability for haemoglobin level should be as for normal whole blood donation. Special considerations as stated in sections 3.6.3, 3.14.1 and 3.15.1 apply to red cell donation by apheresis.

The platelet count should be performed at each visit for plateletpheresis donors.

The full blood count must be carried out at least annually for all component donors and serum albumin and total serum proteins must be measured at least annually for plasma donors. A system must be in operation for regular review of these results, together with a documented protocol of the action to be taken in the light of any abnormal findings.

All Blood Services should perform a risk assessment to evaluate the relative risks and benefits of implementation of leucocyte antibody screening of female platelet donors. If leucocyte antibody screening is implemented, female platelet donors with a subsequent history of pregnancy (regardless of the outcome) should be re-tested (see section 16.8.8).

3.16 Donors of pre-deposit autologous donations

Autologous pre-deposit donations must be collected according to the same requirements as allogeneic donations but the deferral criteria vary. These donations must be clearly identified as such and kept separate from allogeneic donations.

3.16.1 Deferral criteria

The deferral criteria for donors of autologous pre-deposit donations in the UK, originally agreed by the British Committee for Standards in Haematology Blood Transfusion Task Force, were updated in 2007.[4]

The two main deferral criteria are serious cardiac disease (where the clinical setting of the blood collection must be taken into account) and active bacterial infection.

3.17 Donors of immune plasma

Recruitment of donors for specific immune globulins has been suspended in the UK until such time as the UK government decision to use only non-UK source plasma has been rescinded.

3.18 References

1. Joint UKBTS/HPA Professional Advisory Committee's (JPAC) *Donor Selection Guidelines*. Available at www.transfusionguidelines.org.uk.

2. The Mental Capacity Act 2005. Available at www.legislation.gov.uk.

3. Nadler SB, Hidalgo JU, Block T (1962). Prediction of blood volume in normal human adults. *Surgery*, 51, 224–232.

4. British Committee for Standards in Haematology Blood Transfusion Task Force (2007). Guidelines for policies on alternatives to allogeneic blood transfusion. 1. Predeposit autologous blood donation and transfusion. *Transfusion Medicine*, 17, 354–365.

Appendix I Extra-corporeal volume tables

To avoid symptomatic donor hypovolaemia, ECV and final collection volume in millilitres should not exceed 15% TBV (excluding anticoagulant). The maximum safe volume (in mL) is indicated in Table 3.1, after Nadler et al.[3]

Table 3.1 Extra-corporeal volume tables

Note: The bold figures to the top and left are weight (kg) and height (cm) respectively, while those to the bottom and right are weight (stone) and height (feet and inches) respectively.

MALE	Weight											
Height	50	55	60	65	70	75	80	85	90	95	100	
150	518	542	566	590	614	638	663	687	711	735	759	4' 11
153	522	546	570	594	618	642	666	691	715	739	763	5'
155	525	549	574	598	622	646	670	694	718	743	767	5' 1
158	529	553	577	602	626	650	674	698	722	746	771	5' 2
160	533	557	581	605	630	654	678	702	726	750	774	5' 3
163	537	561	585	609	634	658	682	706	730	754	778	5' 4
165	541	565	589	613	638	662	686	710	734	758	782	5' 5
168	545	569	593	617	642	666	690	714	738	762	786	5' 6
170	549	573	597	622	646	670	694	718	742	766	791	5' 7
173	553	577	602	626	650	674	698	722	746	771	795	5' 8
175	557	582	606	630	654	678	702	726	751	775	799	5' 9
178	562	586	610	634	658	682	707	731	755	779	803	5' 10
180	566	590	614	638	663	687	711	735	759	783	807	5' 11
183	570	595	619	643	667	691	715	739	764	788	812	6'
	7.9	8.7	9.5	10.2	11	11.8	12.6	13.4	14.2	15	15.7	

FEMALE	Weight											
Height	50	55	60	65	70	75	80	85	90	95	100	
150	456	481	505	530	555	580	605	630	654	679	704	4' 11
153	460	484	509	534	559	584	608	633	658	683	708	5'
155	463	488	513	538	562	587	612	637	662	686	711	5' 1
158	467	492	517	541	566	591	616	641	665	690	715	5' 2
160	471	495	520	545	570	595	620	644	669	694	719	5' 3
163	475	499	524	549	574	599	623	648	673	698	723	5' 4
165	478	503	528	553	578	602	627	652	677	702	726	5' 5
168	482	507	532	557	582	606	631	656	681	706	730	5' 6
170	486	511	536	561	586	610	635	660	685	710	734	5' 7
173	490	515	540	565	590	614	639	664	689	714	738	5' 8
175	494	519	544	569	594	618	643	668	693	718	742	5' 9
178	499	523	548	573	598	623	647	672	697	722	747	5' 10
180	503	528	552	577	602	627	652	676	701	726	751	5' 11
183	507	532	557	581	606	631	656	681	705	730	755	6'
	7.9	8.7	9.5	10.2	11	11.8	12.6	13.4	14.2	15	15.7	

Appendix II Citrate anticoagulants and the avoidance of citrate toxicity

Based on studies undertaken in 1989–1990 (personal communication, M Gesinde), the following recommendations can be made to avoid citrate toxicity during apheresis procedures.

AII.1 Intermittent flow cell separator machines

The reinfusion rate of citrated blood or plasma should not exceed 0.015 mmol citrate/kg/min.

AII.2 Continuous flow cell separator machines

The continuous reinfusion rate of citrated blood or plasma should not exceed 0.01 mmol citrate/kg/min.

AII.3 Maximum acceptable reinfusion rates (mL/min for a 70 kg donor)

For the four citrate anticoagulants that are commonly used in the UK, recommendations are represented in Table 3.2.

Table 3.2 Citrate anticoagulants

AC	AC:blood ratio	Average plasma citrate (mmol/L)	AC volume in collected plasma (%)	Plasma		Whole blood	
				Int.	Cont.	Int.	Cont.
CPD-50	1+15(1:16)	17	11	60	33	100	60
Acid CPD	1+11(1:12)	19	14	55	29	90	50
ACD-A	1+11(1:12)	16	14	60	33	100	55
ACD-A	1+7(1:8)	23	20	45	24	75	40
AC = anticoagulant, Int. = intermittent flow cell separator, Cont. = continuous flow cell separator							

Packed cells may be reinfused as quickly as the characteristics of the return system and the viscosity will allow, but not normally faster than 130 mL/min.

Packed cells may be reinfused as quickly as the characteristics of the return system and the viscosity will allow, but not normally faster than 130 mL/min.

Note: For donors weighing less than 70 kg, these reinfusion rates need to be suitably adjusted downwards to avoid citrate toxicity occurring. They may also be adjusted upwards for donors above 70 kg in weight.

If anticoagulant formulations or ratios other than those represented above are used, the procedure should be validated to ensure:

- plasma citrate levels are within the required range for fractionation purposes, i.e. 15–25 mmol/L
- the citrate molar reinfusion rate does not exceed these recommended maximum acceptable limits.

Final collection volume must not exceed 15% TBV (excluding anticoagulant).

Appendix III Volume of blood processed per pass

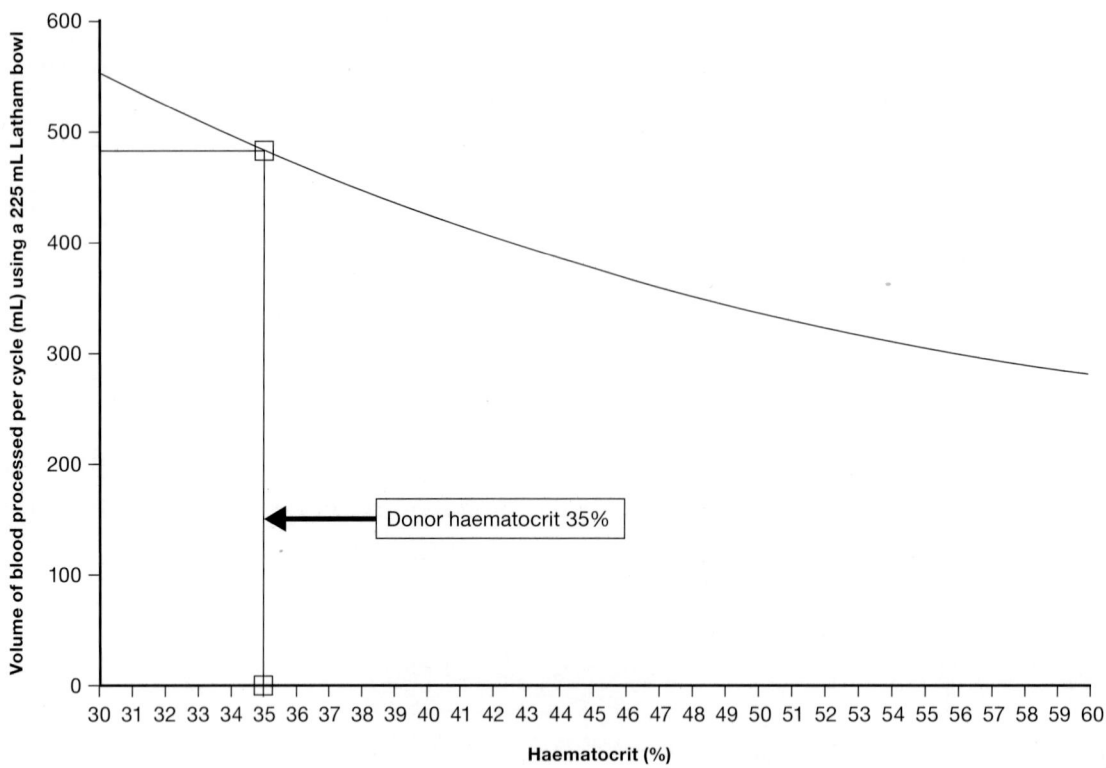

Figure 3.1 Volume of blood processed per cycle vs donor haematocrit. Based on haematocrit of 0.80 in bowl and a flow rate of 60–80 mL/min. Includes harness volume of 35 mL. Source: Haemonetics Corporation.

Figure 3.1 draws attention to the fact that for donors with a low haematocrit an increased volume of blood is processed at each pass. This will influence the ECV accumulating throughout the procedure and this particular group of donors may become symptomatically hypovolaemic.

Chapter 4
Premises and quality assurance at blood donor sessions

This chapter applies to the collection of donations of whole blood and components at permanent sites or by mobile blood collection teams.

4.1 Premises

Premises used for the preparation of components from blood and plasma have been subject to scrutiny by the Competent Authority, the Medicines and Healthcare products Regulatory Agency (MHRA), since 2005. Such facilities must comply with the principles embodied in the *Rules and Guidance for Pharmaceutical Manufacturers and Distributors 2007*.[1]

Notwithstanding the fact that premises used for mobile donor sessions may often be accepted, from necessity, as the only local venue available, they must be of sufficient size, construction and location to allow proper operation, cleaning and maintenance in accordance with accepted rules of hygiene and in compliance with the *WHO Expert Committee on Biological Standardization 43rd Report*.[2]

The designated person in charge of the blood collection team should in all cases be provided with a written plan of action appropriate to each venue. This can be used if conditions on arrival are not found to be acceptable. Care must be taken to avoid disturbances of any other activities within the venue if it is being shared.

4.1.1 Selecting a venue

Whole blood and donor component procedures for the collection of plasma, platelets, red cells or combinations of these may be carried out at fixed or mobile collection sites.

Leucapheresis procedures to collect, for example, granulocytes, lymphocytes or peripheral blood progenitor cells, should only be performed at fixed component units.

In any apheresis unit, or at any blood donor session, a telephone must be immediately available so that the emergency services can be called at any time.

Resuscitation equipment, as required by local and national guidelines for blood donor sessions, must be available at all sessions undertaking routine component procedures.

Account must be taken of the following activities/requirements when selecting a venue:

- registration of donors and all other necessary data processing
- appropriate facilities to assess the fitness of individuals to donate
- withdrawal of blood from donors without risk of contamination or errors
- social and medical care of donors, including those who suffer reactions

- sufficient seating should be provided for donors and staff, with allowance made for possible queues during busy periods

- storage of equipment, reagents and disposables

- storage during the session of blood and components, if they are not to be transferred immediately to the blood processing centre or to appropriate storage in the team vehicle

- access to an adequate electrical supply to support all electrical equipment used for the session

- the space required for these activities will depend on the anticipated workload

- flooring should be non-slip.

4.1.2 Health and safety factors

The requirements of the Health and Safety at Work Act 1974[3] must be taken into account when selecting sessional venues. Each organisation has the responsibility to ensure that venues comply with the Health and Safety at Work Act and that staff are fully aware of their responsibilities under this legislation. It is the responsibility of all staff with supervisory or line management responsibility to ensure that safe systems of work are in place at all times. All venues should be formally assessed for suitability with an appropriate plan to manage risks. Premises should be safe, clean and comfortable for donors and staff. In particular, the following points should be borne in mind:

- The venue should be as close as possible to the centre of population being served. It should be possible for the sessional vehicle(s) to park in close proximity to the access doors, to facilitate off-loading if required. The ground to be covered by staff carrying equipment shall be even and well lit. The space to be used should preferably not entail carriage of equipment on stairs. A similar safe approach should be ensured for donors, with as much provision as possible for car parking. Notices should be displayed, directing donors to the appropriate entry point of the building, and to the room being used.

- Furniture and equipment within the available space should be arranged to minimise crowding (with the increased risk of mistake or accident), enable adequate supervision and ensure a smooth and logical workflow.

- Fire exits must be unobstructed and operational. All sessional staff must be aware of the location of the fire extinguishers and exits.

- Lighting should be adequate for all the required activities. Provision should be made for the use of emergency lighting in the event of interruption of the electricity supply.

- Environmental control may not be within the power of a mobile team, but every effort should be made to ensure that the space does not become too hot, cold or stuffy. Subsidiary cooling fans and heating should be carried on sessional vehicles, and used as necessary. This equipment should be subjected to a planned maintenance programme.

- Facilities for the provision of refreshments for donors and staff should be separated from the other activities of a donor session whenever possible. Every effort should be made to ensure that equipment used in this area poses the minimum threat of danger to all persons.

- Toilet facilities for male and female donors and staff should be provided.

- Separate washing facilities are desirable for those staff involved in 'clean' procedures.

- Adequate facilities must be available for the disposal of waste. On mobile sessions, all waste should be collected and contained in a suitable manner for subsequent disposal in accordance with relevant regulations.

4.2 Staffing and training principles for donation sessions

A consultant with responsibility for the donors in consultation with nursing and operational managers should ensure that there are adequate staffing levels and that staff are properly trained. This consultant may delegate day-to-day clinical responsibility to appropriately trained clinical staff. When donors are undergoing leucapheresis procedures (e.g. granulocyte, lymphocyte and peripheral blood progenitor cell collections) a suitably trained doctor must be immediately available to attend to the donor.

At sessions where component collection is performed one or more suitably trained doctors or registered nurses must be responsible for supervising the performance of venepunctures and for the supervision of machine procedures.

The administration of drugs (e.g. local anaesthetic and citrate) must be supervised by a registered professional in accordance with *Standards for Medicines Management* (2007).[4] During donation, donors should never be left in a room without the presence of an appropriately trained doctor or registered nurse.

Training and certification of registered nurses undertaking donation procedures including training and monitoring of staff, performing venepunctures and obtaining informed consent, must be in accordance with the current *Nursing and Midwifery Council (NMC) Code of Professional Conduct*.[5]

The consultant, in consultation with the nurse manager, must ensure that there is an appropriate staffing level and skill mix to ensure donor safety and adequate monitoring of the equipment in use. They must ensure that, as a minimum requirement, all healthcare professionals involved with component procedures receive basic life-support training annually.

At sessions where component collection is performed planned staffing levels should ensure that normally there is at least one member of suitably trained staff present for every two machines in use. For leucapheresis procedures, higher staffing ratios are required. A programme should be established for initial and continued training to ensure an appropriate level of proficiency.

The consultant with responsibility for donors must ensure that a manual of standard operating procedures (SOPs) is compiled in accordance with local quality assurance systems for whole blood collection and each type of component collection procedure. These SOPs must be regularly reviewed and updated and must take into account the machine manufacturer's operating instructions. A current copy of the relevant manufacturer's manual for each type of machine in use must be available on-site.

4.3 Collection of the donation

The ultimate responsibility for ensuring that every unit of blood and blood components has been collected in accordance with the Blood Safety and Quality Regulations (2005) rests with the 'responsible person' for the Blood Establishment. The advocacy and guardianship of high-quality care for donors is the responsibility of the designated clinical lead in attendance, who must be a registered nurse or medical practitioner.

Guidance for whole blood and component donation procedures is given in Chapter 5. Guidance for laboratory testing procedures is given in Chapters 9 and 12.

4.4 Donor identification

Donors must positively identify themselves at registration by volunteering their name, date of birth and permanent address. Once registered, for subsequent identification their name and date of birth is sufficient. The identity of the donor must be recorded and linked to the donation record.

4.5 Labelling

Session staff must ensure that a set of labels with a unique number is assigned to each donation and that the same unique number appears on the donor session record, the primary and secondary collection packs and all the sample tubes used. Great caution is necessary to avoid crossover or duplication of numbers. The working practice should be designed to minimise the risk of error. Arrangements should be such as to avoid the possibility of errors in the labelling of blood containers and blood samples. The blood or component bags and corresponding samples must not be removed from the donor couch until a satisfactory check on correct labelling has been carried out. It is recommended that each donor couch has its own individual facilities for the handling of samples during donation and labelling.

Packs, sample tubes and the donor session record must never be relabelled. Unused sets of numbers must be accounted for. Labels which have been discarded must not be retrieved.

4.6 Records

It is strongly recommended that all records pertaining to donor and donation identity be entered and maintained in an electronic format which can be accessed readily by approved and qualified personnel, and in a manner which preserves donor confidentiality in accordance with legal requirements. Machine-readable systems for identifying donors and donation derivatives are also recommended. Initial documentation – for example on session records – may be taken manually and archived for the required period in law, with relevant portions transcribed electronically whenever convenient operationally.

4.6.1 Donor session records

A record of the sessional venue, the date, the donation number and the identity of all donors attending must be maintained. For any donors who are deferred, rejected or retired, the full details must be recorded and the reasons given for the action taken.

The records of blood donation sessions should allow identification of each important step associated with the donation. All donations must be recorded including the reason for any unsuccessful donations. All adverse reactions must also be recorded together with the action taken. Full details of any other incidents, including those only involving staff, must be recorded.

These records should be used for the regular compilation of statistics which should be studied monthly by those responsible for activities concerned with the organisation and management of blood collection sessions.

4.7 Control of purchased material and services

4.7.1 Specification and inspection of blood bags

Blood collection shall be by aseptic techniques using a sterile closed system and a single venepuncture. The integrity of the system must be checked prior to use and measures must be taken to prevent non-sterile air entering the system.

Blood shall be collected into containers that are pyrogen free and sterile, containing sufficient licensed anticoagulant for the quantity and purpose of blood to be collected.

The container label shall state the kind and amount of anticoagulant, the amount of blood that can be collected and the required storage temperature.

Manufacturers' directions regarding storage, use and expiry dates of the packs whose outer containers have been opened and resealed must be adhered to.

Batch numbers of the blood packs used shall be recorded.

The donation number on the pack and sample tubes should be checked at the end of the donation to ensure that those for a given donation are identical; that is, the donation number on the donor health and lifestyle questionnaire, the primary and secondary collection packs and the sample tubes must all be identical.

Prior to release from the blood collection session the pack and its associated tubing should be reinspected for defects and its integrity should be checked by applying pressure to the pack to detect any leaks. Any defective pack should be marked for disposal and held separately from intact packs. Details of the defect(s) should be recorded for future analysis and action (see section 5.11).

4.7.2 Specification of apheresis sets

Blood components must be collected by apheresis using sterile, single-use, disposable items that are licensed and CE marked. The apheresis set for collection of components for direct clinical use must have a preconnected access needle to ensure a sterile pathway, and incorporate a bacterial filter in all non-preconnected fluid lines (e.g. saline, SAGM, and the anticoagulant line [not required if the anticoagulant bag is preconnected]). For dual-needle procedures a preconnected needle is only essential for the access venepuncture.

A record must be kept of all lot and/or batch numbers of all the apheresis set components and injectable materials used, in accordance with local quality systems.

4.7.3 Specifications for automated donor apheresis machines (see also section 8.5)

Machines must be correctly installed and commissioned according to each manufacturer's instructions. They must be CE marked.

The environment and operating area for each machine employed and the power supply available must conform to the manufacturer's recommendations for satisfactory machine performance.

Machines must comply with the relevant aspects of the Health and Safety at Work Act 1974[3] and the Good Automated Manufacturing Practice (GAMP) *Guide for Validation of Automated Systems in Pharmaceutical Manufacture.*[6]

Automated apheresis machines must have the following features:

- A manual override system so that the operator can stop the automatic cycle at any time during the procedure.

- A blood flow monitor, to monitor blood flow during blood withdrawal and return. The purpose is to ensure that the selected donor flow rate does not cause collapse of the donor's vein and to monitor the venous pressure during the donor blood return cycle such that if any obstruction to flow occurs the blood pump will automatically reduce speed and/or stop. In either event a visual and audible alarm system should operate.

- An in-line air detector to protect the donor from air embolism. In the event of air entering the extra-corporeal circuit a visible and audible alarm must be activated, the return blood pump must automatically stop and the venous return line must automatically be occluded.

- A blood filter integral with the harness to prevent any aggregates formed during the procedure from being returned to the donor.

- An anticoagulant flow indicator, providing a visible means of monitoring anticoagulant delivery throughout the procedure, and ideally an audible alarm if no anticoagulant is flowing.

- A device for pre-setting the collection volume, monitoring the collection volume during the procedure and automatically ending the procedure. A system with a visual and audible alarm to notify the operator of the completion of the procedure may be provided.

- In the event of a power failure the machine must automatically enter a standby mode once power returns.

Apheresis machines must be serviced in accordance with the manufacturer's instructions. A planned maintenance scheme should be followed. Machine maintenance and servicing must be documented and be in accordance with the procedures outlined in the appropriate Medicines and Healthcare products Regulatory Agency publications: DB 9801, DB 9801 Supplement 1 and DB 2000(02).[7]

Apheresis machines must be routinely cleaned with a suitable decontaminating agent on a daily basis. A standard procedure for dealing immediately with blood spillage must be in operation.

4.7.4 Anticoagulant

A licensed citrate anticoagulant must be used at a ratio which achieves a final plasma citrate concentration of 15–25 mmol/L in the collected component (see Chapter 3, Appendix II).

The anticoagulant must be in date, with no evidence of particles or leakage. Any suspect unit must not be used. The batch number must be recorded on the session record and any defect reported in accordance with local quality systems.

4.8 Protection and preservation of product quality

All whole blood and apheresis components must be transported, tested and stored in accordance with the specifications for blood components in Chapters 7 and 8.

4.9 References

1. Medicines and Healthcare products Regulatory Agency (2007). *Rules and Guidance for Pharmaceutical Manufacturers and Distributors 2007.* London: Pharmaceutical Press. Also available at www.mhra.gov.uk/publications/regulatoryguidance/medicines/othermedicinesregulatoryguidance/CON2030291.

2. World Health Organization (1994). *WHO Expert Committee on Biological Standardization 43rd Report.* Technical Report Series, 840, pp1–218.

3. Health and Safety at Work Act 1974. Available at www.legislation.gov.uk.

4. *Standards for Medicines Management* (2007). Available at www.nmc-uk.org/publications/standards.

5. *Nursing and Midwifery Council (NMC). Code of Professional Conduct.* Available at www.nmc-uk.org.

6. Good Automated Manufacturing Practice (GAMP) *Guide for Validation of Automated Systems in Pharmaceutical Manufacture.* Available at www.ispe.org.

7. Medicines and Healthcare products Regulatory Agency publications, available at www.mhra.gov.uk:

   - DB 9801, *Medical Device and Equipment Management for Hospital and Community-based Organisations*
   - DB 9801 Supplement 1, *Checks and Tests for Newly Delivered Medical Devices*
   - DB 2000(02), *Medical Device and Equipment Management: Repair and Maintenance Provision.*

Chapter 5
Collection of a blood or component donation

This chapter describes the steps involved in the collection of a blood or component donation from the information to be provided to a donor to the information required from the donor post-donation.

Sections 5.1 and 5.2 are closely based on the Blood Safety and Quality Regulations 2005.[1]

5.1 Information to be provided to prospective donors of blood or blood components

The following information must be provided to all donors:

- Accurate educational materials, which are written in terms which can be understood by members of the general public, about the essential nature of blood, the blood donation procedure, blood components and the important benefits to patients.

- For both allogeneic and autologous donations, the reasons for requiring a medical history, the testing of donations and the significance of informed consent.

- For allogeneic donations, the criteria for self-deferral, temporary and permanent deferral, and the reasons why individuals are not to donate blood or blood components if there could be a substantive risk for them or the recipient.

- For autologous donations, the possibility of deferral and the reasons why the donation procedure would not take place in the presence of a health risk to the individual whether as donor or recipient of the autologous blood or blood components.

- Information on the protection of personal data, including confirmation that there will be no disclosure of the identity of the donor, of information concerning the donor's health and of the results of the tests performed, other than in accordance with the requirements of these regulations.

- The reasons why individuals are not to make donations which may be detrimental to their health.

- Specific information on the nature of the procedures involved either in the allogeneic or autologous donation process and their respective associated risks. For autologous donations, the possibility that the autologous blood and blood components may not suffice for the intended transfusion requirements.

- Information on the option for donors to change their mind about donating prior to proceeding further, or the possibility of withdrawing or self-deferring at any time during or after the donation process, without any undue embarrassment or discomfort.

- The reasons why it is important that donors inform the Blood Establishment of any subsequent event that may render any prior donation unsuitable for transfusion.

- Information on the responsibility of the Blood Establishment to inform the donor, through an appropriate mechanism, if test results show any abnormality of significance to the donor's health.

- Information explaining why unused autologous blood and blood components will be discarded and not transfused to other patients.

- Information that test results detecting markers for viruses, such as HIV, HBV, HCV or other relevant blood transmissible microbiologic agents, will result in donor deferral and destruction of the collected unit.

- Information on the opportunity for donors to ask questions at any time.

- If the donated blood is to be used for purposes other than clinical transfusion or uses specified in the general consent materials, specific information must be provided.

5.2 Information to be obtained from donors by Blood Establishments at every donation

5.2.1 Donor identification

Donors must positively identify themselves by volunteering their name, date of birth and permanent address. The identity of the donor must be recorded and linked to the donation record.

5.2.2 Health and medical history of the donor

Health and medical history, provided on a questionnaire and through a confidential personal interview performed by a qualified health professional, must be assessed. This will include relevant factors that may assist in identifying and screening out persons whose donation could present a health risk to others, such as the possibility of transmitting diseases, or health risks to themselves. Donors must be selected in accordance with the current JPAC *Donor Selection Guidelines*[2] which form a constituent part of Chapter 3.

5.2.3 Signature of the donor

The donor must sign the donor questionnaire. This must then be countersigned by the qualified health professional responsible for obtaining the health history confirming that the donor has:

- read and understood the educational materials provided

- had an opportunity to ask questions

- been provided with satisfactory responses to any questions asked

- given informed consent to proceed with the donation process (see Chapter 3)

- been informed, in the case of autologous donations, that the donated blood and blood components may not be sufficient for the intended transfusion requirements

- acknowledged that all the information provided by the donor is true to the best of their knowledge.

5.3 Haemoglobin screening

A validated haemoglobin screen should be applied to all donors prior to donation. The objective is to ensure that prior to each donation the donor has a minimum acceptable haemoglobin concentration (currently at least 125 g/L in females and at least 135 g/L in males, see section 3.15).

5.4 Preparation of the venepuncture site

Blood must be drawn from a suitable vein in the antecubital fossa in an area that is free of skin lesions. The veins can be made more prominent by using appropriate means of venous occlusion.

Although it is not possible to guarantee sterility of the skin surface for venepuncture, a strict standardised and validated procedure for the preparation of the venepuncture site should be in operation (see section 9.5).

The antiseptic solution used must be allowed to dry completely after application to the donor's skin, or the skin must be wiped dry with sterile gauze before venepuncture. Thereafter, the prepared area must not be touched with fingers before the needle is inserted.

5.5 Preparation of the blood pack

5.5.1 Whole blood pack

The blood collection set must be in date and inspected for any defects. These are sometimes obscured by the label attached to the container, so careful inspection is required.

Moisture on the surface of a plastic pack after unpacking should arouse suspicion of a leak and if one or more packs in any packet is found to be abnormally damp, none of the packs in that container can be used. The solution in the set should be checked for clarity and must be clear before accepting the packs for use.

The blood pack is positioned below the level of the donor's arm and the blood collection tube must be clamped off.

The method used for monitoring the volume of blood removed shall be checked to be in working order and the pack placed in the correct position for the method to be effective.

5.5.2 Apheresis sets

The complete apheresis set and individual packaging must be thoroughly inspected for faults prior to use and during the setting up procedure. The set must be in date and a search must be made for set faults such as kinks, occlusions, points of weakness or leaks that may only become detectable during the setting up and priming procedure before the donor is attached to the set.

If an occlusive kink that cannot be remedied or a leak becomes apparent during a procedure then that procedure must be abandoned and any blood constituents remaining in the disposables must not be returned to the donor.

Any faults detected before or during a procedure must be recorded in accordance with local quality systems. Any defects must be reported (see section 5.11).

If there is any doubt about the integrity of any set, it must not be used but should be retained for inspection and returned to the manufacturer if deemed necessary.

5.5.3 Labels

Labelling: Whole blood and apheresis packs and donor sample tubes must be labelled in accordance with local standard operating procedures (SOPs).

All donors' records and labels should be checked for printing errors. Duplicate number sets shall not be used and these and missing numbers shall be reported via a designated senior manager to the printer concerned and to the Chair of the National Working Party or equivalent on machine-readable labels.

5.6 Performance of the venepuncture

Venepuncture should only be undertaken by authorised and trained personnel. If local anaesthetic is used, this should be a licensed medicinal product and injected in a manner which avoids any chance of donor-to-donor cross-infection (e.g. using individual disposable syringes and needles). A record of the batch number(s) should be made at each blood collection session and be capable of being related to individual donors.

Containers of local anaesthetic should be inspected for any leakage and if glass, inspected for cracks. Any suspect containers should be rejected.

Unused material must be discarded at the end of each donor session.

An aseptic technique must be used for drawing up the local anaesthetic into the syringe and the needle must be changed prior to the injection of the local anaesthetic.

Items used for venepuncture must be sterile, single-use and disposable. If the dry outer wrapping of sterile packs becomes wet the contents must not be used. Prior to use, session staff must ensure that the materials used for venepuncture are sterile, in date and suitable for the procedure to be undertaken. The sterile donor needle should not be uncovered and its tamper-proof cover should be checked for integrity immediately prior to the venepuncture.

As soon as the venepuncture has been performed, the clamp on the bleed line must be released.

It is important that a clean, skilful venepuncture is carried out to ensure the collection of a full, clot-free unit of blood suitable for the preparation of labile blood components.

The tubing attached to the needle should be taped to hold the needle in place during the donation.

5.6.1 Sample collection

At the start of the donation 30 mL (up to 45 mL in some circumstances) of blood should be diverted into a pouch. It is recommended that this pouch has a means of access opposite the entry line which allows blood to be sampled for haematological and serological testing without compromising the environmental integrity of the blood in the main pack.

5.7 Whole blood donation

If necessary, the donor should be asked to open and close his/her hand slowly every 10–12 seconds to encourage a free flow of blood.

The donor must never be left unattended during or immediately after donation and should be kept under observation throughout the phlebotomy.

5.7.1 Blood anticoagulation

The blood and anticoagulant should be mixed gently and periodically (at least every 60 seconds) during collection. Mixing should be achieved by manual inversion of the blood pack, or automatically by placing the blood pack on a mechanical agitator or by using a rocking device.

5.7.2 Blood flow

Blood flow should be constantly observed to ensure that the flow is uninterrupted.

The period of donation should not exceed 15 minutes.

5.7.3 Blood volume monitoring

The volume of blood withdrawn must be controlled to protect the donor from excessive loss of blood and to maintain the correct proportion of anticoagulant to blood.

The most efficient way of measuring the blood volume in plastic bags is by weight. The mean weight of 1 mL of blood is 1.06 g, and therefore, for example, a unit containing 470 mL of blood should weigh 470 × 1.06 g plus the weight of the pack(s) and the anticoagulant.

If it is not possible to adjust the weighing device in use for the tare weight of the container and anticoagulant solution it is advisable to record the minimum and maximum weight for the brand of pack in use as products from different manufacturers may vary considerably.

Several kinds of weighing equipment are available and such devices should be used according to the manufacturer's instructions for weighing blood into its plastic pack and periodically calibrated by appropriate techniques.

5.7.4 Completion of the donation

The pressure cuff must be deflated and the needle then removed from the arm. Immediate pressure must then be applied to the venepuncture site through a suitable clean dressing.

The needle must be discarded into a special container designed to minimise risk to personnel.

The pack must be inverted gently several times to ensure the contents are thoroughly mixed.

For pack systems designed for in-line leucodepletion in which the donor line becomes detached from the final red cell pack, and hence unavailable for compatibility testing, the line should be sealed close to the collection pack, according to clearly defined procedures. This sealing may be done without expressing the contents of the line into the main pack if the contents of the line are deemed to be of no further use.

The arm and general well-being of the donor should be checked before the donor leaves the session venue.

5.8 Component donation by apheresis

Guidance for collection procedures is identical to that for normal whole blood donations except for the points listed below.

Performance of the venepuncture: Once the venepuncture is performed subsequent procedures such as releasing clamps on the bleed line should follow the protocol for the particular type of apheresis procedure being undertaken.

Anticoagulation: This occurs automatically in apheresis, but instructions are needed to ensure apheresis machine operators monitor the flow of anticoagulant.

Consideration should be given to withdrawing donors who repeatedly show signs and/or symptoms of citrate toxicity from the apheresis panel. The practice of prophylactic oral supplementation with calcium should be discouraged.

Blood flow and monitoring: Blood flow occurs automatically in apheresis, unless a satisfactory flow rate cannot be maintained.

Instructions are needed for the apheresis operator in the event of a low-flow or no-flow situation. Particular care is needed when monitoring the return flow rate since most apheresis procedures operate with a pumped red cell return such that haematomas can rapidly form unless appropriate action is taken to prevent this from occurring.

Sample collection: In apheresis sampling should take place at the beginning of a donation. The methods employed shall ensure an aseptic technique with no risk of contamination and be clearly defined in the sessional procedures SOP manual.

Completion of the donation and quality control samples: A length of tubing should be left attached to the collection pack(s) as required for laboratory testing purposes. All used disposable equipment must be discarded in such a way as to prevent any risk to personnel, according to Health and Safety regulations.

Final donation inspection: The collected apheresis components must be inspected routinely for the presence of haemolysis, unwanted red cell contamination, other abnormal appearance or evidence of clotting. Such changes may require a review of the apheresis procedure and/or equipment. Any suspected apheresis component abnormality must be recorded, and the donation must be identified and reported in accordance with local quality systems.

5.9 Information to be provided to the donor post-donation

The donor must be provided with information on care of the venepuncture site and requested to report any illness occurring within 14 days of donation. They will already have been made aware of the importance of informing the Blood Establishment of any event that may render their donation unsuitable for clinical transfusion.

5.10 Adverse reactions in donors

The care of all donors at blood collection venues should incorporate research-based therapeutic interventions to reduce the risk of adverse events of donation. An example of the preventative measures that can be implemented are described in 'Points of care' used within one UK Blood Service (see Appendix I at the end of this chapter). This is a donation care pathway designed to minimise vasovagal events, bruising and re-bleeding from the venepuncture site.

All adverse reactions in donors should be documented and reported according to standard protocols. It is recommended that as a minimum data are collected and reviewed on all donor adverse events of donation using the International Haemovigilance Network (IHN) definitions of DAEDs (Appendix II) or similar and a standard data set for Serious Adverse Events of Donation (SAEDs) that is in line with the IHN definitions of SAEDs (Appendix III). This will allow comparison over time and between services of event rates, and monitor the effectiveness of any interventions to reduce event rates. SAEDs should all be fully investigated with a root cause analysis or similar tool to ensure that proper preventative and corrective actions are implemented.

Serious adverse reactions occurring in donors during or post-donation must be reported to the Competent Authority according to the Blood Establishment protocol.

5.11 Adverse events

All adverse events must be documented and reported according to standard protocols.

All bag/harness defects (e.g. pinhole leaks) must be recorded and all defects should be reported to the Quality Assurance Manager. If the defect appears to be batch-related, all packs and blood collected in them must be set aside for further investigation.

Any safety-related defects in equipment, including single-use items, must be reported via the head of department to the Department of Health in accordance with the requirements of the Competent Authority, currently the Medicines and Healthcare products Regulatory Agency (MHRA).

Serious adverse events must be reported to the Competent Authority according to the Blood Establishment protocol.

Online reporting to the MHRA is available at www.mhra.gov.uk.

5.12 Donor compensation

The Blood Transfusion Services should have established procedures to ensure that any claim by a donor for compensation for any injury or loss allegedly attributable to having donated blood or components will be dealt with in a timely manner and within a legal framework.

5.13 References

1. Statutory Instrument 2005 No. 50. The Blood Safety and Quality Regulations 2005. Available at www.legislation.gov.uk.

2. Joint UKBTS/HPA Professional Advisory Committee's (JPAC) *Donor Selection Guidelines*. Available at www.transfusionguidelines.org.uk.

Appendix I Points of care

AI.1 Welcomer

- A principal role of the Welcomer is to reduce potential anxiety in the donor. Observe for donors in a 'hyper-vigilant' state and refer where appropriate.

- Professionalism, including appearance, is crucial in order to assure the donor of a safe and positive experience.

- Greet the donor with a warm welcome and thank them for attending the session and giving up their time to donate blood.

- The Welcomer needs to promote drinks to the donors. Offer the donor 500 mL of fluid to stretch the stomach (gastric dilation) and raise blood pressure (BP), reducing the risk of vasovagal (VV) episodes. This offer or promotion of drinks must be emphasised quite strongly in order for the donor to understand the importance of taking the fluid. Ideally the fluid should be drunk over 5 minutes rather than sipped, and should be taken no longer than 30 minutes prior to donation for best effect. The nurse or supervisor may wish to change the position of the water area on session in line with donor waiting times. An information leaflet for donors is available.

- If possible, donors who are queuing to give their details should be offered fluids along with an explanation of why there is a delay.

- Donors who are waiting to be screened must not be seated facing the pods. The eyes of all waiting donors ideally need to be focused away from clinical activity.

- Ensure all donors are given the Welcome information to read prior to screening.

AI.2 Screening

- Enquire as to whether the donor has had any previous problems when donating blood and try to relieve any anxiety.

- Ask the donor about their preparation for giving blood, e.g. have they had something to eat before attending the session/have they avoided doing any strenuous activity or exercise regime that may increase their risk of an adverse event.

- If a previous adverse event is identified or the donor has an increased risk of an adverse event, a nurse should be asked to speak to the donor. The nurse will also instruct the donor on how to do applied muscle tension (AMT) exercises to raise the BP if appropriate.

- Ask the donor if they have drunk the recommended volumes of fluid prior to the screening. If they have not, it needs to be explained to the donor why drinking fluids is important and offer again. If the donor agrees to drink, give the fluids while talking.

- Ensure new donors and those with a previous history or higher risk of VV episode(s) are indicated in some way. This will help easily identify those with a higher risk of complication or adverse event.

- Once screening is complete, show the donor to the waiting area, which must not have chairs facing the beds. Magazines and reading material should be available as a method of distracting the waiting donors from focusing on the clinical area. It is important to reduce tension and anxiety that will be experienced by many first-time donors and those who may have had a problem donating or an adverse event in the past. Additional fluids could be offered at this point too.

AI.3 Beds

- Prioritise donors and provide appropriate therapeutic attention. Talking to donors will allow you to recognise their coping strategies and how best to put them at their ease.

- If required, in order to raise the donor's BP, once they are on the bed, ask the donor to commence AMT exercises. This keeps their mind occupied as they are counting and their focus away from the venepuncture (VP).

- Where donation chairs are used the donor should be reclined at an angle of 45 degrees from the hip.

- Do not leave the donor before starting VP. Aim to have the pack labelled and VP started promptly to prevent the donor's BP from being affected.

- If an adverse event occurs, a nurse should decide if it is clinically necessary to screen off the donor to ensure privacy for the person involved and to avoid raising anxiety levels in those who are waiting. Screens should be placed around the donor, but initially, if necessary, place your body between the donor and the waiting donors to block their view until screens arrive. Donors should never be left unattended behind a screen.

- Non-donating family/friends are welcome, but must sit by the donor and not stand by the bed.

- Once the donation is complete, remove the needle and cover the VP site with gauze, asking the donor to apply firm pressure with three fingers to the dressing.

- Sit the donor up, extending their legs out in front of them if possible.

- Stay with the donor until they leave the bed. Use the time to complete any observations, give advice to the donor, assess pallor and ensure the donor is applying the correct pressure to their arm.

- After 1 minute the donor can move their legs over the side of the bed. After a further minute if the site is observed, do so by lifting the gauze without removing it, to protect the donor from any blood splash. This also shields the donor from seeing the VP site. If there is no new bleeding, apply the dressing.

AI.4 Appointments and teas

- Ensure the computer does not obscure your direct vision of the donors.

- Ensure there is adequate space around the tea table and chairs in case of falls and potential head injury.

- Stress to donors who refuse a drink, the importance of having a post-donation drink to replace fluid depletion.

- Encourage new donors and those with a previous VV episode to have cold drinks.

- Deal with re-bleeds promptly. Try to ensure nearby donors see as little as possible.

- If a donor becomes unwell, stay with them and call for assistance.

- When giving post-donation advice, take care not to embarrass donors or trigger other donors to listen in to the conversation.

Appendix II   International Haemovigilance Network categories for donor adverse events

AII.1 Complications mainly with local symptoms

AII.1.1 Complications mainly characterised by the occurrence of blood outside the vessels

Haematoma
A haematoma is an accumulation of blood in the tissues outside the vessels.

Arterial puncture
Arterial puncture is a puncture of the brachial artery or of one of its branches by the needle used for bleeding of the donor.

Delayed bleeding
Delayed bleeding is spontaneous recommencement of bleeding from the venepuncture site, which occurs after the donor has left the donation site.

AII.1.2 Complications mainly characterised by pain

Nerve irritation

Irritation of a nerve by pressure from a haematoma.

Nerve injury

Injury of a nerve by the needle at insertion or withdrawal.

Tendon injury

Injury of a tendon by the needle.

Painful arm

Cases characterised mainly by severe local and radiating pain in the arm used for the donation and arising during or within hours following donation, but without further details to permit classification in one of the already more specific categories mentioned above.

AII.1.3 Other kinds of categories with local symptoms

Thrombophlebitis

Inflammation in a vein associated with a thrombus.

Allergy (local)

Allergic type skin reaction at the venepuncture site caused by allergens in solutions used for disinfection of the arm or allergens from the needle.

AII.2 Complications mainly with generalised symptoms

AII.2.1 Vasovagal reaction

A vasovagal reaction is a general feeling of discomfort and weakness with anxiety, dizziness and nausea, which may progress to loss of consciousness (faint).

AII.2.2 Immediate vasovagal reaction

Symptoms occurred before donor has left the donation site.

AII.2.3 Immediate vasovagal reaction with injury

Injury caused by falls or accidents in donors with a vasovagal reaction and unconsciousness before donor has left the donation site.

AII.2.4 Delayed vasovagal reaction

Symptoms occurred after donor has left the donation site.

AII.2.5 Delayed vasovagal reaction with injury

Injury caused by falls or accidents in donors with a vasovagal reaction and unconsciousness after donor has left the donation site.

AII.3 Complications related to apheresis

AII.3.1 Citrate reaction

AII.3.2 Haemolysis

AII.3.3 Generalised allergic reaction

AII.3.4 Air embolism

AII.4 Other complications related to blood donation

Appendix III International Haemovigilance Network definition of severe donor adverse events

Conditions which define a case as severe are:

- Hospitalisation: If it was attributable to the complication.

- Intervention:
  - to preclude permanent damage or impairment of a body function
  - to prevent death (life-threatening).

- Symptoms: Causing significant disability or incapacity following a complication of blood donation and persisted for more than a year after the donation (long-term morbidity).

- Death: If it follows a complication of blood donation and the death was possibly, probably or definitely related to the donation.

For the purpose of consistent reporting of SAEDs the UK Blood Transfusion Services have adopted these categories:

- death within 7 days of donation

- hospital admission within 24 hours of donation

- injury resulting in a fracture within 24 hours

- road traffic collision (RTC) within 24 hours of donation

- acute coronary syndrome (ACS) diagnosed within 24 hours of donation

- problems relating to needle insertion persisting for more than a year

- anaphylaxis, haemolysis or air embolism (component donors).

Chapter 6
Evaluation and manufacture of blood components

6.1 Scope of the guidelines

These guidelines provide a framework on which Blood Establishments should assemble standard operating procedures (SOPs) for the manufacture of blood components.

These guidelines apply to single-donor and small-pool components (<12 donors) prepared from units of whole blood or by apheresis.

Blood Establishments should ensure that the hospital blood banks that they supply are informed of these component production guidelines, and should consult with them on proposed changes to existing component processing and on the adoption of new components.

Technologies for pathogen inactivation of blood components are now being used in Europe. Within the UK, methylene blue treated plasma and the medicinal product solvent detergent treated pooled plasma are in use. Treatment of plasma and of platelets with amotosalen ultraviolet (UV) treatment or riboflavin UV treatment is CE marked and may be used in the UK in the future. Specifications for these and similar products will be considered as and when they are adopted. At present no CE-marked technology exists for pathogen inactivation of red cells, although some companies are working on suitable approaches.

Filters suitable for the removal of abnormal prion from red cells have been CE marked and have been under clinical assessment in the UK. Recommendations on their use have recently been submitted to ministers and the outcome on this is awaited. As part of the validation and clinical assessment, specifications for these products have been drafted and are available in the Trial component (Annex 3) section of the online version of these guidelines.[1]

6.2 Setting and maintaining specifications

The wide variability of the source material from which blood components are prepared makes it difficult to set stringent limits. Nevertheless, realistic minimum specifications should be set and complied with.

Table 6.1 Discard limits

Blood component	Parameter	LOWER LIMIT (less than)
Red Cells in Additive Solution	Haemoglobin (g/unit)	30
Red Cells for Intrauterine Transfusion	Haemoglobin (g/unit)	30
Red Cells for Exchange Transfusion (not Whole Blood)	Haemoglobin (g/unit)	30
Platelets, Pooled	Platelet yield ($\times 10^9$/unit)	160
Platelets, Apheresis	Platelet yield ($\times 10^9$/unit)	160

Discard limits are also set for certain components that are subject to non-destructive quality monitoring, such that components that are excessively out of specification are not used therapeutically (Table 6.1).

Component and process quality monitoring results should be subjected to statistical analysis so that trends can be identified. Guidance on appropriate approaches to statistical process monitoring is given in the Council of Europe guide,[2] and in Beckman et al. (2009).[3] A flowchart adapted from Beckman et al., to aid in selection of appropriate methods, is reproduced as Figure 6.1.

If the results of analyses show a consistent trend towards the minimum requirements specified in Chapter 7, the cause should be investigated. The criteria to be investigated must be detailed in the relevant SOP together with the corrective action to be taken. The steps to be considered should include the following:

- An investigation of the collection, testing, production and distribution procedures as appropriate.
- Checking that procedures are up to date and are not being deviated from.
- Checking the operation of equipment and storage conditions (this may include reviewing validation documentation and/or revalidation).

The person responsible for quality assurance and/or production may initiate investigations beyond the scope of written procedures.

6.3 Component and process monitoring tests

These guidelines also indicate the minimum level of other process monitoring tests necessary to ensure components are prepared to specification.

Any assay used for blood component quality monitoring should be validated and documented before introduction and before any changes to methodology or manufacture are brought into use. Blood Establishments should ensure that they participate in the National External Quality Assessment Scheme (NEQAS) or other available external quality assurance schemes for the assays used to assess component quality.

Each component should be visually inspected at each stage of processing and immediately prior to issue. The component must be withdrawn if there is evidence of leakage, damage to or fault in the container, excessive air, suspicion of microbial contamination or any other contraindications such as platelet clumping, unusual turbidity, haemolysis or other abnormal colour change.

6: EVALUATION AND MANUFACTURE OF BLOOD COMPONENTS

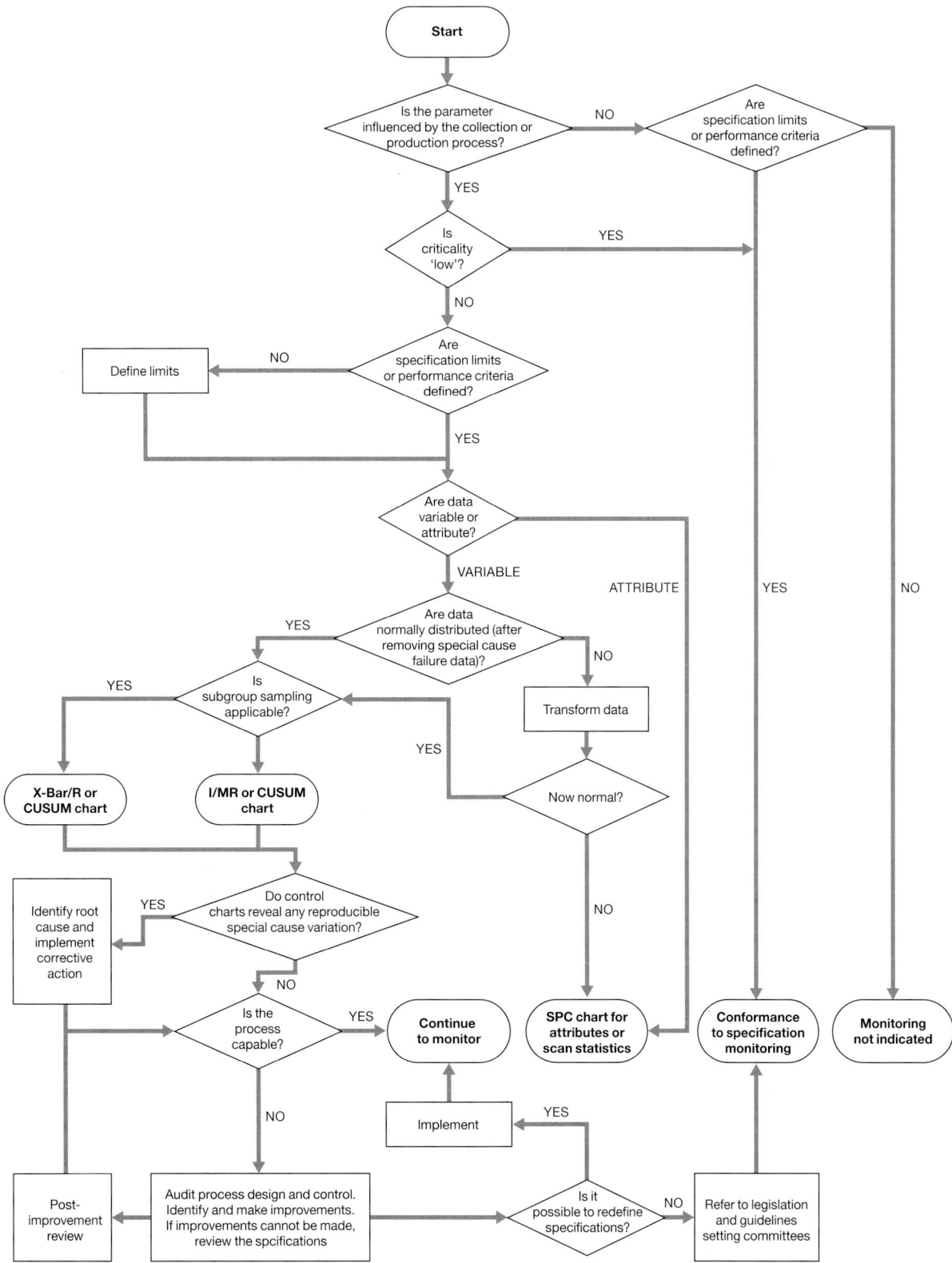

Figure 6.1 Algorithm for the selection of quality monitoring methods

6.3.1 Sampling procedures

Sampling procedures should be designed and validated, prior to acceptance as standard practice, to ensure the sample truly reflects the contents of the component pack.

Validation of sampling procedures should be repeated before application to new components, relevant changes to blood pack design or different quality parameters, or before the introduction of new sampling equipment. Also there should be a procedure for continuous assessment of staff competence/sampling techniques.

Where test samples are removed from a component to be issued for transfusion, the sampling procedure should be designed and validated to ensure that the sterility and essential properties of the component are not adversely affected.

Samples for leucocyte counting must be taken and tested within 48 hours of donation, unless the sampling and testing times used have been validated to yield equivalent results.

6.3.2 Frequency of tests

The regularity with which components are made and the extent of their compliance with specification influences the frequency with which component and process monitoring tests are required.

If there is a trend towards the minimum requirements specified in Chapter 7, the frequency of quality monitoring tests should be increased according to defined procedures until the relevant component attributes have been brought under control.

The testing protocol should take into account all major production variables and ensure samples are representative of these.

6.3.3 Component weight:volume

To provide information that is useful for clinicians, the component specifications given in Chapter 7 generally require the component label to indicate a volume. This may be either the calculated volume or nominal volume, and the nominal volume may be based on a national or locally established volume specification.

Since volume generally is calculated by dividing the component weight by its specific gravity, the following conventions should apply in order to ensure some element of standardisation:

- Whole blood volume is most appropriately calculated by deducting the weight of the pack assembly and dividing the resulting weight by the nominal specific gravity of 1.06.

- To provide quality monitoring data that demonstrate the capability of the blood collection process, deduct the weight of the anticoagulant before converting to volume.

- To provide quality monitoring data that reflect the provision of whole blood as a component, the volume given on the component label should include whole blood and anticoagulant.

- For red cell components, volume is calculated by weighing the pack, deducting the weight of the pack assembly only, and dividing the resultant weight by the nominal specific gravity 1.06. The weight of anticoagulant and, if relevant, additive solution are not deducted when calculating the volume of red cell components.

- For platelets and plasma components, volume is calculated by weighing the pack, deducting the weight of the pack assembly and dividing the resulting weight by the nominal specific gravity of 1.03.

6.4 Component processing

6.4.1 Premises

Component production areas should satisfy the requirements defined in the current *Rules and Guidance for Pharmaceutical Manufacturers and Distributors 2007*.[4] In addition:

- the ambient temperature of blood component processing areas should be maintained within a range that would not be expected to adversely affect component viability/shelf life

- where appropriate, steps should be taken to ensure that air quality in the blood component processing environment does not increase the bioburden to which blood components are exposed.

6.4.2 The starting material

The starting material for component preparation is whole blood or the products of apheresis collected from donors who satisfy current donor selection criteria. Components must be collected into blood packs/apheresis harness assemblies that are CE marked.

Before use, packs/apheresis harness assemblies that have not previously been validated, or contain component parts that have not previously been validated, should be subject to validation or process qualification as appropriate according to the protocols set out in Chapter 8.

Starting material for component preparation should be transported as described in section 6.11.2.

As a route to reducing the incidence of transfusion-related acute lung injury (TRALI), large plasma volume products (clinical fresh frozen plasma; platelet concentrates stored in plasma) should be made using plasma from male donors (or non-parous or antibody screened parous female donors) wherever feasible.

Unless subjected to a validated pathogen inactivation process, components for use in intrauterine transfusion, neonates and infants under 1 year must be prepared from previously tested donors who have given at least one donation in the last 2 years. This donation must have been either negative for all mandatory markers, or if repeat reactive, confirmed to be non-specific reactive and the donor reinstated in accordance with section 9.4 (on reinstatement of blood donors).

All components prepared in the UK have been leucodepleted since 1999.

6.4.3 Prevention of microbial contamination

Infections associated with the microbial contamination of blood and blood components still occur. While there is no evidence to suggest that routine, retrospective sterility testing of blood components diminishes or eliminates such instances of infection, the following measures will minimise the risks:

- Creating and maintaining the highest level of awareness among all personnel of the constant care and attention to detail needed to minimise microbial contamination, e.g. validation and periodic monitoring of the effectiveness of venepuncture site preparation.

- Using validated procedures designed to minimise microbial contamination of the environment and prevent microbial contamination of components.

- Diverting the first part of the donation into a sample pouch, to avoid entry into the primary donation. This may be used for mandatory screening tests.

- Monitoring the microbial load in equipment and in the environment of component preparation areas. Assessing the contamination rate in outdated components may provide additional, indirect evidence of processing cleanliness.

It is important that data derived from such monitoring exercises are accumulated and regularly examined with a view to taking appropriate action.

Screening of platelet components for bacterial contamination has been evaluated and implemented by some Blood Establishments to help reduce the risks associated with bacterial contamination. However, it does not eliminate this problem, at least with current testing technologies.

6.4.4 Closed system

The term 'closed system' refers to a system in which the blood pack assembly is manufactured under clean conditions, sealed to the external environment and sterilised by an approved method.

6.4.4.1 Venting

With the exception of the venepuncture procedure and strict requirements for open processing (see section 6.4.5), the blood pack system and its contents must not be vented to the external environment at any stage during blood collection or processing.

6.4.4.2 Sealing

Blood pack and apheresis harness fluid pathways must at all times be protected from the external environment by:

- hermetic seal(s) incorporated during manufacture or Blood Establishment use
- other validated devices for effecting a permanent seal
- break seal closure(s)*
- port(s) incorporating a tamper-proof closure and pierceable membrane*
- microbial filter(s).*

*These devices must comply with the requirements of relevant standards for medical devices, including ISO 3826 Parts 1 (blood bags, 2010), 2 (graphic symbols, 2008) and 3 (blood bags with integrated features, 2006), must be validated by the manufacturer and must be provided with clear instructions for use.

Before severing any sub-component of the pack assembly, the pack contents must first be protected from the external environment by a minimum of one permanent seal made using a validated hermetic sealer cleaned and maintained according to SOP.

Temporary sealing clamps/clips must be used only to control the flow of fluid within a closed system. They must not be used as the sole means of protection from the external environment.

When a device for making a sterile connection is used the system can be regarded as closed provided that the process of joining and sealing has been validated and shown not to lead to an increased risk of microbial contamination of the component. The procedure for use should ensure that the operator carefully checks the suitability of every weld and also pays particular attention to effective cleaning of the working parts of the equipment.

Cleaning should be by validated procedure with regular checks to ensure conformance to procedures.

Pressure or tensile testing the strength of welds should be performed during the validation or qualification of equipment.[5,6]

Where a sterile connecting device has been used to add satellite packs, the components must not be issued with the weld in place.

6.4.4.3 Pre-donation sampling

Pre-donation sampling must only be carried out using blood pack assemblies that incorporate a device to prevent the return of blood and/or air from the sample pouch towards the donor and donation. The procedure must be validated by the Blood Establishment and documented in blood collection SOP.

After filling, the sample pouch must be permanently sealed from the donation before collecting blood samples.

In the event of inadvertent contamination of the donation by blood or air from the sample pouch, the donation must be discarded.

6.4.5 Open system

The term 'open system' refers to a system in which the integrity of the closed system must be breached but where every effort is made to prevent microbial contamination by operating in a clean environment, using sterilised materials and aseptic handling techniques. In such circumstances, positive pressure should be exerted on the original container and maintained until the container is sealed. Open system processing should be undertaken in a designated clean environment as defined in the current *Rules and Guidance for Pharmaceutical Manufacturers and Distributors 2007*.[4]

The sterility of components prepared in an open system should be monitored using validated methods.

Blood components prepared by an open system should be used as soon as possible. If storage is unavoidable, components with a recommended storage temperature of 22 ±2°C should be used within 6 hours. Components with a recommended storage temperature of 4 ±2°C should be used within 24 hours.

Components are rendered unsuitable for clinical use when breached and the requirements defined for an open system have not been observed, unless issued under medical concession.

Any new development in component preparation by an open procedure must be validated to ensure the maintenance of sterility before the procedure can be used to produce components for therapeutic use.

Procedures for collecting samples for sterility testing must not adversely affect the sterility of components intended for subsequent transfusion.

6.5 Component shelf life

Component storage specifications are given in Chapter 7.

Where components are pooled or undergo procedures that influence the shelf life, the maximum shelf life of the component must not exceed the expiry date of the oldest constituent component or the expiry date of the new component produced by the procedure, whichever is the shorter.

For all other components the date of collection will be assigned Day 0 of the shelf life. Day 1 of storage will commence at one minute past midnight on the day after collection.

6.6 Labelling

6.6.1 Component labelling

Barcoded labels and on-demand printing must be used whenever possible.

The design, content and use of labels for blood components should conform to specifications set out in Chapters 23 and 26. It is planned that a more extensive library of relevant blood component labels will be available within the electronic component portfolio being developed for the website for the *Guidelines for the Blood Transfusion Services in the United Kingdom*.[1]

Procedures should be established to ensure labels are satisfactory for their intended use.

Pre-printed labels to be attached to blood donations, documentation and components should be stored under secure conditions.

6.6.2 Donation/donor identification

The use of a unique barcoded/eye-readable donation number links the donation to its donor. Donation numbers must be attached to all integral packs, sample tubes and corresponding documents at the time of donation.

When component production requires the use of subsidiary packs which are not an integral part of the pack assembly (e.g. filtration, pooling, freezing), a secure system must be in place to ensure that the correct eye-readable and barcoded donation number is placed on each additional pack used.

When components are pooled there should be a system that ensures that the pool carries a unique barcoded and eye-readable identification number(s). This barcode must be able to be read by component manufacturers and blood banks.

When a component is divided a secure system must be in place to ensure that all sub-batches can be traced.

6.7 Component storage

6.7.1 Specifications for component storage areas

Storage areas for blood components must operate within a specified temperature range and should provide adequate space and suitable lighting, and be arranged and equipped to allow dry, clean and orderly storage.

Good manufacturing practice requires that components of different status are appropriately identified and effectively separated.

Recognised status categories are noted below.

6.7.1.1 Quarantine

Procedures should ensure that untested components are not quarantined with components which have produced, or are likely to produce, repeatably reactive results in mandatory microbiological screening tests.

Secure and exclusive quarantine storage should be available for known biohazard material awaiting disposal (see section 6.8.2).

6.7.1.2 Non-conforming

Components which do not comply with the specification for mandatory tests or are otherwise unsuitable for transfusion should be categorised as non-conforming. Normally, such components would be discarded. However, if they are to be issued for therapeutic, reagent or research use, a concessionary release procedure must be used (see section 6.10).

6.7.1.3 Returned

Components that have been returned from areas outside the direct control of the blood supplier should not normally be returned to stock.

Components that have been returned to the blood supplier with substantive evidence that they have been stored appropriately and within specification, should be held securely pending possible reinstatement to stock by a designated person.

6.7.1.4 Stock

Only those components which have been deemed satisfactory for issue by a designated person should be held in stock (see section 6.9).

Appropriate security and status labelling of component storage areas are essential.

A current inventory should be maintained of components in each storage category/area.

Areas/equipment in which components are to be stored should be validated before their introduction into routine use and checked for calibration to a documented schedule thereafter.

A permanent, continuous record of storage temperatures should be made, reviewed and stored. There should be a log of alarm events that describes the corrective actions taken.

6.7.2 Procedures for component storage

Written procedures must be established for the storage of blood components. These should include the following:

- a procedure to ensure components are not released to stock unless authorised by a designated person (see section 6.7.1.4)

- definitions of the designated storage areas including the storage specification, the status of components to be stored in each area and the persons who are authorised to access each specific area

- procedures for validating and monitoring the conditions of storage

- procedures for ensuring the good order and cleanliness of storage areas

- procedures to ensure the storage of blood components does not jeopardise their identity, integrity or quality

- a procedure which ensures appropriate stock rotation.

6.8 Non-conforming components and biohazards

6.8.1 Discard of non-conforming components (including outdated components)

Procedures for the discard of non-conforming components should ensure that an appropriate record of discard is maintained. This includes:

- the donation number
- the component identity
- the reason for discard
- the date of discard
- the identity of the person effecting the discard.

If the discard process involves recording as a discard on computer software and physically discarding, then adequate records are required for both steps.

6.8.2 Biohazards

Components from donations that are repeatably reactive in mandatory microbiological screening tests or from donors whose records indicate their components should be destroyed because they are on a high-risk deferral registry or because of previous mandatory test results are classified as biohazards.

Secure and effective procedures are required to ensure that all components and samples from biohazard donations are retrieved for safe disposal in accordance with Blood Service policies and with the Department of Health's *Safe Management of Healthcare Waste*.[7] Procedures should include:

- a system which ensures all components prepared from any donation can be traced
- maintaining a record of the person who retrieves each biohazard component, including laboratory samples.

When biohazard material (e.g. plasma) is retained for laboratory use, it must be appropriately labelled to prevent it ever being used for therapeutic purposes and must be stored in a secure freezer or other storage unit that is clearly labelled to prohibit the storage of material for therapeutic use. An inventory of freezer (or other storage unit) contents of such samples, record of 'sample' retention, reason for retention and fate should be maintained.

6.9 Component release

All components must be appropriately labelled in accordance with these guideline specifications including those general guidelines outlined in section 6.5 and Chapters 23 and 26.

Standard procedures must ensure that blood and blood components cannot be released to stock until all the required laboratory tests, mandatory and additional, have been completed, documented and approved within a validated system of work and it has been ascertained that conditions of production and storage have been satisfactory. Compliance with these requirements may be achieved by the use of a computer program, or suite of programs, which requires the input of valid and acceptable test results for all the mandatory and discretionary laboratory tests before permitting, or withholding, the release of each individual unit.

Where a computer-based system is not used or is temporarily unavailable, documented approval for the release of each individual unit should be by a designated person.

All biohazard donations and components otherwise unsuitable for issue should be reconciled and accounted for, preferably prior to releasing accompanying 'usable' blood components to stock.

6.10 Release of components which do not conform to specified requirements

Blood and/or blood components may be issued for research, for reagent and, in exceptional cases, for therapeutic use when they do not conform to specified requirements. Each Blood Establishment must have written instructions detailing the circumstances under which such concessionary issues can be made and the procedures to be followed.

For major non-conformances in components intended for therapeutic use (e.g. an HLA-matched platelet that is significantly below specified cell counts, extension of shelf life for an autologous donation or, in extreme circumstances, a donor sample not tested for mandatory microbiological marker etc.) the instructions should, as a minimum, include the following:

- that such component issues are authorised by a Blood Establishment consultant to the relevant registered medical practitioner

- that the reason for the issue is fully documented

- that a verbal and written warning indicating an increased level of risk is given by a Blood Establishment consultant to the receiving registered medical practitioner who should sign a statement indicating that he/she is willing to accept these risks

- that the name of the recipient is entered on the issue documentation

- that the component is clearly identified with a label indicating that it does not conform to specification, the details of the non-conformance, the name of the recipient and that it must not be used for any other patient.

Issues of non-conforming components should be subjected to a formal review process.

Minor non-conformances in components intended for therapeutic use (e.g. non-critical blood pack faults, minor label issues) should be referred for assessment by the quality manager.

6.11 Transportation of blood components

6.11.1 General considerations

Donated blood and blood components should be transported by a secure system using transit containers, packing materials and procedures which have been validated for the purpose to ensure the component surface temperature can be maintained within the correct ranges during transportation (Chapter 7).

Monitoring of routine transport temperatures should be performed periodically.

Revalidation should be performed if changes are made to the transport containers, packing materials or procedures.

As far as is practicable, transit containers should be equilibrated to a component's storage temperature prior to filling.

Transport containers should be appropriately labelled and should be secure and protect components and samples from damage during transit.

Documentation should accompany components in transit to permit their identification.

Transport containers should not be exposed to temperatures beyond the range and time for which they have been validated.

Where melting ice is used to achieve an appropriate storage temperature, it should not come into direct contact with the components.

Dead air space in packaging containers should be minimised.

Written procedures for the transportation of components should be established and should ensure compliance with the guidance given above. In addition, written procedures should include the following:

- definition of approved systems of packaging, transportation and transport conditions required for each component

- a requirement for monitoring the performance of approved systems of packaging and transportation.

6.11.2 Transportation from collection site to processing centre

Blood and samples from donor sessions must be transported to the receiving blood supplier under appropriate conditions of temperature, security and hygiene.

Donations from which it is intended to prepare platelets should be transported in conditions that ensure the surface temperature of the blood packs does not drop below 18°C.

Blood and samples being transported from donor sessions must be accompanied by documentation, which ensures that all donations in the consignment can be accounted for. (Note: 'Documentation' includes information in writing or in electronic format.)

6.11.3 Transport of components from Blood Establishments to hospital blood banks/users

Blood components should be transported under conditions which are as close as possible to their specific storage requirements and comply with the requirements of Chapter 7. Transport time should be kept to a minimum.

It should be noted that, occasionally, red cell components are issued before they have been cooled to their storage temperature (4 ±2°C). In such circumstances, it may be neither possible nor necessary to maintain the transport temperature within the range 2–10°C and local judgement should be exercised.

Components dispatched from a blood supplier should be accompanied by a dispatch note detailing as a minimum:

- the donation number of each component

- if relevant, the component's ABO and RhD blood group

- the signature(s) and designation of the person(s) responsible for the issue

- space for the signature(s) and designation of the person(s) receiving the consignment.

A copy of the signed and annotated dispatch note (either paper or an electronic equivalent acceptable to the quality director) should be returned to the blood supplier for storage.

6.12 Component recall and traceability

There must be a documented system available in each Blood Establishment whereby adverse effects caused by the administration of any component, or the identification of a component quality problem, can enable the recall, if appropriate, of all unused components derived from that donation or all donations which are a constituent of a component pool. Similarly, there must be a documented system in each Blood Centre for the recall of any component or constituent of a component pool where reasonable grounds exist for believing it could cause adverse effects.

Any recall of a component should lead to a thorough investigation with a view to preventing a recurrence.

A system must be in place that ensures that any transfused (or discarded) blood component can be linked to the original donation and donor from which it was derived.[8]

6.13 References

1. *Guidelines for the Blood Transfusion Services in the United Kingdom* (The Red Book). Available at www.transfusionguidelines.org.uk.

2. Council of Europe (2010). *Guide for the Preparation, Use and Quality Assurance of Blood Components*, 16th edition. Council of Europe Publishing.

3. Beckman N, Nightingale MJ, Pamphilon D (2009). Practical guidelines for applying statistical process control to blood component production. *Transfusion Medicine*, 19, 329–339.

4. Medicines and Healthcare products Regulatory Agency (2007). *Rules and Guidance for Pharmaceutical Manufacturers and Distributors 2007* (the 'Orange Guide'). London: Pharmaceutical Press.

5. Nightingale MJ, Lees B, Biset R, Mertens W (2006). Use of a (proposed) standard protocol to validate Terumo TSCD-II connections between dissimilar blood bag tubing. *Vox Sanguinis*, 91, 241–269.

6. Nightingale MJ, De Korte D, Chabenel A, Hughes W, Rowe GP, Nicholson G (2011). Eurobloodpack: a common European design for blood bag systems with integral leucodepletion filters. *Vox Sanguinis*, 101, 250–254.

7. Department of Health: Health Technical Memorandum 07-01: *Safe Management of Healthcare Waste*. Published by TSO (The Stationery Office) November 2006.

8. UK Blood Safety and Quality Regulations (BSQR). Available at www.legislation.gov.uk/uksi/2005/50. BSQR amendments available at www.legislation.gov.uk/uksi/2005/2898 and www.legislation.gov.uk/uksi/2006/2013

Chapter 7
Specifications for blood components

This chapter details process, product, quality monitoring, labelling, discard, storage and transport specifications.

7.1 Leucocyte depletion

With very few stated exceptions (e.g. granulocytes), from November 1999 all allogeneic blood components produced in the UK have been subjected to a leucocyte depletion process. The term 'LD' may be used where necessary instead of 'leucocyte depleted' or 'leucocyte depletion' although component names will state 'Leucocyte Depleted' where appropriate. The UK specification for leucodepletion is that more than 90% of leucocyte-depleted components from relevant processes should have less than 1×10^6 leucocytes and more than 99% of components should contain less than 5×10^6 leucocytes, both with 95% confidence. Process performance should be assessed against the 1×10^6 limit when using statistical process control (statistical process monitoring) measurements.

Leucocyte depletion can be achieved by a number of methods, which must be validated before use. If filtration is used the recommended capacity of the filter must not be exceeded.

Currently, it is not feasible to assess all components for the effectiveness of the leucodepletion process. Therefore, the UK Blood Transfusion Services (UKBTS) should apply recognised statistical process monitoring methodologies such as those proposed by the International Society of Blood Transfusion Biomedical Excellence for Safer Transfusion (ISBT) BEST Expert Working Party, published in *Transfusion*,[1] to ensure the following:

- conformance of the process to the LD process specification

- identification of LD component specified limit failures

- stability of the process over time.

The residual leucocyte testing schedule should be defined in process monitoring and conformance checking procedures.

It is advisable to identify results to a production run or 'batch' and to ensure conformance of components to relevant specifications before release of components to stock or to ensure that a monitored filter batch is producing components that conform to specification.

A leucocyte depletion process is controlled if a control chart or equivalent is in use and does not currently display control limit or trend warnings.

A leucocyte depletion process is uncontrolled if a control chart or equivalent is not in operation for the process or if a current control chart or equivalent displays control limit or trend warnings.

Where statistical process monitoring methodology is not judged appropriate due to an inability to control the process or the production of small numbers of components, all components routinely issued to stock must have been shown to contain less than 1×10^6 leucocytes.

Issue (to stock) of components, which do not meet the leucocyte depletion specified limit, must follow a concessionary release procedure (see section 6.10).

Patient-designated components should not be discarded before referral to a clinician.

Secondary components or split components produced from primary components do not require a leucocyte count provided the primary process is controlled or the individual primary component is tested and found to be acceptable.

Plasma components derived from whole blood filtration do not require residual leucocytes to be monitored provided the associated red cell process is controlled.

Leucocyte or platelet counts on components produced from frozen and thawed material should be made, where necessary, prior to the initial freezing process unless otherwise validated.

If the leucodepletion process transfers the final component into a pack that was not part of the original pack assembly, a secure system must be in place to ensure the correct identification number is put on the final component pack.

Leucocyte depletion of components should take place before the end of Day 2 (Day 0 is the day of collection).

Once a red cell component has been cooled to its storage temperature (i.e. 4 ±2°C) prior to leucodepletion, and when leucodepletion by filtration is to take place at ambient temperature, the ambient temperature of the room in which filtration takes place should not exceed 26°C (see also section 6.4).

If components are removed from their designated storage temperature to undergo a leucodepletion process, they must be returned to their storage temperature as soon as possible and in any event within 3 hours (see also section 6.4).

7.2 Other component specifications

Other component and process monitoring specifications are detailed later in this chapter. As far as possible, all parameters tested should be derived from a single component. Because of biological variability, it is acceptable if a minimum of 75% of the results from component and process monitoring tests (other than leucocyte depletion specifications, platelets for intrauterine transfusion, washed red cells, and prion-reduced red cell components) achieve the specifications.

Yield specifications (e.g. platelet yield/unit, total haemoglobin/unit) for components produced by splitting primary components should be the indicated specification for the primary component divided by the number of split components produced.

Haemolysis measurements on red cell components are performed at the end of the component shelf life. Due to intermittent availability of outdated red cell components, each primary process should be validated to give haemolysis of <0.8% of the red cell mass at the end of component shelf life in >75% of components with a minimum of 20 components tested. Revalidation of the red cell preparation processes for red cell haemolysis must be performed at least annually and after any alteration to the production method.

For mandatory microbiology screening and blood grouping tests, all components must conform to the requirements specified in Chapter 9. Concessionary procedures for release of components that do not conform to these requirements are given in section 6.10.

7.3 Production advice

The timing and method of separation depends on the components to be prepared from a given donation.

If the production, washing or splitting process transfers the final component into a pack that was not part of the original pack assembly, a secure system must be in place to ensure the correct identification number is put on the final component pack.

Where a production process amends the expiry date of the component, there are different consequences, dependent on the process.

Further processing or irradiation may reduce the expiry date of the component. Here the expiry date of the new component must not exceed that of the primary component or the expiry date limitations conferred by the process.

Components produced by pooling primary components must have an expiry date of the shortest dated component used.

When remanufacturing neonatal or paediatric red cell components into adult components, to avoid unnecessary wastage, the expiry date may be extended.

Processing of a red cell component to allow frozen storage will result in a lengthened expiry date.

The method of preparation should ensure that plasma components have the maximum level of labile coagulation factors with minimum cellular contamination.

Donations from donors with clinically significant human platelet antigen (HPA) and/or human leucocyte antigen (HLA) antibodies should not be used for the production of plasma-rich blood products (e.g. fresh frozen plasma, platelet concentrate, whole blood, cryoprecipitate). Red cells suspended in additive solution can be produced from such donations.

Platelet and plasma components should not be produced from lipaemic or icteric donations or be contaminated with red cells. Procedures should exist for assessing these findings.

An upper platelet concentration should be assigned for each platelet component type based on pack validation data or the pack manufacturer's recommendations.

pH measurements on platelet components should be made between 20 and 24°C or the measurements corrected to 22°C.

Unless a validated pathogen inactivation process is used, blood components for use in intrauterine transfusion, neonates and infants (see also section 7.21), and plasma components for direct clinical use must be derived from selected donors who fulfil the following criteria:

- Have given at least one donation in the last 2 years, which was either negative for all mandatory markers, or if repeat reactive, has been confirmed to be non-specifically reactive and the donor reinstated in accordance with section 9.4 (on reinstatement of blood donors).
- Negative results were obtained for mandatory microbiology markers with the current donation.

Each component should be visually inspected at each stage of processing and immediately prior to issue. The component must be withdrawn if there is evidence of leakage, damage to or fault in the container, excessive air, suspicion of microbial contamination or any other contraindications such as platelet clumping, unusual turbidity, haemolysis or other abnormal colour change.

7.4 Whole Blood, Leucocyte Depleted

A unit of blood collected into an anticoagulant, containing less than 1×10^6 leucocytes.

7.4.1 Technical information

- A unit of whole blood collected in the UK currently consists of 450 mL ±10% of blood from a suitable donor (see Chapter 3), plus 63 mL of anticoagulant, which is then leucocyte depleted, and stored in an approved container. The Eurobloodpack contains 66.5 mL of anticoagulant and is suitable for the collection of 475 mL ±10%, although in the UK a volume of 495 mL will not be exceeded.

- Whole Blood, Leucocyte Depleted should be transfused through a 170–200 μm filter.

7.4.2 Labelling

For general guidelines, see section 6.6.

The following shall be included on the label:

(* = in eye-readable and UKBTS approved barcode format)

- Whole Blood, Leucocyte Depleted* and volume
- the blood component producer's name*
- the donation number*
- the ABO group*
- the RhD group stated as positive or negative*
- the name, composition and volume of the anticoagulant solution
- the date of collection
- the expiry date*
- the temperature of storage
- the blood pack lot number.*

In addition, the following statements should be made:

INSTRUCTION

Always check patient/component compatibility/identity

Inspect pack and contents for signs of deterioration or damage

Risk of adverse reaction/infection, including vCJD

7.4.3 Storage

For general guidelines, see section 6.7.

- The component may be stored for a maximum of 35 days at a core temperature of 4 ±2°C if an adenine-supplemented anticoagulant is used, otherwise the maximum period of storage is 28 days at a core temperature of 4 ±2°C.

- Variation from the core temperature of 4 ±2°C must be kept to a minimum during storage and restricted to any short period necessary for examining, labelling or issuing the component.

- Exceptionally, i.e. due to equipment failure at a Blood Centre, red cell components which have been exposed to a core temperature not exceeding 10°C and not less than 1°C may be released for transfusion provided that:

  - the component has been exposed to such a temperature change on one occasion only
  - the duration of the temperature excursion has not exceeded 5 hours
  - a documented system is available in each Blood Centre to cover such eventualities
  - adequate records of the incident are compiled and retained.

7.4.4 Testing

In addition to the mandatory and other tests required for blood donations described in Chapter 9, and leucocyte counting (see sections 6.3 and 7.1), a minimum of 75% of those components tested for the parameters shown in Table 7.1 shall meet the specified values.

Table 7.1 Whole Blood, Leucocyte Depleted – additional tests

Parameter	Frequency of test	Specification
Volume*	1% or as determined by statistical process control (if ≤10 components produced per month then test every available component)	470 ±50 mL
Haemolysis	As per section 7.2	<0.8% of red cell mass
Haemoglobin content	1% or as determined by statistical process control (if ≤10 components produced per month then test every available component)	≥40 g/unit
Leucocyte count**	As per sections 6.3 and 7.1	$<1 \times 10^6$/unit
* After volume losses resulting from leucodepletion			
** Methods validated for counting low numbers of leucocytes must be used			

7.4.5 Transportation

For general guidelines, see section 6.11.

For red cell components, transit containers, packing materials and procedures should have been validated to ensure the component surface temperature can be maintained between 2°C and 10°C during transportation. Additionally:

- the validation exercise should be repeated periodically
- if melting ice is used, it should not come into direct contact with the components
- dead air space in packaging containers should be minimised
- as far as is practicable, transit containers should be equilibrated to their storage temperature prior to filling with components
- transport time normally should not exceed 12 hours.

In some instances it is necessary to issue red cell components that have not been cooled to their storage temperature prior to placing in the transit container. The transport temperature specified above is not applicable for such consignments.

7.5 Red Cells, Leucocyte Depleted

A red cell component containing less than 1×10^6 leucocytes.

7.5.1 Technical information

- A red cell component prepared by removing a proportion of the plasma from leucocyte-depleted whole blood or by leucodepleting plasma reduced red cells.
- Red Cells, Leucocyte Depleted should be transfused through a 170–200 μm filter.

7.5.2 Labelling

For general guidelines, see section 6.6.

The following shall be included on the label:

(* = in eye-readable and UKBTS approved barcode format)

- Red Cells, Leucocyte Depleted* and volume
- the blood component producer's name*
- the donation number*
- the ABO group*
- the RhD group stated as positive or negative*
- the name, composition and volume of the anticoagulant solution
- the date of collection
- the expiry date*
- the temperature of storage
- the blood pack lot number.*

In addition, the following statements should be made:

INSTRUCTION

Always check patient/component compatibility/identity

Inspect pack and contents for signs of deterioration or damage

Risk of adverse reaction/infection, including vCJD

7.5.3 Storage

For general guidelines, see section 6.7.

- The component may be stored for a maximum of 35 days at a core temperature of 4 ±2°C if an adenine supplemented anticoagulant is used, otherwise the maximum period of storage is 28 days at a core temperature of 4 ±2°C.

- Variation from the core temperature of 4 ±2°C must be kept to a minimum during storage and restricted to any short period necessary for examining, labelling or issuing the component.

- Exceptionally, i.e. due to equipment failure at a Blood Centre, red cell components which have been prepared in a closed system and exposed to a core temperature not exceeding 10°C and not less than 1°C may be released for transfusion provided that:

  - the component has been exposed to such a temperature change on one occasion only
  - the duration of the temperature change has not exceeded 5 hours
  - a documented system is available in each Blood Centre to cover such eventualities
  - adequate records of the incident are compiled and retained.

7.5.4 Testing

In addition to the mandatory and other tests required for blood donations described in Chapter 9, and leucocyte counting (see sections 6.3 and 7.1), a minimum of 75% of those components tested for the parameters shown in Table 7.2 shall meet the specified values.

Table 7.2 Red Cells, Leucocyte Depleted – additional tests

Parameter	Frequency of test	Specification
Volume	1% or as determined by statistical process control (if ≤10 components produced per month then test every available component)	280 ±60 mL
Haemoglobin content		≥40 g/unit
Haemolysis	As per section 7.2	<0.8% of red cell mass
Leucocyte count*	As per sections 6.3 and 7.1	$<1 \times 10^6$/unit
* Methods validated for counting low levels of leucocytes must be used		

7.5.5 Transportation

For general guidelines, see section 6.11.

For red cell components, transit containers, packing materials and procedures should have been validated to ensure the component surface temperature can be maintained between 2°C and 10°C during transportation. Additionally:

- the validation exercise should be repeated periodically
- if melting ice is used, it should not come into direct contact with the components
- dead air space in packaging containers should be minimised
- as far as is practicable, transit containers should be equilibrated to their storage temperature prior to filling with components
- transport time normally should not exceed 12 hours.

In some instances it is necessary to issue red cell components that have not been cooled to their storage temperature prior to placing in the transit container. The transport temperature specified above is not applicable for such consignments.

7.6 Red Cells in Additive Solution, Leucocyte Depleted

A red cell component containing less than 1×10^6 leucocytes and suspended in an approved additive solution.

7.6.1 Technical information

- A red cell component prepared by removing a proportion of the plasma from leucocyte-depleted whole blood and suspending in an approved additive solution. Leucodepletion may be carried out on either the whole blood starting material or on the final component.

- Red Cells in Additive Solution, Leucocyte Depleted should be transfused through a 170–200 µm filter.

- May be produced by remanufacture of Red Cells for Exchange Transfusion, Leucocyte Depleted (section 7.24) up to 6 days after donation.

7.6.2 Labelling

For general guidelines, see section 6.6.

The following shall be included on the label:

(* = in eye-readable and UKBTS approved barcode format)

- Red Cells in Additive Solution, Leucocyte Depleted* and volume
- the blood component producer's name*
- the donation number*
- the ABO group*
- the RhD group stated as positive or negative*
- the name, composition and volume of the additive solution
- the date of collection
- the expiry date*
- the temperature of storage
- the blood pack lot number.*

In addition, the following statements should be made:

INSTRUCTION

Always check patient/component compatibility/identity

Inspect pack and contents for signs of deterioration or damage

Risk of adverse reaction/infection, including vCJD

7.6.3 Storage

For general guidelines, see section 6.7.

- The component may be stored for a maximum of 35 days at a core temperature of 4 ±2°C.

- Variation from the core temperature of 4 ±2°C must be kept to a minimum during storage and restricted to any short period necessary for examining, labelling or issuing the component.

- Exceptionally, i.e. due to equipment failure at a Blood Centre, red cell components which have been prepared in a closed system and exposed to a core temperature not exceeding 10°C and not less than 1°C may be released for transfusion provided that:

  - the component has been exposed to such a temperature change on one occasion only
  - the duration of the temperature excursion has not exceeded 5 hours
  - a documented system is available in each Blood Centre to cover such eventualities
  - adequate records of the incident are compiled and retained.

7.6.4 Testing

In addition to the mandatory and other tests required for blood donations described in Chapter 9, and leucocyte counting (see sections 6.3 and 7.1), a minimum of 75% of those components tested for the parameters shown in Table 7.3 shall meet the specified values.

Table 7.3 Red Cells in Additive Solution, Leucocyte Depleted – additional tests

Parameter	Frequency of test	Specification
Volume	1% or as determined by statistical process control (if ≤10 components produced per month then test every available component)	280 ±60 mL
Haemoglobin content		≥40 g/unit**
Haemolysis	As per section 7.2	<0.8% of red cell mass
Leucocyte count*	As per sections 6.3 and 7.1	<1 × 10^6/unit
* Methods validated for counting low numbers of leucocytes must be used		
** Units tested and found to have <30 g/unit should not be issued for transfusion		

7.6.5 Transportation

For general guidelines, see section 6.11.

For red cell components, transit containers, packing materials and procedures should have been validated to ensure the component surface temperature can be maintained between 2°C and 10°C during transportation. Additionally:

- the validation exercise should be repeated periodically
- if melting ice is used, it should not come into direct contact with the components
- dead air space in packaging containers should be minimised

- as far as is practicable, transit containers should be equilibrated to their storage temperature prior to filling with components
- transport time normally should not exceed 12 hours.

In some instances it is necessary to issue red cell components that have not been cooled to their storage temperature prior to placing in the transit container. The transport temperature specified above is not applicable for such consignments.

7.7 Red Cells, Washed, Leucocyte Depleted

A red cell component, containing less than 1×10^6 leucocytes, which has been washed with 0.9% w/v sodium chloride for injection (BP) or other validated solution. The Red Cells, Washed, Leucocyte Depleted may then be suspended in an approved solution.

7.7.1 Technical information

- The amount of residual protein will depend on the washing protocol. Washing can be performed by interrupted or continuous flow centrifugation.
- The use of validated washing procedures that incorporate chilled saline or other validated solution for suspension is recommended. This will minimise the risk of bacterial growth and help to produce a component that meets the transit temperature requirements. Use of an automated, closed washing system would be preferable.
- If the washing process results in the transfer of the final component into a pack that was not part of the original pack assembly, a secure system must be in place to ensure the correct donation identification number is put on the component pack of Red Cells, Washed, Leucocyte Depleted.
- Red Cells, Washed, Leucocyte Depleted should be transfused through a 170–200 μm filter.

7.7.2 Labelling

For general guidelines, see section 6.6.

The following shall be included on the label:

(* = in eye-readable and UKBTS approved barcode format)

- Red Cells, Washed, Leucocyte Depleted* and volume
- the blood component producer's name*
- the donation number*
- the ABO group*
- the RhD group stated as positive or negative*
- the name, composition and volume of the suspending solution
- the date and time of preparation
- the expiry date and time*

- the temperature of storage
- the blood pack lot number.*

In addition, the following statements should be made:

INSTRUCTION

Always check patient/component compatibility/identity

Inspect pack and contents for signs of deterioration or damage

Risk of adverse reaction/infection, including vCJD

7.7.3 Storage

For general guidelines, see section 6.7.

The component should be used as soon as possible if produced in an open system. Where the component has been produced in a closed system and storage is required the component should be stored at a core temperature of 4 ±2°C and used within 24 hours of production if suspended in saline or a defined validated period if suspended in an approved additive solution.

7.7.4 Testing

In addition to the mandatory and other tests required for blood donations described in Chapter 9, and leucocyte counting (see sections 6.3 and 7.1), a minimum of 75% of those components tested for the parameters shown in Table 7.4 shall meet the specified values. Provided the component is prepared from a process that is validated for leucocyte removal, testing of washed red cells for residual leucocytes is not required.

7.7.5 Transportation

For general guidelines, see section 6.11.

For red cell components, transit containers, packing materials and procedures should have been validated to ensure the component surface temperature can be maintained between 2°C and 10°C during transportation. Additionally:

- the validation exercise should be repeated periodically
- if melting ice is used, it should not come into direct contact with the components
- dead air space in packaging containers should be minimised
- as far as is practicable, transit containers should be equilibrated to their storage temperature prior to filling with components
- transport time normally should not exceed 12 hours.

In some instances it is necessary to issue red cell components that have not been cooled to their storage temperature prior to placing in the transit container. The transport temperature specified above is not applicable for such consignments.

Table 7.4 Red Cells, Washed, Leucocyte Depleted – additional tests

Parameter	Frequency of test	Specification
Volume	1% or as determined by statistical process control (if ≤10 components produced per month then test every available component)	Within locally specified volume range
Haemoglobin content		≥40 g/unit
Residual protein		<0.5 g/unit
Leucocyte count* (pre-wash)	As per sections 6.3 and 7.1	$<1 \times 10^6$/unit
* Methods validated for counting low numbers of leucocytes must be used		

7.8 Red Cells, Thawed and Washed, Leucocyte Depleted

A red cell component, that contains less than 1×10^6 leucocytes, frozen in the presence of a cryoprotectant (preferably within 5 days of collection), and washed before use. Red Cells, Thawed and Washed, Leucocyte Depleted may then be suspended in an approved additive solution.

7.8.1 Technical information

- The concentration and nature of the cryoprotectant must provide appropriate protection of the red cells at the intended storage temperature. The entire process of freezing, thawing and washing must be validated and documented.

- The use of validated washing procedures that incorporate chilled saline or other validated solution for suspension is recommended. This will minimise the risk of bacterial contamination and helps to produce a component that meets the transit temperature requirements. Use of an automated, closed washing system would be preferable.

- The target minimum haemoglobin content is 36 g.

- If the washing process results in the transfer of the final component into a pack that was not part of the original pack assembly, a secure system must be in place to ensure the correct donation identification number is put on the pack in which the component is frozen and the pack in which the final component is presented.

- Red Cells, Thawed and Washed, Leucocyte Depleted should be transfused through a 170–200 µm filter.

7.8.2 Labelling

For general guidelines, see section 6.6.

The following shall be included on the label:

(* = in eye-readable and UKBTS approved barcode format)

- Red Cells, Thawed and Washed, Leucocyte Depleted* and volume

- the blood component producer's name*

- the donation number*

- the ABO group*

- the RhD group stated as positive or negative*

- the name, composition and volume of the suspending solution
- the date and time of preparation
- the expiry date and time*
- the temperature of storage
- the blood pack lot number.*

In addition, the following statements should be made:

INSTRUCTION

Always check patient/component compatibility/identity

Inspect pack and contents for signs of deterioration or damage

Risk of adverse reaction/infection, including vCJD

7.8.3 Storage

For general guidelines, see section 6.7.

- Maintenance of a constant storage temperature is important, particularly if a low-glycerol cryoprotectant system is used. Storage should be controlled to ensure the temperature is:
  - −60°C to −80°C if stored in an electrical freezer, when a high-glycerol method is used
  - −140°C to −150°C if stored in vapour phase liquid nitrogen, when a low-glycerol method is used.
- The storage may be extended to at least 10 years, if the correct storage temperature is guaranteed.
- The thawed component should be used as soon as possible if produced in an open system. Where the component has been produced in a closed system and storage is required the component should be stored at a core temperature of 4 ±2°C and used within 24 hours of production if suspended in saline or a defined validated period if suspended in an approved additive solution.

7.8.4 Testing

In addition to the mandatory and other tests required for blood donations described in Chapter 9, and leucocyte counting (see sections 6.3 and 7.1), a minimum of 75% of those components tested for the parameters shown in Table 7.5 shall meet the specified values. Provided the component is prepared from a process that is validated for leucocyte removal, testing of washed red cells for residual leucocytes is not required.

Table 7.5 Red Cells, Thawed and Washed, Leucocyte Depleted – additional tests

Parameter	Frequency of test	Specification
Volume	All	Within locally defined nominal volume range
Supernatant haemoglobin	1% or as determined by statistical process control (if ≤10 components produced per month then test every available component)	≤2 g/unit
Red cell haemoglobin		≥36 g/unit
Leucocyte count*	As per sections 6.3 and 7.1	$<1 \times 10^6$/unit**
*Methods validated for counting low numbers of leucocytes must be used		
**Pre-freeze		

7.8.5 Transportation

For general guidelines, see section 6.11.

- The transport requirements for red cells in the frozen state will be influenced by the nature and concentration of cryoprotectant used: e.g. a component containing <20% glycerol requires a refrigerant colder than dry ice, such as the vapour phase of liquid nitrogen.

- For thawed red cell components, transit containers, packing materials and procedures should have been validated to ensure the component surface temperature can be maintained between 2°C and 10°C during transportation. Additionally:

  - the validation exercise should be repeated periodically
  - if melting ice is used, it should not come into direct contact with the components
  - dead air space in packaging containers should be minimised
  - as far as is practicable, transit containers should be equilibrated to their storage temperature prior to filling with components
  - transport time normally should not exceed 12 hours.

In some instances it is necessary to issue red cell components that have not been cooled to their storage temperature prior to placing in the transit container. The transport temperature specified above is not applicable for such consignments.

7.9 Platelets, Pooled, Buffy Coat Derived, Leucocyte Depleted

A pool of platelets, derived from buffy coats, which contains less than 1×10^6 leucocytes.

7.9.1 Technical information

- Donations of whole blood where the bleed time exceeded 15 minutes are not suitable for platelet production.

- The buffy coats must be prepared at ambient temperature before the whole blood is cooled to below 20°C.

- Initial separation of buffy coat must occur within 24 hours of venepuncture (unless supported by additional validation), with a minimum buffy coat rest period of 2 hours before secondary pooling and processing of buffy coats to produce the final component, which is generally completed before the end of Day 1.

- The volume of suspension medium must be sufficient to maintain the pH within the range 6.4–7.4 at the end of the shelf life of the component.

- The production process transfers the final component into a pack that was not part of the original pack assembly. Therefore a secure system must be in place to ensure a full audit trail and that the correct identification number is put on the final component pack.

- Where the production method requires the use of a single unit of plasma for resuspension, the plasma from group O donors should be tested for high-titre anti-A and anti-B and 'high-titre negative' units labelled. The testing method and acceptable limits should be defined (see also Chapter 9). Plasma should be selected from male donors as a TRALI risk reduction strategy.

- Platelets, Pooled, Buffy Coat Derived, Leucocyte Depleted, should be transfused through a 170–200 µm filter.

7.9.2 Labelling

For general guidelines, see section 6.6.

The following shall be included on the label:

(* = in eye-readable and UKBTS approved barcode format)

- Platelets, Pooled, Buffy Coat Derived, Leucocyte Depleted* and volume

- the blood component producer's name*

- a unique pool or batch number or the donation number of all contributing platelet units*

- the ABO group*

- the RhD group stated as positive or negative*

- the expiry date*

- the temperature of storage and a comment that continuous gentle agitation throughout storage is recommended

- the blood pack lot number*

- the name, composition and volume of the anticoagulant or additive solution.

In addition, the following statements should be made:

INSTRUCTION

Always check patient/component compatibility/identity

Inspect pack and contents for signs of deterioration or damage

Risk of adverse reaction/infection, including vCJD

7.9.3 Storage

For general guidelines, see section 6.7.

- The storage period depends on a number of factors including the nature of the container, the concentration of platelets and on whether an open or closed system is used.

- Packs currently in use for this purpose allow for storage at a core temperature of 22 ±2°C with continuous gentle agitation for up to 5 days in a closed system. Appropriate pack and platelet concentration combinations may allow storage up to 7 days, but due to concerns over bacterial contamination requires either an assay to exclude bacterial contamination prior to transfusion or application of a licensed pathogen inactivation procedure.

- If any production stage involves an open system, after preparation the component should be used as soon as possible. If storage is unavoidable, the component should be stored at a core temperature of 22 ±2°C with continuous agitation and used within 6 hours.

- Platelets should be gently agitated during storage. If agitation is interrupted, for example due to equipment failure or prolonged transportation, the components are suitable for use, retaining the same shelf life, provided the interruptions are for no longer than a total of 24 hours.

7.9.4 Testing

In addition to the mandatory and other tests required for blood donations described in Chapter 9, and leucocyte counting (see sections 6.3 and 7.1), a minimum of 75% of those components tested for the parameters shown in Table 7.6 shall meet the specified values.

Table 7.6 Platelets, Pooled, Buffy Coat Derived, Leucocyte Depleted – additional tests

Parameter	Frequency of test	Specification
Volume	1% or as determined by statistical process control (if ≤10 components produced per month then test every available component)	Within locally defined nominal volume range
Platelet count		$\geq 240 \times 10^9$/pool**
pH at end of shelf life		6.4–7.4
Leucocyte count*	As per sections 6.3 and 7.1	$<1 \times 10^6$/pool
* Methods validated for counting low numbers of leucocytes must be used		
** Units tested and found to have $<160 \times 10^9$/pool should not be issued for transfusion		

Note: Visual inspection of platelet components for the swirling phenomenon, clumping, excessive red cell contamination and abnormal volume is a useful pre-issue check.

7.9.5 Transportation

For general guidelines, see section 6.11.

- Containers for transporting platelets should be equilibrated at room temperature before use. During transportation the temperature of platelets must be kept as close as possible to the recommended storage temperature and, on receipt, unless intended for immediate therapeutic use, the component should be transferred to storage at a core temperature of 22 ±2°C with continuous gentle agitation.

- Plastic overwraps should be removed prior to storage.

7.10 Platelets, Apheresis, Leucocyte Depleted

A single-donor platelet component containing less than 1×10^6 leucocytes.

7.10.1 Technical information

- Platelets, Apheresis, Leucocyte Depleted may be collected by a variety of apheresis systems using different protocols. Since platelet yields may vary, each procedural protocol must be fully validated, documented and specifications set accordingly.

- If filtration is used the recommended capacity of the filter should not be exceeded.

- The volume of suspension medium must be sufficient to maintain the pH within the range 6.4–7.4 at the end of the shelf life of the component.

- If the leucodepletion process transfers the final component into a pack that was not part of the original pack assembly, a secure system must be in place to ensure the correct identification number is put on the final component pack.

- The plasma from group O donors should be tested for high-titre anti-A and anti-B, and 'high-titre negative' units labelled. The testing method and acceptable limits should be defined (see also Chapter 9). Screening of female donors for HLA/HNA antibodies should be considered as a TRALI risk reduction strategy.

- Platelets, Apheresis, Leucocyte Depleted should be transfused through a 170–200 µm filter.

7.10.2 Labelling

For general guidelines, see section 6.6.

The following shall be included on the label:

(* = in eye-readable and UKBTS approved barcode format)

- Platelets, Apheresis, Leucocyte Depleted* and volume
- the blood component producer's name*
- the donation number and, if divided, sub-batch number*
- the ABO group*
- the RhD group stated as positive or negative*
- the expiry date*
- the temperature of storage and a comment that continuous gentle agitation throughout storage is recommended
- the blood pack lot number*
- the name, composition and volume of the anticoagulant or additive solution.

In addition, the following statements should be made:

INSTRUCTION

Always check patient/component compatibility/identity

Inspect pack and contents for signs of deterioration or damage

Risk of adverse reaction/infection, including vCJD

7.10.3 Storage

For general guidelines, see section 6.7.

- The storage period depends on a number of factors including the nature of the container, the concentration of platelets and whether an open or closed system is used.

- Packs currently in use for this purpose allow for storage at a core temperature of 22 ±2°C with continuous gentle agitation for up to 5 days in a closed system. Appropriate pack and platelet concentration combinations may allow storage up to 7 days, but due to concerns over bacterial contamination requires either an assay to exclude bacterial contamination prior to transfusion or application of a licensed pathogen inactivation procedure.

- Where any manufacturing step involves an open system the platelets should be used as soon as possible after collection. If storage is unavoidable, the component should be stored at a core temperature of 22 ±2°C with continuous agitation and used within 6 hours.

- Platelets should be gently agitated during storage. If agitation is interrupted, for example due to equipment failure or prolonged transportation, the components are suitable for use, retaining the same shelf life, provided the interruption is for no longer than a total of 24 hours.

7.10.4 Testing

In addition to the mandatory and other tests required for blood donations described in Chapter 9, and leucocyte counting (see sections 6.3 and 7.1), a minimum of 75% of those components tested for the parameters shown in Table 7.7 shall meet the specified values.

Table 7.7 Platelets, Apheresis, Leucocyte Depleted – additional tests

Parameter	Frequency of test	Specification
Volume	1% or as determined by statistical process control (if ≤10 components produced per month then test every available component)	Within locally defined nominal volume range
Platelet count		$\geq 240 \times 10^9$/unit**
pH at end of shelf life		6.4–7.4
Leucocyte count*	As per sections 6.3 and 7.1	$<1 \times 10^6$/unit
* Methods validated for counting low numbers of leucocytes must be used		
** Units tested and found to have $<160 \times 10^9$/pool should not be issued for transfusion		

Note: Visual inspection of platelet components for the swirling phenomenon, clumping, excessive red cell contamination and abnormal volume is a useful pre-issue check.

7.10.5 Transportation

For general guidelines, see section 6.11.

- Containers for transporting platelets should be equilibrated at room temperature before use. During transportation the temperature of platelets must be kept as close as possible to the recommended storage temperature and, on receipt, unless intended for immediate therapeutic use, the component should be transferred to storage at a core temperature of 22 ±2°C with continuous gentle agitation.

- Plastic overwraps should be removed prior to storage.

7.11 Platelets in Additive Solution and Plasma, Leucocyte Depleted

A platelet concentrate, derived from buffy coats or apheresis, which contains less than 1×10^6 leucocytes and where the suspending medium comprises approximately 30% plasma and 70% additive solution.

7.11.1 Technical Information

- The component is manufactured as a primary component and not as a remanufactured secondary component.

- Donations of whole blood where the bleed time exceeded 15 minutes are not suitable for platelet production.

- Where prepared from buffy coats, the buffy coats must be prepared at ambient temperature before the whole blood is cooled to below 20°C.

- Where prepared from buffy coats, initial separation of buffy coat must occur within 24 hours of venepuncture (unless supported by additional validation), with a minimum buffy coat rest period of 2 hours before secondary pooling and processing of buffy coats to produce the final component, which is generally completed before the end of Day 1.

- Screening of female apheresis donors for HLA/HNA antibodies should be considered as a TRALI risk reduction strategy.

- The volume of suspension medium must be sufficient to maintain the pH within the range 6.4–7.4 at the end of the shelf life of the component.

- Where the production process transfers the final component into a pack that was not part of the original pack assembly, a secure system must be in place to ensure the audit trail and the correct identification number is put on the final component pack.

- Platelets in Additive Solution and Plasma, Leucocyte Depleted, should be transfused through a 170–200 µm filter.

7.11.2 Labelling

For general guidelines, see section 6.6.

The following shall be included on the label:

(* = in eye-readable and UKBTS approved barcode format)

- Platelets in Additive Solution and Plasma, Leucocyte Depleted * and volume

- the blood component producer's name*

- a unique pool or batch number or the donation number of all contributing platelet units*

- the RhD group stated as positive or negative*

- the name, composition and volume of the anticoagulant and platelet additive solution

- the expiry date*

- the temperature of storage and a comment that continuous gentle agitation throughout storage is recommended
- the blood pack lot number*

In addition, the following statements should be made:

INSTRUCTION

Always check patient/component compatibility/identity

Inspect pack and contents for signs of deterioration or damage

Risk of adverse reaction/infection, including vCJD

7.11.3 Storage

For general guidelines, see section 6.7.

- The storage period depends on a number of factors including the nature of the container, the concentration of platelets and on whether an open or closed system is used.
- Packs currently in use for this purpose allow for storage at a core temperature of 22 ±2°C with continuous gentle agitation for up to 5 days in a closed system. Appropriate pack and platelet concentration combinations may allow storage up to 7 days, but due to concerns over bacterial contamination would require either an assay to exclude bacterial contamination prior to transfusion or application of a licensed pathogen reduction procedure.
- If any production stage involves an open system, after preparation the component should be used as soon as possible. If storage is unavoidable, the component should be stored at a core temperature of 22 ±2°C with continuous agitation and used within 6 hours.

7.11.4 Testing

In addition to the mandatory and other tests required for blood donations described in Chapter 9 and leucocyte counting (see section 6.3 and 7.1), a minimum of 75% of those components tested for the parameters shown at Table 7.8 shall meet the specified values.

Table 7.8 Platelets in Additive Solution and Plasma – additional tests

Parameter	Frequency of test	Specification
Volume	1% or as determined by statistical process control (if ≤10 components produced per month then test every available component)	Within locally defined nominal volume range
Platelet count		$\geq 240 \times 10^9$/pool
pH at end of shelf life	If less than 10 per month, every available component	6.4–7.4
Leucocyte count*	As per sections 6.3 and 7.1	$<1 \times 10^6$/pool*
* Methods validated for counting low levels of leucocytes must be used		

Note: Visual inspection of platelet components for the swirling phenomenon, clumping, excessive red cell contamination and abnormal volume is a useful pre-issue check.

7.11.5 Transportation

For general guidelines, see section 6.11.

Containers for transporting platelets should be equilibrated at room temperature before use. During transportation the temperature of platelets must be kept as close as possible to the recommended storage temperature and, on receipt, unless intended for immediate therapeutic use, the component should be transferred to storage at a core temperature of 22 ±2°C with continuous gentle agitation. Plastic overwraps should be removed prior to storage.

7.12 Platelets in Additive Solution, Leucocyte Depleted

A platelet concentrate derived from buffy coats or apheresis, which contains less than 1×10^6 leucocytes and where the suspending medium is additive solution. This component is indicated for patients with reactions to plasma-containing components.

7.12.1 Technical information

- Donations of whole blood where the bleed time exceeded 15 minutes are not suitable for platelet production.

- Where prepared from buffy coats, the buffy coats must be prepared at ambient temperature before the whole blood is cooled to below 20°C.

- Where prepared from buffy coats, initial separation of buffy coat must occur within 24 hours of venepuncture (unless supported by additional validation), with a minimum buffy coat rest period of 2 hours before secondary pooling and processing of buffy coats to produce the final component, which is generally completed before the end of Day 1.

- The volume of suspension medium must be sufficient to maintain the pH within the range 6.4–7.4 at the end of the shelf life of the component.

- Where the production process transfers the final component into a pack that was not part of the original pack assembly, a secure system must be in place to ensure a full audit trail and that the correct identification number is put on the final component pack.

- Platelets in Additive Solution, Leucocyte Depleted, should be transfused through a 170–200 µm filter.

7.12.2 Labelling

For general guidelines, see section 6.6.

The following shall be included on the label:

(* = in eye-readable and UKBTS approved barcode format)

- Platelets in Additive Solution, Leucocyte Depleted* and volume

- the blood component producer's name*

- a unique pool or batch number or the donation number of all contributing platelet units*

- the ABO group*

- the RhD group stated as positive or negative*

- the expiry date and time*

- the temperature of storage and a comment that continuous gentle agitation throughout storage is recommended

- the blood pack lot number*
- the name, composition and volume of the additive solution.

In addition, the following statements should be made:

INSTRUCTION

Always check patient/component compatibility/identity

Inspect pack and contents for signs of deterioration or damage

Risk of adverse reaction/infection, including vCJD

7.12.3 Storage

For general guidelines, see section 6.7.

- The storage period depends on a number of factors including the nature of the container, the concentration of platelets, the additive solution used and whether an open or closed system is used.

- Platelets in Additive Solution, Leucocyte Depleted, should be used within 24 hours of production.

- If any production stage involves an open system, after preparation the component should be used as soon as possible. If storage is unavoidable, the component should be stored at a core temperature of 22 ±2°C with continuous agitation and used within 6 hours.

7.12.4 Testing

In addition to the mandatory and other tests required for blood donations described in Chapter 9, and leucocyte counting (see sections 6.3 and 7.1), a minimum of 75% of those components tested for the parameters shown in Table 7.9 shall meet the specified values.

Table 7.9 Platelets in Additive Solution, Leucocyte Depleted – additional tests

Parameter	Frequency of test	Specification
Volume	1% or as determined by statistical process control (if ≤10 components produced per month then test every available component)	Within locally defined nominal volume range
Platelet count		$\geq 200 \times 10^9$/unit
pH at end of shelf life		6.4–7.4
Leucocyte count*	As per sections 6.3 and 7.1	$<1 \times 10^6$/unit
* Methods validated for counting low levels of leucocytes must be used		

Note: Visual inspection of platelet components for the swirling phenomenon, clumping, excessive red cell contamination and abnormal volume is a useful pre-issue check.

7.12.5 Transportation

For general guidelines, see section 6.11.

- Containers for transporting platelets should be equilibrated at room temperature before use. During transportation the temperature of platelets must be kept as close as possible to the recommended storage temperature and, on receipt, unless intended for immediate therapeutic use, the component should be transferred to storage at a core temperature of 22 ±2°C with continuous gentle agitation.

- Plastic overwraps should be removed prior to storage.

7.13 Granulocytes, Apheresis

A component prepared from anticoagulated blood, which is separated into components by a suitable apheresis machine with retention of granulocytes as the major cellular product, suspended in a portion of the plasma. The remaining elements may be returned to the donor.

7.13.1 Technical information

- The component is not leucocyte depleted.

- The component contains red cells and requires compatibility testing.

- Granulocytes may be collected by a variety of apheresis systems using different protocols. Since yields may vary, each procedural protocol must be fully validated, documented and specifications set accordingly.

- Cytomegalovirus (CMV) seronegative granulocytes should be considered for CMV seronegative recipients.

- The component must not be agitated during storage.

- The component must be irradiated before use.

- Granulocytes, Apheresis should be transfused through a 170–200 μm filter.

7.13.2 Labelling

For general guidelines, see section 6.6.

The following shall be included on the label:

(* = in eye-readable and UKBTS approved barcode format)

- Granulocytes, Apheresis* and volume

- the blood component producer's name*

- the donation number*

- the ABO group*

- the RhD group stated as positive or negative*

- the date of collection

- the expiry date and time*

- the temperature of storage

- the statement 'Do not agitate'

- the blood pack lot number*

- the name, composition and volume of the anticoagulant solution.

In addition, the following statements should be made:

INSTRUCTION

Always check patient/component compatibility/identity

Inspect pack and contents for signs of deterioration or damage

Risk of adverse reaction/infection, including vCJD

7.13.3 Storage

For general guidelines, see section 6.7.

- Granulocytes, apheresis should be used as soon as possible after their preparation. If storage is unavoidable, provided the component has been prepared using a closed system, the component should be stored, without agitation, at a core temperature of 22 ±2°C and used within 24 hours of collection.

7.13.4 Testing

In addition to the mandatory and other tests required for blood donations described in Chapter 9, all components tested for the parameters shown in Table 7.10 shall meet the specified values.

Table 7.10 Granulocytes, Apheresis – additional tests

Parameter	Frequency of test	Specification
Volume	1% or as determined by statistical process control (if ≤10 components produced per month then test every available component)	Within locally defined nominal volume range (≤500 mL)
Total granulocyte count		$>1 \times 10^{10}$/unit

7.13.5 Transportation

For general guidelines, see section 6.11.

- Containers for transporting Granulocytes, Apheresis should be equilibrated at room temperature before use. During transportation the temperature of the component must be kept as close as possible to the recommended storage temperature and, on receipt, unless intended for immediate therapeutic use, the component should be transferred to storage at a core temperature of 22 ±2°C.

- Plastic overwraps should be removed prior to storage.

7.14 Granulocytes, Pooled, Buffy Coat Derived, in Platelet Additive Solution and Plasma

A pool of granulocytes, derived from buffy coats, with retention of neutrophils as the major cellular product, suspended in a portion of the plasma and platelet additive solution.

7.14.1 Technical information

- The component is not leucodepleted.

- The component contains red cells and requires compatibility testing.

- CMV seronegative granulocytes should be considered for CMV seronegative recipients.

- The component contains 2.0 adult transfusion doses (ATDs) of platelets[2] and additional platelet transfusion is therefore unlikely to be required.

- The component must not be agitated during storage.

- The component must be irradiated before use.

- Granulocytes should be transfused through a 170–200 µm filter.

- The component must be stored in a pack that allows gas exchange (i.e. a platelet pack).

- The production process transfers the final component into a pack that was not part of the original pack assembly. Therefore a secure system must be in place to ensure a full audit trail and that the correct identification number is put on the final component pack.

- Recommended dose for adults is 1–2 packs daily and for a child 10–20 mL/kg.

- A clinical study has been undertaken in 30 human patients using this component. Leucocyte antibody formation occurred at a rate similar to historical multiply transfused controls[3] of 29 patients assessed).[4]

7.14.2 Labelling

For general guidelines, see section 6.6.

The following should be included on the label:

(* = in eye-readable and UKBTS approved barcode format)

- Granulocytes, Pooled, Buffy Coat Derived, in Platelet Additive Solution and Plasma* and volume

- the blood component producer's name*

- a unique pool or batch number or the donation number of all contributing units*

- the ABO group*

- the RhD group stated as positive or negative*

- the date of collection

- the expiry date and time*

- the temperature of storage

- the statement 'Do not agitate'

- the blood pack lot number*

- the name, composition and volume of the anticoagulant solution

- the name, composition and volume of the platelet additive solution.

In addition, the following statements should be made:

INSTRUCTION

Always check patient/component compatibility/identity

Inspect pack and contents for signs of deterioration or damage

Risk of adverse reaction/infection, including vCJD

7.14.3 Storage

For general guidelines, see section 6.7.

- Granulocytes should be used as soon as possible after their preparation. If storage is unavoidable, provided the component is produced using a closed system, the component should be stored, without agitation, at a core temperature of 22 ±2°C and transfusion should commence by midnight on Day 1 (the day following donation).

7.14.4 Testing

In addition to the mandatory and other tests required for blood donations described in Chapter 9, all components tested for the parameters shown in Table 7.11 shall meet the specified values.

Table 7.11 Granulocytes, Pooled, Buffy Coat Derived, in Additive Solution and Plasma – additional tests

Parameter	Frequency of test	Specification
Volume	1% or as determined by statistical process control (if ≤10 components produced per month then test every available component)	175–250 mL*
Total granulocyte count		$>5 \times 10^9$/unit*
* Based on production from ten whole blood donations		

7.14.5 Transportation

For general guidelines, see section 6.11.

- Containers for transporting granulocytes should be equilibrated at room temperature before use. During transportation the temperature of the component must be kept as close as possible to the recommended storage temperature and, on receipt, unless intended for immediate therapeutic use, the component should be transferred to storage at a core temperature of 22 ±2°C without agitation.

- Plastic overwraps should be removed prior to storage.

7.15 Fresh Frozen Plasma, Leucocyte Depleted

Plasma that has been obtained from whole blood or by apheresis from a previously tested donor (as defined in section 7.3). The plasma contains less than 1×10^6 leucocytes per component and has been rapidly frozen to a temperature that will maintain the activity of labile coagulation factors.

7.15.1 Technical information

- Donations of whole blood where the bleed time exceeded 15 minutes are not suitable for the production of plasma components for direct clinical use.

- Plasma should be selected from male donors or consideration should be given to screening female donors for HLA/HNA antibodies, as a TRALI risk reduction measure.

- The plasma should be separated before the red cell component is cooled to its storage temperature. Greater FVIII:C yields will be obtained when the plasma is separated as soon as possible after venepuncture and rapidly frozen to –25°C or below.

- The method of preparation should ensure the component has the maximum level of labile coagulation factors with minimum cellular contamination. The production process should be validated to ensure that components meet the specified limits for FVIII:C concentration.

- Component samples collected for the quality monitoring assessment of FVIII:C should be from an equal mix of group O and non-O donations due to the difference in FVIII:C levels between ABO blood groups.

- Fresh Frozen Plasma, Leucocyte Depleted should be transfused through a 170–200 μm filter.

7.15.2 Labelling

For general guidelines, see section 6.6.

The following shall be included on the label:

(* = in eye-readable and UKBTS approved barcode format)

- Fresh Frozen Plasma, Leucocyte Depleted* and volume
- the blood component producer's name*
- the donation number and, if divided, sub-batch number*
- the ABO group*
- the RhD group stated as positive or negative*
- the date of collection
- the expiry date of the frozen component*
- the temperature of storage
- the blood pack lot number*
- a warning that the component must be used within 4 hours of thawing if maintained at 22 ±2°C, or 24 hours of thawing if stored at 4 ±2°C
- the name, composition and volume of the anticoagulant.

In addition, the following statements should be made:

INSTRUCTION

Always check patient/component compatibility/identity

Inspect pack and contents for signs of deterioration or damage

Risk of adverse reaction/infection, including vCJD

7.15.3 Storage

For general guidelines, see section 6.7.

- The component should be stored at a core temperature of −25°C or below for a maximum of 24 months.

- Although a storage temperature below −25°C improves the preservation of labile coagulation factors, lower temperatures increase the fragility of plastic. Particular care must be taken when handling such packs.

- The component should be thawed in a waterbath or other equipment designed for the purpose, within a vacuum-sealed overwrap bag according to a validated procedure. The optimal temperature at which the component should be thawed is 37°C; temperatures between 33°C and 37°C are acceptable.

- Protocols must be in place to ensure that the equipment is cleaned daily and maintained to minimise the risk of bacterial contamination. After thawing, the content should be inspected to ensure that no insoluble cryoprecipitate is visible and that the container is intact.

- Once thawed, the component must not be refrozen and should be transfused as soon as possible. If delay is unavoidable, the component may be stored and should be used within 4 hours if maintained at 22 ±2°C or 24 hours if stored at 4 ±2°C, but it should be borne in mind that extended post-thaw storage will result in a decline in the content of labile coagulation factors.

7.15.4 Testing

In addition to the mandatory and other tests required for blood donations described in Chapter 9, and leucocyte counting (see sections 6.3 and 7.1), a minimum of 75% of those components tested for the parameters shown in Table 7.12 shall meet the specified values.

Table 7.12 Fresh Frozen Plasma, Leucocyte Depleted – additional tests

Parameter	Frequency of test	Specification
Volume	1% or as determined by statistical process control (if ≤10 components produced per month then test every available component)	Stated volume ±10%
Total protein		≥50 g/L
Platelet count		$<30 \times 10^9/L$**
Red cell count		$<6 \times 10^9/L$**
FVIII:C		≥0.70 IU/mL
Leucocyte count*	As per sections 6.3 and 7.1	$<1 \times 10^6$/unit**
* Methods validated for counting low numbers of leucocytes must be used		
** Pre-freeze in starting component		

7.15.5 Transportation

For general guidelines, see section 6.11.

Every effort should be made to maintain the core storage temperature during transportation. Unless the component is to be thawed and used straightaway it should be transferred immediately to storage at the recommended temperature.

7.16 Fresh Frozen Plasma, Methylene Blue Treated and Removed, Leucocyte Depleted

This component is intended for use in children and is made from plasma from a country with a low risk of variant Creutzfeldt-Jakob Disease (vCJD).

Fresh Frozen Plasma, Methylene Blue Treated (MBT) and Removed, Leucocyte Depleted, is plasma that has been obtained from whole blood or by apheresis from a previously tested donor (as defined in section 7.3), contains less than 1×10^6 leucocytes and has been treated with methylene blue and exposure to visible light to inactivate pathogens.

Following methylene blue treatment and removal, the plasma is rapidly frozen to a temperature that will maintain the activity of labile coagulation factors.

7.16.1 Technical information

- Where the starting component is sourced outside the UK, a detailed and agreed specification must be available.
- Donations of whole blood where the bleed time exceeded 15 minutes are not suitable for the production of plasma components for direct clinical use.
- Plasma should be selected from male donors or consideration should be given to screening female donors for HLA/HNA antibodies, as a TRALI risk reduction measure.
- The plasma should be separated before the red cell component is cooled to its storage temperature. Greater FVIII:C yields will be obtained when the plasma is separated as soon as possible after venepuncture, methylene blue treated and rapidly frozen to –25°C or below.
- The method of preparation should ensure the component has the maximum level of labile coagulation factors with minimum cellular contamination. The production process should be validated to ensure that components meet the specified limits for FVIII:C concentration.
- Component samples collected for the quality monitoring assessment of FVIII:C should be from an equal mix of group O and non-O donations due to the difference in FVIII levels between ABO blood groups.
- The MBT process reduces the FVIII:C content by approximately 30% when compared to standard fresh frozen plasma.
- Intact white blood cells in the plasma should be reduced to less than 1×10^6 per unit prior to exposure to methylene blue and visible light.
- The process for methylene blue removal should be validated to give components with a methylene blue concentration ≤0.30 µmol/L (less than approximately 30 µg per unit).
- Fresh Frozen Plasma, Methylene Blue Treated and Removed, Leucocyte Depleted should be transfused through a 170–200 µm filter.

7.16.2 Labelling

For general guidelines, see section 6.6.

The following shall be included on the label:

(* = in eye-readable and UKBTS approved barcode format)

- Fresh Frozen Plasma, Methylene Blue Treated and Removed, Leucocyte Depleted* and volume
- the blood component producer's name*
- the donation number*
- the ABO group*
- the RhD group stated as positive or negative*
- the date of collection
- the expiry date of the frozen component*

- the temperature of storage
- the blood pack lot number*
- a warning that the component should be used within 4 hours of thawing if maintained at 22 ±2°C and 24 hours if maintained at 4 ±2°C
- the name, composition and volume of the anticoagulant.

In addition, the following statements should be made:

INSTRUCTION

Always check patient/component compatibility/identity

Inspect pack and contents for signs of deterioration or damage

Risk of adverse reaction/infection

7.16.3 Storage

For general guidelines, see section 6.7.

- The component should be stored at a core temperature of –25°C or below for a maximum of 24 months.
- Although a storage temperature below –25°C improves the preservation of labile coagulation factors, lower temperatures increase the fragility of plastic. Particular care must be taken when handling such packs.
- The component should be thawed in a waterbath or other equipment designed for the purpose, within a vacuum-sealed overwrap bag according to a validated procedure. The optimal temperature at which the component should be thawed is 37°C; temperatures between 33°C and 37°C are acceptable.
- Protocols must be in place to ensure that the equipment is cleaned daily and maintained to minimise the risk of bacterial contamination. After thawing, the content should be inspected to ensure that no insoluble cryoprecipitate is visible and that the container is intact.
- Once thawed, the component must not be refrozen and should be transfused as soon as possible. If delay is unavoidable, the component may be stored and should be used within 4 hours if maintained at 22 ±2°C or 24 hours if stored at 4 ±2°C, but it should be borne in mind that extended post-thaw storage will result in a decline in the content of labile coagulation factors.

7.16.4 Testing

In addition to the mandatory and other tests required for blood donations described in Chapter 9, and leucocyte counting (see sections 6.3 and 7.1), a minimum of 75% of those components tested for the parameters shown in Table 7.13 shall meet the specified values.

Table 7.13 Fresh Frozen Plasma, Methylene Blue Treated and Removed, Leucocyte Depleted – additional tests

Parameter	Frequency of test	Specification
Volume	1% or as determined by statistical process control (if ≤10 components produced per month then test every available component)	Within locally defined nominal volume range and within any limits specified for the MBT process used
Platelet count		$<30 \times 10^9$/L**
FVIII:C		≥0.50 IU/mL
Leucocyte count*	As per sections 6.3 and 7.1	$<1 \times 10^6$/unit**
* Methods validated for counting low numbers of leucocytes must be used		
** Pre-freeze in starting component		

7.16.5 Transportation

For general guidelines, see section 6.11.

Every effort should be made to maintain the core storage temperature during transportation. Unless the component is to be thawed and used straightaway it should be transferred immediately to storage at the recommended temperature.

7.17 Cryoprecipitate, Leucocyte Depleted

The component represents a source of concentrated FVIII:C, and von Willebrand factor, fibrinogen, FXIII and fibronectin from a unit of fresh frozen plasma. The plasma from which the cryoprecipitate was produced contains less than 1×10^6 leucocytes per component and is derived from a previously tested donor (as defined in section 7.3).

7.17.1 Technical information

- Donations of whole blood where the bleed time exceeded 15 minutes are not suitable for the production of plasma components for direct clinical use.

- Cryoprecipitate, Leucocyte Depleted is the cryoglobulin fraction of plasma obtained by thawing a single donation of Fresh Frozen Plasma, Leucocyte Depleted (see section 7.15) at 4 ±2°C.

- Plasma should be selected from male donors or consideration should be given to screening female donors for HLA/HNA antibodies, as a TRALI risk reduction measure.

- For storage, Cryoprecipitate, Leucocyte Depleted should be rapidly frozen to a core temperature of –25°C or below within 2 hours of preparation.

- Component samples collected for the quality monitoring assessment of FVIII:C should be from an equal mix of group O and non-O donations due to the difference in FVIII:C levels between ABO blood groups.

- Cryoprecipitate, Leucocyte Depleted should be transfused through a 170–200 µm filter.

7.17.2 Labelling

For general guidelines, see section 6.6.

The following shall be included on the component label:

(* = in eye-readable and UKBTS approved barcode format)

- Cryoprecipitate, Leucocyte Depleted* and volume
- the blood component producer's name*
- the donation number*
- the ABO group*
- the RhD group stated as positive or negative*
- the date of collection
- the expiry date of the frozen component*
- the temperature of storage
- the blood pack lot number*
- a warning that the component must be used within 4 hours of thawing
- the name, composition and volume of the anticoagulant.

In addition, the following statements should be made:

INSTRUCTION

Always check patient/component compatibility/identity

Inspect pack and contents for signs of deterioration or damage

Risk of adverse reaction/infection, including vCJD

7.17.3 Storage

For general guidelines, see section 6.7.

- The component should be stored at a core temperature of −25°C or below for a maximum of 24 months.
- Although a storage temperature below −25°C improves the preservation of labile coagulation factors, lower temperatures increase the fragility of plastic. Particular care must be taken when handling such packs.
- The component should be thawed in a waterbath or other equipment designed for the purpose, within a vacuum-sealed overwrap bag according to a validated procedure. The optimal temperature at which the component should be thawed is 37°C; temperatures between 33°C and 37°C are acceptable.
- Protocols must be in place to ensure that the equipment is cleaned daily and maintained to minimise the risk of bacterial contamination. After thawing, the content should be inspected to ensure that no insoluble cryoprecipitate is visible and that the container is intact.
- Once thawed, the component must not be refrozen and should be used immediately. If delay is unavoidable, the component should be stored at ambient temperature and used within 4 hours.

7.17.4 Testing

In addition to the mandatory and other tests required for blood donations described in Chapter 9, and leucocyte counting (see sections 6.3 and 7.1), a minimum of 75% of those components tested for the parameters shown in Table 7.14 shall meet the specified values.

Table 7.14 Cryoprecipitate, Leucocyte Depleted – additional tests

Parameter	Frequency of test	Specification
Volume	1% or as determined by statistical process control (if ≤10 components produced per month then test every available component)	Within locally defined nominal range
Fibrinogen		≥140 mg/unit
FVIII:C		≥70 IU/unit
Leucocyte count*	As per sections 6.3 and 7.1	$<1 \times 10^6$/unit**
* Methods validated for counting low numbers of leucocytes must be used		
** Pre-freeze in starting component		

7.17.5 Transportation

For general guidelines, see section 6.11.

Every effort should be made to maintain the core storage temperature during transportation. Unless the component is to be thawed and used straightaway it should be transferred immediately to storage at the recommended temperature.

7.18 Cryoprecipitate Pooled, Leucocyte Depleted

The pooled component represents a source of concentrated FVIII:C, von Willebrand factor, fibrinogen, FXIII and fibronectin from primary cryoprecipitate components derived from units of fresh frozen plasma. The plasma from which the cryoprecipitate was produced was derived from a previously tested donor (as defined in section 7.3) and contains less than 1×10^6 leucocytes per primary component.

7.18.1 Technical information

- Donations of whole blood where the bleed time exceeded 15 minutes are not suitable for the production of plasma components for direct clinical use.

- Cryoprecipitate Pooled, Leucocyte Depleted is the cryoglobulin fraction of plasma obtained by thawing and pooling five single cryoprecipitate components or pooling five single cryoprecipitate components immediately after production from thawed fresh frozen plasma.

- Plasma should be selected from male donors or consideration should be given to screening female donors for HLA/HNA antibodies, as a TRALI risk reduction measure.

- For storage, Cryoprecipitate Pooled, Leucocyte Depleted should be rapidly frozen to a core temperature of –25°C or below within 2 hours of preparation.

- Component samples collected for the quality monitoring assessment of FVIII:C should be from an equal mix of group O and non-O donations due to the difference in FVIII levels between ABO blood groups.

- Initial process validation must ensure that for a minimum of 20 tested Cryoprecipitate Pooled, Leucocyte Depleted components a minimum of 75% of those components tested for the parameters shown in Table 7.15 shall meet the specified values.

- Annual process validation is acceptable for quality monitoring purposes, provided that the primary components, Fresh Frozen Plasma, Leucocyte Depleted and/or Cryoprecipitate, Leucocyte Depleted are separately monitored as part of monthly testing. If this is not the case, test monthly 1% or as determined by statistical process control (if ≤10 components produced per month then test every available component), of Cryoprecipitate Pooled, Leucocyte Depleted components. A minimum of 75% of those components tested for the parameters shown in Table 7.15 shall meet the specified values.

- A secure system must be in place to ensure a full audit trail and that the correct identification number is put on the final component pack.

- Cryoprecipitate Pooled, Leucocyte Depleted should be transfused through a 170–200 µm filter.

7.18.2 Labelling

For general guidelines, see section 6.6.

The following shall be included on the component label:

(* = in eye-readable and UKBTS approved barcode format)

- Cryoprecipitate Pooled, Leucocyte Depleted* and volume
- the blood component producer's name*
- a unique pool or batch number or the donation number of all contributing units*
- the ABO group*
- the RhD group stated as positive or negative*
- the date of collection
- the expiry date of the frozen component*
- the temperature of storage
- the blood pack lot number*
- a warning that the component must be used within 4 hours of thawing
- the name, composition and volume of anticoagulant.

In addition, the following statements should be made:

INSTRUCTION

Always check patient/component compatibility/identity

Inspect pack and contents for signs of deterioration or damage

Risk of adverse reaction/infection, including vCJD

7.18.3 Storage

For general guidelines, see section 6.7.

- The component should be stored at a core temperature of –25°C or below for a maximum of 24 months.

- Although a storage temperature below –25°C improves the preservation of labile coagulation factors, lower temperatures increase the fragility of plastic. Particular care must be taken when handling such packs.

- The component should be thawed in a waterbath or other equipment designed for the purpose, within a vacuum-sealed overwrap bag according to a validated procedure. The optimal temperature at which the component should be thawed is 37°C; temperatures between 33°C and 37°C are acceptable.

- Protocols must be in place to ensure that the equipment is cleaned daily and maintained to minimise the risk of bacterial contamination. After thawing, the content should be inspected to ensure that no insoluble cryoprecipitate is visible and that the container is intact.

- Once thawed, the component must not be refrozen and should be transfused as soon as possible. If delay is unavoidable, the component should be stored at ambient temperature and used within 4 hours.

7.18.4 Testing

In addition to the mandatory and other tests required for blood donations described in Annex 4, and leucocyte counting (see sections 6.3 and 7.1), a minimum of 75% of those components tested for the parameters shown at Table 7.15 shall meet the specified values.

Table 7.15 Cryoprecipitate Pooled, Leucocyte Depleted – additional tests

Parameter	Frequency of test	Specification
Volume	1% or as determined by statistical process control (if ≤10 components produced per month then test every available component)	100–250 mL
Fibrinogen	Refer to Technical information (section 17.18.1) above	≥700 mg/unit
FVIII:C		≥350 IU/unit
Leucocyte count	As per sections 6.3 and 7.1	<1 × 10^6/unit* in the starting component

* Pre-freeze methods validated for counting low numbers of leucocytes must be used

7.18.5 Transportation

For general guidelines, see section 6.11.

Every effort should be made to maintain the core storage temperature during transportation. Unless the component is to be thawed and used straightaway it should be transferred immediately to storage at the recommended temperature.

7.19 Cryoprecipitate, Methylene Blue Treated and Removed, Leucocyte Depleted

This component is made for neonatal use – refer to section 7.28.

7.20 Plasma, Cryoprecipitate Depleted, Leucocyte Depleted

The supernatant plasma removed during the preparation of Cryoprecipitate, Leucocyte Depleted. The plasma from which the Plasma, Cryoprecipitate Depleted, Leucocyte Depleted was made contains less than 1×10^6 leucocytes per component and is derived from a previously tested donor (as defined in section 7.3).

7.20.1 Technical information

- Donations of whole blood where the bleed time exceeded 15 minutes are not suitable for the production of plasma components for direct clinical use.

- Plasma should be selected from male donors or consideration should be given to screening female donors for HLA/HNA antibodies, as a TRALI risk reduction measure.

- Plasma, Cryoprecipitate Depleted, Leucocyte Depleted should be frozen to a core temperature of –25°C or below within 2 hours of separation from its Cryoprecipitate, Leucocyte Depleted.

- Plasma, Cryoprecipitate Depleted, Leucocyte Depleted should be transfused through a 170–200 μm filter.

7.20.2 Labelling

For general guidelines, see section 6.6.

The following shall be included on the component label:

(* = in eye-readable and UKBTS approved barcode format)

- Plasma, Cryoprecipitate Depleted, Leucocyte Depleted* and volume
- the blood component producer's name*
- the donation number*
- the ABO group*
- the RhD group stated as positive or negative*
- the date of collection
- the expiry date of the frozen component*
- the temperature of storage
- the blood pack lot number*
- a warning that the component must be used within 4 hours of thawing if maintained at 22 ±2°C, or 24 hours of thawing if stored at 4 ±2°C
- the name, composition and volume of the anticoagulant.

In addition, the following statements should be made:

INSTRUCTION

Always check patient/component compatibility/identity

Inspect pack and contents for signs of deterioration or damage

Risk of adverse reaction/infection, including vCJD

7.20.3 Storage

For general guidelines, see section 6.7.

- The component should be stored at a core temperature of –25°C or below for a maximum of 24 months.

- Although a storage temperature below –25°C improves the preservation of labile coagulation factors, lower temperatures increase the fragility of plastic. Particular care must be taken when handling such packs.

- The component should be thawed in a waterbath or other equipment designed for the purpose, within a vacuum-sealed overwrap bag according to a validated procedure. The optimal temperature at which the component should be thawed is 37°C; temperatures between 33°C and 37°C are acceptable.

- Protocols must be in place to ensure that the equipment is cleaned daily and maintained to minimise the risk of bacterial contamination. After thawing, the content should be inspected to ensure that no insoluble cryoprecipitate is visible and that the container is intact.

- Once thawed, the component must not be refrozen and should be transfused as soon as possible. If delay is unavoidable, the component may be stored and should be used within 4 hours if maintained at 22 ±2°C or 24 hours if stored at 4 ±2°C, but it should be borne in mind that extended post-thaw storage will result in a decline in the content of labile coagulation factors.

7.20.4 Testing

In addition to the mandatory and other tests required for blood donations described in Chapter 9, and leucocyte counting (see sections 6.3 and 7.1), a minimum of 75% of those components tested for the parameters shown in Table 7.16 shall meet the specified values.

Table 7.16 Plasma, Cryoprecipitate Depleted, Leucocyte Depleted – additional tests

Parameter	Frequency of test	Specification
Volume	1% or as determined by statistical process control (if ≤10 components produced per month then test every available component)	Stated volume ±10%
Platelet count		$<30 \times 10^9/L$**
Red cell count		$<6 \times 10^9/L$**
Leucocyte count*	As per sections 6.3 and 7.1	$<1 \times 10^6/unit$**
* Methods validated for counting low numbers of leucocytes must be used		
** Pre-freeze in starting component (fresh frozen plasma)		

7.20.5 Transportation

For general guidelines, see section 6.11.

Every effort should be made to maintain the core storage temperature during transportation. Unless the component is to be thawed and used straightaway it should be transferred immediately to storage at the recommended temperature.

7.21 Components suitable for use in intrauterine transfusion, neonates and infants under 1 year

7.21.1 General requirements

- Unless they are subjected to a validated pathogen inactivation process, components for use in intrauterine transfusion, neonates and infants under 1 year must be prepared from previously tested donors who fulfil the following criteria:

  - have given at least one donation in the last 2 years, which was either negative for all mandatory markers, or if repeat reactive, has been confirmed to be non-specifically reactive and the donor reinstated in accordance with section 9.4, Reinstatement of blood donors

  - negative results were obtained for mandatory microbiology markers with the current donation.

- Red cell and platelet components should be negative for CMV antibodies although leucodepleted components may be used if CMV antibody negative components are not available.

- Components should be tested and shown to be free of clinically significant, irregular blood group antibodies including high-titre anti-A and anti-B.

- It is good practice to provide neonates, who are likely to be repeatedly transfused, with components in which the original donation has been split, thereby providing the potential to reduce donor exposures in this vulnerable group of recipients.

- When a component is to be split for neonatal use, the original pack must first be mixed thoroughly by a validated procedure to ensure that the contents are homogeneous.

- When a component is split for neonatal use, it is sufficient to undertake leucocyte counting on the parent pack or process.

- When a component is split for neonatal use, each 'split' must be identified by a unique number to ensure all splits can be accounted for.

7.22 Red Cells for Intrauterine Transfusion (IUT), Leucocyte Depleted

A component for intrauterine transfusion, prepared by removing a proportion of the plasma from fresh whole blood. The component should be leucocyte depleted to less than 1×10^6 leucocytes per unit.

7.22.1 Technical information

- The component must be prepared and used for IUT by the end of Day 5, should be free from clinically significant irregular blood group antibodies including high-titre anti-A and anti-B (see Chapter 12), and should be negative for antibodies to CMV.

- The component must be irradiated and should be transfused within 24 hours of irradiation. See the British Committee for Standards in Haematology (BCSH) 'Transfusion guidelines for neonates and older children'.[5]

- Unless the Blood Centre recommends screening is unnecessary, the donor should be Haemoglobin S screen negative.
- Red Cells for Intrauterine Transfusion, Leucocyte Depleted should be transfused through a 170–200 µm filter.

7.22.2 Labelling

For general guidelines, see section 6.6.

The following shall be included on the label:

(* = in eye-readable and UKBTS approved barcode format)

- Red Cells for Intrauterine Transfusion, Leucocyte Depleted* and volume
- the blood component producer's name*
- the donation number*
- the ABO group*
- the RhD group stated as positive or negative*
- the name, composition and volume of the anticoagulant solution
- the date of collection
- the expiry date*
- the temperature of storage
- the blood pack lot number.*

In addition, the following statements should be made:

INSTRUCTION

Always check patient/component compatibility/identity

Inspect pack and contents for signs of deterioration or damage

Risk of adverse reaction/infection, including vCJD

7.22.3 Storage

For general guidelines, see section 6.7.

- The component may be stored for a maximum of 5 days at a core temperature of 4 ±2°C.
- The component must be used within 24 hours of irradiation and within the overall maximum 5-day shelf life.
- Variation from the core temperature of 4 ±2°C must be kept to a minimum during storage and restricted to any short period necessary for examining, labelling or issuing the component.
- Exceptionally, i.e. due to equipment failure at a Blood Centre, red cell components which have been prepared by a closed system and exposed to a core temperature not exceeding 10°C and not less than 1°C may be released for transfusion provided that:
  - the component has been exposed to such a temperature change on one occasion only

- the duration of the temperature excursion has not exceeded 5 hours
- a documented system is available in each Blood Centre to cover such eventualities
- adequate records of the incident are compiled and retained.

7.22.4 Testing

In addition to the mandatory and other tests required for blood donations described in Chapter 9, and leucocyte counting (see sections 6.3 and 7.1), the component shall be free from clinically significant irregular blood group antibodies and high-titre anti-A and/or anti-B, and antibodies to CMV. Furthermore, a minimum of 75% of those components tested for the other parameters shown in Table 7.17 shall meet the specified values.

Table 7.17 Red Cells for Intrauterine Transfusion (IUT), Leucocyte Depleted – additional tests

Parameter	Frequency of test	Specification
Volume	1% or as determined by statistical process control (if ≤10 components produced per month then test every available component)	Within locally defined nominal volume range
Haematocrit		0.70–0.85
Haemoglobin content		Locally defined**
Leucocyte count*	As per sections 6.3 and 7.1	$<1 \times 10^6$/unit
* Methods validated for counting low levels of leucocytes must be used		
** Units tested and found to have <30 g/unit should not be issued for transfusion		

7.22.5 Transportation

For general guidelines, see section 6.11.

For red cell components, transit containers, packing materials and procedures should have been validated to ensure the component surface temperature can be maintained between 2°C and 10°C during transportation. Additionally:

- the validation exercise should be repeated periodically
- if melting ice is used, it should not come into direct contact with the components
- dead air space in packaging containers should be minimised
- as far as is practicable, transit containers should be equilibrated to their storage temperature prior to filling with components
- transport time normally should not exceed 12 hours.

In some instances it is necessary to issue red cell components that have not been cooled to their storage temperature prior to placing in the transit container. The transport temperature specified above is not applicable for such consignments.

7.23 Whole Blood for Exchange Transfusion, Leucocyte Depleted

A component for exchange or large-volume transfusion of neonates, containing less than 1×10^6 leucocytes per unit.

7.23.1 Technical information

- The component must be prepared and used for exchange transfusion by the end of Day 5, should be free from clinically significant irregular blood group antibodies including high-titre anti-A and anti-B (see Chapter 12) and should be negative for antibodies to CMV.

- The component should be irradiated and transfused within 24 hours of irradiation. See the BCSH 'Transfusion guidelines for neonates and older children'.[5]

- Unless the Blood Centre recommends screening is unnecessary, the donor should be Haemoglobin S screen negative.

- Whole Blood for Exchange Transfusion, Leucocyte Depleted should be transfused through a 170–200 µm filter.

- If not required for exchange transfusion, the component may be remanufactured into Red Cells in Additive Solution, Leucocyte Depleted (see section 7.6), up to 6 days after donation, with a shelf life of up to 35 days in total.

7.23.2 Labelling

For general guidelines, see section 6.6.

The following shall be included on the label:

(* = in eye-readable and UKBTS approved barcode format)

- Whole Blood for Exchange Transfusion, Leucocyte Depleted* and volume
- the blood component producer's name*
- the donation number*
- the ABO group*
- the RhD group stated as positive or negative*
- the name, composition and volume of the anticoagulant solution
- the date of collection
- the expiry date*
- the temperature of storage
- the blood pack lot number.*

In addition, the following statements should be made:

INSTRUCTION

Always check patient/component compatibility/identity

Inspect pack and contents for signs of deterioration or damage

Risk of adverse reaction/infection, including vCJD

7.23.3 Storage

For general guidelines, see section 6.7.

- The component may be stored for a maximum of 5 days at a core temperature of 4 ±2°C.

- The component should be used within 24 hours of irradiation and within the overall maximum 5-day shelf life.

- Variation from the core temperature of 4 ±2°C must be kept to a minimum during storage and restricted to any short period necessary for examining, labelling or issuing the component.

- Exceptionally, i.e. due to equipment failure at a Blood Centre, red cell components which have been prepared in a closed system and exposed to a core temperature not exceeding 10°C and not less than 1°C may be released for transfusion provided that:

  - the component has been exposed to such a temperature change on one occasion only
  - the duration of the temperature excursion has not exceeded 5 hours
  - a documented system is available in each Blood Centre to cover such eventualities
  - adequate records of the incident are compiled and retained.

- If Whole Blood for Exchange Transfusion, Leucocyte Depleted is unused within its specified shelf life, the Blood Centre may return the component to stock provided that:

  - the component was stored within specification
  - the component is appropriately relabelled as Whole Blood Leucocyte Depleted and, if necessary, 'irradiated'
  - the storage restrictions of irradiated red cells are observed, i.e. use within 14 days of irradiation.

7.23.4 Testing

In addition to the mandatory and other tests required for blood donations described in Chapter 9, and leucocyte counting (see sections 6.3 and 7.1), the component shall be free from clinically significant irregular blood group antibodies and high-titre anti-A and/or anti-B, and antibodies to CMV. Furthermore, a minimum of 75% of those components tested for the other parameters shown in Table 7.18 shall meet the specified values.

Table 7.18 Whole Blood for Exchange Transfusion, Leucocyte Depleted – additional tests

Parameter	Frequency of test	Specification
Volume	1% or as determined by statistical process control (if ≤10 components produced per month then test every available component)	Within locally defined nominal volume range
Haematocrit		0.4–0.5
Haemoglobin content		≥40 g/unit
Leucocyte count*	As per sections 6.3 and 7.1	$<1 \times 10^6$/unit
* Methods validated for counting low levels of leucocytes must be used		

7.23.5 Transportation

For general guidelines, see section 6.11.

For red cell components, transit containers, packing materials and procedures should have been validated to ensure the component surface temperature can be maintained between 2°C and 10°C during transportation. Additionally:

- the validation exercise should be repeated periodically
- if melting ice is used, it should not come into direct contact with the components
- dead air space in packaging containers should be minimised
- as far as is practicable, transit containers should be equilibrated to their storage temperature prior to filling with components
- transport time normally should not exceed 12 hours.

In some instances it is necessary to issue red cell components that have not been cooled to their storage temperature prior to placing in the transit container. The transport temperature specified above is not applicable for such consignments.

7.24 Red Cells for Exchange Transfusion, Leucocyte Depleted

A component for exchange or large-volume transfusion of neonates prepared by leucodepleting fresh whole blood to less than 1×10^6 leucocytes per component and removing a proportion of the plasma.

7.24.1 Technical information

- The component must be prepared and used by the end of Day 5, should be free from clinically significant irregular blood group antibodies including high-titre anti-A and anti-B (see Chapter 12), and should be negative for antibodies to CMV.
- The component should be irradiated and transfused within 24 hours of irradiation. See the BCSH 'Transfusion guidelines for neonates and older children'.[3]
- Unless the Blood Centre recommends screening is unnecessary, the donor should be Haemoglobin S screen negative.
- Red Cells for Exchange Transfusion, Leucocyte Depleted should be transfused through a 170–200 μm filter.
- If not required for exchange transfusion, the component may be remanufactured into Red Cells in Additive Solution, Leucocyte Depleted (see section 7.6), up to 6 days after donation, with a shelf life of up to 35 days in total.

7.24.2 Labelling

For general guidelines, see section 6.6.

The following shall be included on the label:

(* = in eye-readable and UKBTS approved barcode format)

- Red Cells for Exchange Transfusion, Leucocyte Depleted* and volume
- the blood component producer's name*
- the donation number*
- the ABO group*
- the RhD group stated as positive or negative*

- the name, composition and volume of the anticoagulant solution
- the date of collection
- the expiry date*
- the temperature of storage
- the blood pack lot number.*

In addition, the following statements should be made:

INSTRUCTION

Always check patient/component compatibility/identity

Inspect pack and contents for signs of deterioration or damage

Risk of adverse reaction/infection, including vCJD

7.24.3 Storage

For general guidelines, see section 6.7.

- The component may be stored for a maximum of 5 days at a core temperature of 4 ±2°C.
- Transfusion of this component should commence within 24 hours of irradiation and within the overall maximum 5-day shelf life.
- Variation from the core temperature of 4 ±2°C must be kept to a minimum during storage and restricted to any short period necessary for examining, labelling or issuing the component.
- Exceptionally, i.e. due to equipment failure at a Blood Centre, red cell components which have been prepared in a closed system and exposed to a core temperature not exceeding 10°C and not less than 1°C may be released for transfusion provided that:
  - the component has been exposed to such a temperature change on one occasion only
  - the duration of the temperature excursion has not exceeded 5 hours
  - a documented system is available in each Blood Centre to cover such eventualities
  - adequate records of the incident are compiled and retained.
- If Red Cells for Exchange Transfusion, Leucocyte Depleted are unused within their specified shelf life, the Blood Centre may return them to stock provided that:
  - the component was stored within specification
  - the component is appropriately relabelled as Red Cells, Leucocyte Depleted and, if necessary, 'irradiated'
  - the storage restrictions of irradiated red cells are observed, i.e. use within 14 days of irradiation.

7.24.4 Testing

In addition to the mandatory and other tests required for blood donations described in Chapter 9, and leucocyte counting (see sections 6.3 and 7.1), the component shall be free from clinically significant irregular blood group antibodies and high-titre anti-A and/or anti-B, and antibodies to CMV. Furthermore, a minimum of 75% of those components tested for the other parameters shown in Table 7.19 shall meet the specified values.

Table 7.19 Red Cells for Exchange Transfusion, Leucocyte Depleted – additional tests

Parameter	Frequency of test	Specification
Volume	1% or as determined by statistical process control (if ≤10 components produced per month then test every available component)	Within locally defined nominal volume range
Haematocrit		0.50–0.60
Haemoglobin content		≥40 g/unit**
Leucocyte count*	As per sections 6.3 and 7.1	$<1 \times 10^6$/unit
* Methods validated for counting low levels of leucocytes must be used		
** Units tested and found to have <30 g/unit should not be issued for transfusion		

7.24.5 Transportation

For general guidelines, see section 6.11.

For red cell components, transit containers, packing materials and procedures should have been validated to ensure the component surface temperature can be maintained between 2°C and 10°C during transportation. Additionally:

- the validation exercise should be repeated periodically
- if melting ice is used, it should not come into direct contact with the components
- dead air space in packaging containers should be minimised
- as far as is practicable, transit containers should be equilibrated to their storage temperature prior to filling with components
- transport time normally should not exceed 12 hours.

In some instances it is necessary to issue red cell components that have not been cooled to their storage temperature prior to placing in the transit container. The transport temperature specified above is not applicable for such consignments.

7.25 Red Cells for Neonates and Infants, Leucocyte Depleted

A red cell component suitable for neonates and infants under 1 year that contains less than 1×10^6 leucocytes (per starting component). The Red Cells for Neonates and Infants, Leucocyte Depleted may be divided into approximately equal volumes using a closed system.

7.25.1 Technical information

- The component should be free from clinically significant irregular blood group antibodies including high-titre anti-A and anti-B and should be negative for antibodies to CMV.

- Red Cells for Neonates and Infants, Leucocyte Depleted should be transfused through a 170–200 μm filter.
- Unless the Blood Centre recommends screening is unnecessary, the donor should be Haemoglobin S screen negative.

7.25.2 Labelling

For general guidelines, see section 6.6.

The following shall be included on the label:

(* = in eye-readable and UKBTS approved barcode format)

- Red Cells for Neonates and Infants, Leucocyte Depleted* and volume
- the blood component producer's name*
- the donation number and, if divided, sub-batch number*
- the ABO group*
- the RhD group stated as positive or negative*
- the name, composition and volume of the anticoagulant solution
- the date of collection
- the expiry date*
- the temperature of storage
- the blood pack lot number.*

In addition, the following statements should be made:

INSTRUCTION

Always check patient/component compatibility/identity

Inspect pack and contents for signs of deterioration or damage

Risk of adverse reaction/infection, including vCJD

7.25.3 Storage

For general guidelines, see section 6.7.

- For top-up transfusions of neonates and infants under 1 year, this component may be stored for a maximum of 35 days at a core temperature of 4 ±2°C if an adenine-supplemented anticoagulant is used, otherwise (e.g. with CPD anticoagulant) the maximum period of storage is 28 days at a core temperature of 4 ±2°C.
- Variation from the core temperature of 4 ±2°C must be kept to a minimum during storage and restricted to any short period necessary for examining, labelling or issuing the component.
- For large-volume transfusion of neonates, this component should be used within 24 hours of irradiation and before the end of Day 5.

- Exceptionally, i.e. due to equipment failure at a Blood Centre, red cell components which have been prepared in a closed system and exposed to a core temperature not exceeding 10°C and not less than 1°C may be released for transfusion provided that:
  - the component has been exposed to such a temperature change on one occasion only
  - the duration of the temperature excursion has not exceeded 5 hours
  - a documented system is available in each Blood Centre to cover such eventualities
  - adequate records of the incident are compiled and retained.

7.25.4 Testing

In addition to the mandatory and other tests required for blood donations described in Chapter 9, and leucocyte counting (see sections 6.3 and 7.1), the component shall be free from clinically significant irregular blood group antibodies and high-titre anti-A and/or anti-B, and antibodies to CMV. Furthermore, a minimum of 75% of those components tested for the other parameters shown in Table 7.20 shall meet the specified values.

Table 7.20 Red Cells for Neonates and Infants, Leucocyte Depleted – additional tests

Parameter	Frequency of test	Specification
Volume	1% or as determined by statistical process control (if ≤10 components produced per month then test every available component)	Within locally defined nominal volume range
Haemoglobin content		Locally defined
Haemolysis (only required if produced as a primary component)	As per section 7.2	<0.8% of red cell mass
Leucocyte count*	As per sections 6.3 and 7.1	$<1 \times 10^6$/starting component
* Methods validated for counting low levels of leucocytes must be used		

7.25.5 Transportation

For general guidelines, see section 6.11.

For red cell components, transit containers, packing materials and procedures should have been validated to ensure the component surface temperature can be maintained between 2°C and 10°C during transportation. Additionally:

- the validation exercise should be repeated periodically
- if melting ice is used, it should not come into direct contact with the components
- dead air space in packaging containers should be minimised
- as far as is practicable, transit containers should be equilibrated to their storage temperature prior to filling with components
- transport time normally should not exceed 12 hours.

In some instances it is necessary to issue red cell components that have not been cooled to their storage temperature prior to placing in the transit container. The transport temperature specified above is not applicable for such consignments.

7.26 Red Cells in Additive Solution for Neonates and Infants, Leucocyte Depleted

A red cell component suitable for top-up or large-volume transfusion of neonates and infants under 1 year containing less than 1×10^6 leucocytes (per starting component). The red cells are suspended in an additive solution and may be divided into approximately equal volumes using a closed system.

7.26.1 Technical information

- The component should be free from clinically significant irregular blood group antibodies including high-titre anti-A and anti-B and should be negative for antibodies to CMV.
- Red Cells in Additive Solution for Neonates and Infants, Leucocyte Depleted should be transfused through a 170–200 μm filter.
- Unless the Blood Centre recommends screening is unnecessary, the donor should be Haemoglobin S screen negative.

7.26.2 Labelling

For general guidelines, see section 6.6.

The following shall be included on the label:

(* = in eye-readable and UKBTS approved barcode format)

- Red Cells in Additive Solution for Neonates and Infants, Leucocyte Depleted* and volume
- the blood component producer's name*
- the donation number and, if divided, sub-batch number*
- the ABO group*
- the RhD group stated as positive or negative*
- the name, composition and volume of the additive solution
- the date of collection
- the expiry date*
- the temperature of storage
- the blood pack lot number.*

In addition, the following statements should be made:

INSTRUCTION

Always check patient/component compatibility/identity

Inspect pack and contents for signs of deterioration or damage

Risk of adverse reaction/infection, including vCJD

7.26.3 Storage

For general guidelines, see section 6.7.

- Red Cells in Additive Solution for Neonates and Infants, Leucocyte Depleted for top-up transfusion of neonates and infants under 1 year may be stored for a maximum of 35 days at a core temperature of 4 ±2°C.

- Variation from the core temperature of 4 ±2°C must be kept to a minimum during storage and restricted to any short period necessary for examining, labelling or issuing the component.

- For large-volume transfusion of neonates and infants under 1 year, this component should be transfused within 24 hours of irradiation and before the end of Day 5.

- Exceptionally, i.e. due to equipment failure at a Blood Centre, red cell components which have been prepared in a closed system and exposed to a core temperature not exceeding 10°C and not less than 1°C may be released for transfusion provided that:

  - the component has been exposed to such a temperature change on one occasion only
  - the duration of the temperature excursion has not exceeded 5 hours
  - a documented system is available in each Blood Centre to cover such eventualities
  - adequate records of the incident are compiled and retained.

7.26.4 Testing

In addition to the mandatory and other tests required for blood donations described in Chapter 9, and leucocyte counting (see sections 6.3 and 7.1), the component shall be free from clinically significant irregular blood group antibodies and high-titre anti-A and/or anti-B, and antibodies to CMV. Furthermore, a minimum of 75% of those components tested for the other parameters shown in Table 7.21 shall meet the specified values.

Table 7.21 Red Cells in Additive Solution for Neonates and Infants, Leucocyte Depleted – additional tests

Parameter	Frequency of test	Specification
Volume	1% or as determined by statistical process control (if ≤10 components produced per month then test every available component)	280 ±60 mL
Haemoglobin content		≥40 g/unit
Haemolysis (only required if produced as a primary component)	As per section 7.2	<0.8% of red cell mass
Leucocyte count*	As per sections 6.3 and 7.1	$<1 \times 10^6$/starting component
* Methods validated for counting low numbers of leucocytes must be used		

7.26.5 Transportation

For general guidelines, see section 6.11.

For red cell components, transit containers, packing materials and procedures should have been validated to ensure the component surface temperature can be maintained between 2°C and 10°C during transportation. Additionally:

- the validation exercise should be repeated periodically
- if melting ice is used, it should not come into direct contact with the components

- dead air space in packaging containers should be minimised

- as far as is practicable, transit containers should be equilibrated to their storage temperature prior to filling with components

- transport time normally should not exceed 12 hours.

In some instances it is necessary to issue red cell components that have not been cooled to their storage temperature prior to placing in the transit container. The transport temperature specified above is not applicable for such consignments.

7.27 Fresh Frozen Plasma, Neonatal Use, Methylene Blue Treated and Removed, Leucocyte Depleted

Fresh Frozen Plasma, Neonatal Use, Methylene Blue Treated (MBT) and Removed, Leucocyte Depleted is plasma that has been obtained from whole blood or by apheresis from a country with a low risk of vCJD, contains less than 1×10^6 leucocytes and has been treated with methylene blue and exposure to visible light to inactivate pathogens, and processed to remove residual methylene blue.

Using a closed system the component may be subdivided into approximately equal volumes and rapidly frozen to a temperature that will maintain the activity of labile coagulation factors.

7.27.1 Technical information

- Where the starting component is sourced outside the UK, a detailed and agreed specification must be available.

- Donations of whole blood where the bleed time exceeded 15 minutes are not suitable for the production of plasma components for direct clinical use.

- The component should be free from clinically significant irregular blood group antibodies including high-titre anti-A and anti-B. Testing for CMV antibodies is not required.

- Plasma should be selected from male donors or consideration should be given to screening female donors for HLA/HNA antibodies, as a TRALI risk reduction measure.

- The plasma should be separated before the red cell component is cooled to its storage temperature. Greater FVIII:C yields will be obtained when the plasma is separated as soon as possible after venepuncture and rapidly frozen to −25°C or below.

- The method of preparation should ensure the component has the maximum level of labile coagulation factors with minimum cellular contamination. The production process should be validated to ensure that components meet the specified limits for FVIII:C concentration.

- Component samples collected for the quality monitoring assessment of FVIII:C should be from an equal mix of group O and non-O donations due to the difference in FVIII levels between ABO blood groups.

- The MBT process reduces the FVIII:C content by approximately 30% when compared to standard fresh frozen plasma.

- Intact white blood cells in the plasma should be reduced to less than 1×10^6 per unit prior to exposure to methylene blue and visible light.

- The process for methylene blue removal should be validated to give components with a methylene blue concentration ≤0.30 µmol/L. The methylene blue content of the final component is the initial content of the unsplit starting component (less than approximately 30 µg per unit) divided by the number of split components produced.

- Fresh Frozen Plasma, Neonatal Use, Methylene Blue Treated and Removed, Leucocyte Depleted should be transfused through a 170–200 µm filter.

7.27.2 Labelling

For general guidelines, see section 6.6.

The following shall be included on the label:

(* = in eye-readable and UKBTS approved barcode format)

- Fresh Frozen Plasma, Neonatal Use, Methylene Blue Treated and Removed, Leucocyte Depleted* and volume
- the blood component producer's name*
- the donation number*
- the ABO group*
- the RhD group stated as positive or negative*
- the date of collection
- the expiry date of the frozen component*
- the temperature of storage
- the blood pack lot number*
- a warning that the component should be used within 4 hours of thawing
- the name, composition and volume of the anticoagulant.

In addition, the following statements should be made:

INSTRUCTION

Always check patient/component compatibility/identity

Inspect pack and contents for signs of deterioration or damage

Risk of adverse reaction/infection

7.27.3 Storage

For general guidelines, see section 6.7.

- The component should be stored at a core temperature of –25°C or below for a maximum of 24 months.
- Although a storage temperature below –25°C improves the preservation of labile coagulation factors, lower temperatures increase the fragility of plastic. Particular care must be taken when handling such packs.

- The component should be thawed in a waterbath or other equipment designed for the purpose, within a vacuum-sealed overwrap bag according to a validated procedure. The optimal temperature at which the component should be thawed is 37°C; temperatures between 33°C and 37°C are acceptable.

- Protocols must be in place to ensure that the equipment is cleaned daily and maintained to minimise the risk of bacterial contamination. After thawing, the content should be inspected to ensure that no insoluble cryoprecipitate is visible and that the container is intact.

- Once thawed, the component must not be refrozen and should be transfused as soon as possible. If delay is unavoidable, the component may be stored and should be used within 4 hours if maintained at 22 ±2°C or 24 hours if stored at 4 ±2°C, but it should be borne in mind that extended post-thaw storage will result in a decline in the content of labile coagulation factors.

7.27.4 Testing

In addition to the mandatory and other tests required for blood donations described in Chapter 9, and leucocyte counting (see sections 6.3 and 7.1), the component shall be free from clinically significant irregular blood group antibodies and high-titre anti-A and/or anti-B. Furthermore, a minimum of 75% of those components tested for the other parameters shown in Table 7.22 shall meet the specified values.

Table 7.22 Fresh Frozen Plasma, Neonatal Use, Methylene Blue Treated and Removed, Leucocyte Depleted – additional tests

Parameter	Frequency of test	Specification
Volume	1% or as determined by statistical process control (if ≤10 components produced per month then test every available component)	Within locally defined nominal volume range and within any limits specified for the MBT process used
Platelet count		$<30 \times 10^9$/L**
FVIII:C		≥0.50 IU/mL
Leucocyte count*	As per sections 6.3 and 7.1	$<1 \times 10^6$/unit**
* Methods validated for counting low numbers of leucocytes must be used		
** Pre-freeze in starting component		

7.27.5 Transportation

For general guidelines, see section 6.11.

Every effort should be made to maintain the core storage temperature during transportation. Unless the component is to be thawed and used straightaway it should be transferred immediately to storage at the recommended temperature.

7.28 Cryoprecipitate, Methylene Blue Treated and Removed, Leucocyte Depleted

The component represents a source of concentrated FVIII:C, and von Willebrand factor, fibrinogen, FXIII and fibronectin from a unit of Fresh Frozen Plasma, Methylene Blue Treated and Removed. The plasma from which the Cryoprecipitate, Methylene Blue Treated and Removed, Leucocyte Depleted was produced contains less than 1×10^6 leucocytes per component and is from a country with a low risk of vCJD.

7.28.1 Technical information

- Where the starting component is sourced outside the UK, a detailed and agreed specification must be available.

- Donations of whole blood where the bleed time exceeded 15 minutes are not suitable for the production of plasma components for direct clinical use.

- Plasma should be selected from male donors or screening of female donors for HLA/HNA antibodies should be considered, as a TRALI risk reduction strategy.

- Cryoprecipitate, Methylene Blue Treated and Removed, Leucocyte Depleted is the cryoglobulin fraction of plasma obtained by thawing a single donation of Fresh Frozen Plasma, Neonatal Use, Methylene Blue Treated and Removed, Leucocyte Depleted (see section 7.27) at 4 ±2°C.

- The process for methylene blue removal should be validated to give components with a methylene blue concentration ≤0.30 µmol/L (less than approximately 30 µg per unit) in the starting component.

- For storage, Cryoprecipitate, Methylene Blue Treated and Removed, Leucocyte Depleted should be rapidly frozen to a core temperature of –25°C or below within 2 hours of preparation.

- Component samples collected for the quality monitoring assessment of FVIII:C should be from an equal mix of group O and non-O donations due to the difference in FVIII levels between ABO blood groups.

- Cryoprecipitate, Methylene Blue Treated and Removed, Leucocyte Depleted should be transfused through a 170–200 µm filter.

7.28.2 Labelling

For general guidelines, see section 6.6.

The following shall be included on the component label:

(* = in eye-readable and UKBTS approved barcode format)

- Cryoprecipitate, Methylene Blue Treated and Removed, Leucocyte Depleted* and volume
- the blood component producer's name*
- the donation number*
- the ABO group*
- the RhD group stated as positive or negative*

- the date of collection
- the expiry date of the frozen component*
- the temperature of storage
- the blood pack lot number*
- a warning that the component must be used within 4 hours of thawing
- the name, composition and volume of the anticoagulant or additive solution.

In addition, the following statements should be made:

INSTRUCTION

Always check patient/component compatibility/identity

Inspect pack and contents for signs of deterioration or damage

Risk of adverse reaction/infection

7.28.3 Storage

For general guidelines, see section 6.7.

- The component should be stored at a core temperature of –25°C or below for a maximum of 24 months.
- Although a storage temperature below –25°C improves the preservation of labile coagulation factors, lower temperatures increase the fragility of plastic. Particular care must be taken when handling such packs.
- The component should be thawed in a waterbath or other equipment designed for the purpose, within a vacuum-sealed overwrap bag according to a validated procedure. The optimal temperature at which the component should be thawed is 37°C; temperatures between 33°C and 37°C are acceptable.
- Protocols must be in place to ensure that the equipment is cleaned daily and maintained to minimise the risk of bacterial contamination. After thawing, the content should be inspected to ensure that no insoluble cryoprecipitate is visible and that the container is intact.
- Once thawed, the component must not be refrozen and should be used immediately. If delay is unavoidable, the component should be stored at ambient temperature and used within 4 hours.

7.28.4 Testing

In addition to the mandatory and other tests required for blood donations described in Chapter 9, and leucocyte counting (see sections 6.3 and 7.1), a minimum of 75% of those components tested for the parameters shown in Table 7.23 shall meet the specified values.

Table 7.23 Cryoprecipitate, Methylene Blue Treated and Removed, Leucocyte Depleted – additional tests

Parameter	Frequency of test	Specification
Volume	1% or as determined by statistical process control (if ≤10 components produced per month then test every available component)	Within locally defined nominal range
Fibrinogen		>140 mg/unit
FVIII:C		≥50 IU/unit
Leucocyte count*	As per sections 6.3 and 7.1	$<1 \times 10^6$/unit**
* Methods validated for counting low numbers of leucocytes must be used		
** Pre-freeze in starting component		

7.28.5 Transportation

For general guidelines, see section 6.11.

Every effort should be made to maintain the core storage temperature during transportation. Unless the component is to be thawed and used straightaway it should be transferred immediately to storage at the recommended temperature.

7.29 Platelets for Intrauterine Transfusion, Leucocyte Depleted

A hyperconcentrated platelet component for intrauterine transfusion, prepared by apheresis, that contains less than 1×10^6 leucocytes per donation.

7.29.1 Technical information

- The component should be free from clinically significant irregular blood group antibodies including high-titre anti-A and anti-B and should be negative for antibodies to CMV.

- The component must be used by the end of Day 1.

- The component must be irradiated. See the BCSH 'Transfusion guidelines for neonates and older children'.[5]

- The component should contain a concentration of platelets between 2 and 4×10^{12}/L in a collected volume generally in the range of 50–100 mL.

- All components should be quality monitored and achieve the specified requirements. The testing need not necessarily be performed before component release.

- Screening of female donors for HLA/HNA antibodies should be considered as a TRALI risk reduction strategy. If platelets are to be issued as HPA-matched (e.g. HPA-1a or HPA-5b negative) then donors should be screened and found negative for all clinically significant HLA and HPA antibodies (as defined in Chapters 16 and 18). This screening can be done on an initial sample and does not need repeating at each donation unless the donor has been transfused or pregnant since the last antibody screen.

- A record which demonstrates that the donor has not been transfused since the initial negative screen for antibodies and in case of female donors that the donor has not been pregnant since the initial negative screen for antibodies needs to be maintained.

- Platelets for Intrauterine Transfusion, Leucocyte Depleted should be transfused through a 170–200 µm filter.

7.29.2 Labelling

For general guidelines, see section 6.6.

The following shall be included on the label:

(* = in eye-readable and UKBTS approved barcode format)

- Platelets for Intrauterine Transfusion, Leucocyte Depleted* and volume
- the blood component producer's name*
- the donation number*
- the ABO group*
- the RhD group stated as positive or negative*
- the relevant HPA and HLA type, if necessary
- the date of collection
- the expiry date and time*
- the temperature of storage and a comment that continuous gentle agitation during storage is recommended
- the blood pack lot number*
- the name, composition and volume of the anticoagulant.

In addition, the following statements should be made:

INSTRUCTION

Always check patient/component compatibility/identity

Inspect pack and contents for signs of deterioration or damage

Risk of adverse reaction/infection, including vCJD

7.29.3 Storage

For general guidelines, see section 6.7.

- The component should be stored at a core temperature of 22 ±2°C for use up to the end of Day 1.
- The component should be gently and continuously agitated during storage.

7.29.4 Testing

In addition to the mandatory and other tests required for blood donations described in Chapter 9, and leucocyte counting (see sections 6.3 and 7.1), the component shall be free from clinically significant irregular blood group antibodies and high-titre anti-A and/or anti-B and antibodies to CMV. Furthermore, all components tested for the other parameters shown in Table 7.24 shall meet the specified values.

Table 7.24 Platelets for Intrauterine Transfusion, Leucocyte Depleted – additional tests

Parameter	Frequency of test	Specification
Volume	Every component	Within locally defined range
Platelet concentration		$2–4 \times 10^{12}/L$
pH at end of shelf life*		6.4–7.4
Leucocyte count**	As per sections 6.3 and 7.1	$<1 \times 10^6$/unit
* The shelf life of this hyperconcentrated platelet component has been set to reflect validation data. Therefore, once this has been validated locally, there is no need to measure pH at expiry on a routine basis		
** Methods validated for counting low numbers of leucocytes must be used		

Note: Visual inspection of platelet components for the swirling phenomenon, clumping, excessive red cell contamination and abnormal volume is a useful pre-issue check.

7.29.5 Transportation

For general guidelines, see section 6.11.

- Containers for transporting platelets should be equilibrated at room temperature before use. During transportation the temperature of platelets must be kept as close as possible to the recommended storage temperature and, on receipt, unless intended for immediate therapeutic use, the component should be transferred to storage at a core temperature of 22°C with continuous gentle agitation.

- Plastic overwraps should be removed prior to storage.

7.30 Platelets for Neonatal Use, Leucocyte Depleted

An apheresis platelet component for neonatal use that contains less than 1×10^6 leucocytes per starting component.

7.30.1 Technical information

- The component should be free from clinically significant irregular blood group antibodies including high-titre anti-A and anti-B and should be negative for antibodies to CMV.

- The component may be prepared by splitting Platelets, Apheresis, Leucocyte Depleted (see section 7.10) using a closed system.

- The component should contain $>40 \times 10^9$ platelets in sufficient plasma to maintain the pH between 6.4 and 7.4 at the end of the shelf life of the component.

- The component may be leucodepleted as part of an apheresis process or by subsequent filtration of the platelet component.

- Screening of female donors for HLA/HNA antibodies should be considered as a TRALI risk reduction strategy. If platelets are to be issued as HPA-matched (e.g. HPA-1a or HPA-5b negative) then donors should be screened and found negative for all clinically significant HLA and HPA antibodies (as defined in Chapters 16 and 18). This screening can be done on an initial sample and does not need repeating at each donation unless the donor has been transfused or pregnant since the last antibody screen.

- A record which demonstrates that the donor has not been transfused since the initial negative screen for antibodies and in the case of female donors that the donor has not been pregnant since the initial negative screen for antibodies needs to be maintained.

- Platelets for Neonatal Use, Leucocyte Depleted should be transfused through a 170–200 μm filter.

7.30.2 Labelling

For general guidelines, see section 6.6.

The following shall be included on the label:

(* = in eye-readable and UKBTS approved barcode format)

- Platelets for Neonatal Use, Leucocyte Depleted* and volume
- the blood component producer's name*
- the donation number and, if divided, sub-batch number*
- the ABO group*
- the RhD group stated as positive or negative*
- the date of collection
- the expiry date*
- the temperature of storage and a comment that continuous gentle agitation throughout storage is recommended
- the blood pack lot number*
- the name, composition and volume of the anticoagulant or additive solution.

In addition, the following statements should be made:

INSTRUCTION

Always check patient/component compatibility/identity

Inspect pack and contents for signs of deterioration or damage

Risk of adverse reaction/infection, including vCJD

7.30.3 Storage

For general guidelines, see section 6.7.

- The component should be stored at a core temperature of 22 ±2°C for up to 5 days. Appropriate pack and platelet concentration combinations may allow storage up to 7 days, but due to concerns over bacterial contamination would require either an assay to exclude bacterial contamination prior to transfusion or application of a licensed pathogen inactivation procedure.

- Platelets should be agitated during storage. If agitation is interrupted, for example due to equipment failure or prolonged transportation, the components are suitable for use, retaining the same shelf life, provided the interruption is for no longer than a total of 24 hours.

7.30.4 Testing

In addition to the mandatory and other tests required for blood donations described in Chapter 9, and leucocyte counting (see sections 6.3 and 7.1), the component shall be free from clinically significant irregular blood group antibodies and high-titre anti-A and/or anti-B, and antibodies to CMV. Furthermore, a minimum of 75% of those components tested for the other parameters shown in Table 7.25 shall meet the specified values.

Table 7.25 Platelets for Neonatal Use, Leucocyte Depleted – additional tests

Parameter	Frequency of test	Specification
Volume	1% or as determined by statistical process control (if ≤10 components produced per month then test every available component)	Within locally defined range
Platelet count		$\geq 40 \times 10^9$/unit
pH at end of shelf life*		6.4–7.4
Leucocyte count**	As per sections 6.3 and 7.1	$<1 \times 10^6$/starting component
* If producing low numbers, use of most units is likely to make testing of outdated units impossible. In this situation periodic checks to ensure end-of-shelf-life quality should be undertaken with the combination of blood pack platelet concentration and storage conditions in routine use.		
** Methods validated for counting low levels of leucocytes must be used.		

Note: Visual inspection of platelet components for the swirling phenomenon, clumping, excessive red cell contamination and abnormal volume is a useful pre-issue check.

7.30.5 Transportation

For general guidelines, see section 6.11.

- Containers for transporting platelets should be equilibrated at room temperature before use. During transportation the temperature of platelets must be kept as close as possible to the recommended storage temperature and, on receipt, unless intended for immediate therapeutic use, the component should be transferred to storage at a core temperature of 22°C with continuous gentle agitation.

- Plastic overwraps should be removed prior to storage.

7.31 Irradiated components

- For the whole of this section X-irradiation may be regarded as equivalent to gamma irradiation. Times when irradiation should be undertaken and the permitted post-irradiation storage times are the same, as are the required labelling and dosing (recommended minimum dose achieved in the irradiation field is 25 Gy, with no part receiving >50 Gy).

- Note that the X-ray equipment should be dose-mapped prior to release from the factory and at installation, and the manufacturers recommend routine dosimetry at 6-monthly intervals (gamma-irradiation equipment requires annual dosimetry). A radiation-sensitive label specifically for use with X-irradiation is available.

- It is not necessary to irradiate the following components:
  - cryopreserved red cells after washing
  - plasma components.

- For more information, refer to the BCSH *Guidelines on the Use of Irradiated Blood Components*.[3]

- Irradiated components not used for the intended recipient can safely be used for recipients who do not require irradiated components provided the other requirements of Chapters 6 and 7 have been satisfied. However, any reduction in shelf life resulting from the irradiation process must be observed.

- Irradiated components should conform to their appropriate specification previously given in this chapter. In addition, the guidelines shown below should be observed.

7.31.1 Description

Irradiated components are components that have been irradiated by a validated procedure.

7.31.2 Technical information

- Other than for use in intrauterine transfusion, exchange transfusion, or large-volume transfusion of neonates, red cells can be irradiated at any time up to 14 days after collection.

- Platelets can be irradiated at any stage in their storage.

- Granulocytes should be irradiated as soon as possible after production.

- For red cells, platelets and granulocytes the recommended minimum dose achieved in the irradiation field is 25 Gy, with no part receiving >50 Gy.

- Laboratories performing irradiation of blood components must work to a clearly defined specification and are strongly recommended to work closely with a medical physicist. The defined irradiation procedure must be validated and there must be regular monitoring of the blood component dosimetry and the laboratory equipment.

- It is recommended that irradiation of blood components is carried out using dedicated blood irradiation machines. If radiotherapy machines are used, equivalent protocols should be developed.

- Appropriate radiation-sensitive labels should be used as an aid to differentiating irradiated from non-irradiated components. However, it may not be necessary to attach a radiation-sensitive label to every component pack, provided that the irradiation procedure follows a validated, documented and well-controlled system of work that is integrated with the component labelling and release mechanism and permits retrospective audit of each stage of the irradiation process.

- There should be a permanent record of all units irradiated. This should include details of irradiation batch and donation numbers, component type, the site of irradiation, when irradiation was performed and by whom.

7.31.3 Labelling

- Irradiated components must be identified by the applied labelling and include the date of irradiation and any reduction in shelf life.

- Labels which are sensitive to irradiation and change from 'NOT IRRADIATED' to 'IRRADIATED' are available and are considered a useful indicator of exposure to irradiation. The dose at which the label changes to 'IRRADIATED' must be marked on the label. It must be remembered that such labels simply reflect that the unit has been exposed to radiation and their use does not replace the need for regular and precise dosimetry nor carefully controlled working procedures.

7.31.4 Storage

For general guidelines, see section 6.7.

- Red cell components, other than for intrauterine transfusion, exchange transfusion, or large-volume transfusion of neonates and infants can be irradiated at any time up to 14 days after collection and stored for up to 14 days thereafter, provided the other requirements of this section are adhered to.

- Where irradiated red cells are intended for intrauterine or exchange transfusion or where the patient is at particular risk from hyperkalaemia, red cells should be transfused within 24 hours of irradiation. Furthermore, red cells intended for intrauterine transfusion, exchange transfusion, or large-volume transfusion of neonates or infants should be transfused within 5 days of collection.

- Irradiated platelets can be stored up to their normal shelf life of 5 days after collection, or 7 days if appropriately tested or pathogen inactivated.

- Granulocytes must be irradiated and should be used with minimum delay after irradiation but within the shelf life specified earlier in this chapter.

7.32 References

1. Dumont L, Dzik W, Rebulla P, Brandwein H and members of the BEST Expert Working Party of the ISBT (1996). Practical guidelines for process validation and process control of white cell-reduced blood components: report of the Biomedical Excellence for Safer Transfusion (BEST) Working Party of the International Society of Blood Transfusion (ISBT). *Transfusion*, 36, 11–20.

2. Bashir S, Stanworth S, Massey E, Goddard F, Cardigan R. (2008). Neutrophil function is preserved in a pooled granulocyte component prepared from whole blood donations. *British Journal of Haematology*, 140, 701–711.

3. British Committee for Standards in Haematology Blood Transfusion Task Force (2010). *Guidelines on the Use of Irradiated Blood Components*. Available at www.bcshguidelines.com/documents/Irradiation_BJH_2011.pdf.

4. Massey E, Harding K, Kahan BC, Llewelyn C, Wynn R, Moppett J, Robinson SP, Green A, Lucas G, Sadani D, Liakopoulou E, Bolton-Maggs P, Marks DI, Stanworth S (2012). The granulocytes in neutropenia 1 (GIN 1) study: a safety study of granulocytes collected from whole blood and stored in additive solution and plasma. *Transfusion Medicine*, 22, 277–284.

5. British Committee for Standards in Haematology Blood Transfusion Task Force (2004). Transfusion guidelines for neonates and older children. *British Journal of Haematology*, 124, 433–453.

Chapter 8
Evaluation of novel blood components, production processes and blood packs: generic protocols

8.1 Aims and introduction

This chapter aims to describe how a proposed novel blood component, production process or blood pack is to be evaluated to:

- gain sufficient data to validate the component and production method

- gain sufficient data to support the clinical use of the component

- allow the Standing Advisory Committee on Blood Components (SACBC) to recommend to the Joint UKBTS/HPA Professional Advisory Committee (JPAC) that the component should be included in the Red Book

- provide sufficient information to prevent all Blood Transfusion Centres (other than those performing a full evaluation) from having to complete a full validation of the novel component before it enters routine production. They will only need to undertake installation and process qualification.

The chapter starts by identifying the steps that a group of investigators will need to undertake to submit a novel blood component for inclusion in the Red Book (see Table 8.1), thereby allowing it to be produced on a routine basis throughout the UK.

It is recognised that some novel components may be developed by a group of investigators in conjunction with a commercial company undertaking speculative research. As a result, the group of investigators may wish to enter the process at Step 9. In this case the SACBC will expect any requirements for data collection in the preceding steps to be complied with when the protocols and reports are submitted to the SACBC Chair for consideration. If sufficient data are not included then a request for extra data will be made (Step 11).

Guidance on how specific novel components should be tested is included in sections 8.2–8.4, and is followed by information on generic protocols for the evaluation of apheresis equipment (section 8.5) and blood packs (section 8.6).

Table 8.1 Steps for evaluation of novel components

Step	Details	Information
1. Investigators identify requirement for a novel blood component.	The requirement must be derived from R&D work or as the result of clinical discussions. The blood component needs: • to fulfil an unmet clinical need OR • provide production benefit and have a Blood Service proposer. Investigators will need preliminary data to support their application.	The new component may be derived from a commercially available product. In this case data to support the submission may be derived from the manufacturer. Investigators must critically appraise data already available. All data must be maintained on file. Data will be used to demonstrate validation has been completed in support of Blood Transfusion Centre licensing activities. Data required may include clinical outcome.
2. Investigators may obtain initial advice from the SACBC Chair as to whether the component should be treated as novel.	Yes: Go to Step 3. No: Undertake local validation and produce the component locally under the general principles of good manufacturing practice and the Red Book.	The proposed new component may require evaluation even if it complies with existing Red Book guidelines if: • a new production technique is involved (e.g. leucocyte-depleted red cells produced by apheresis) • there are different steps in the production process (e.g. white-cell filtration immediately following collection). • Definitive advice about the need for full-scale evaluation will be provided from the SACBC following a written submission.
Characterise the new blood component		
3. Apply to the Standing Advisory Committee on Information Technology (SACIT) Chair for a development barcode (via the UKBTS Component Portfolio when available).	Allocated by the SACIT.	Allows component production, discard and use to be tracked using the Blood Transfusion Centre's IT system. This will allow the evaluation to be integrated within the Centre's quality system.
4. Investigators define the intended specification for the blood component.	Written specification to include: • expected characteristics (e.g. leucocyte count) • testing characteristics (blood grouping, microbiology etc.) • sampling time, sampling method and sample handling conditions to confirm that the component meets specification. Reference should also be made to the research papers from which the specification is derived.	Specify all key points which will allow subsequent production of the component to be well controlled.

Step	Details	Information
5. Write the protocol for component evaluation.	Investigators' group writes procedures for: • component production • monitoring of performance • clinical use • outcome measurement • adverse incidents in production/use of the blood component or uses manufacturer's documentation to produce 'in-house' protocols.	Principles of good clinical and good manufacturing practice should apply. Comply with generic protocols (sections 8.2–8.5). Laboratory studies should comply with local standards. Must include in the procedure the sampling regimes, data analysis and expected ranges, which will be used to confirm that production of the component is under control. Must include detail of the data analysis methods.
6. Investigators should ensure their protocol complies with Chapter 8 and may seek advice from the SACBC.		
7. **Obtain ethics committee approval, if required.**		Must comply with local consenting and ethics policies for the use of donated material.
8. Investigators apply protocol.	Document evidence of protocol being implemented. Investigation should be subject to independent quality audit.	Audit may be carried out on behalf of collaborating manufacturers even though this may be confidential regarding the data collected. A summary outlining non-compliances against good clinical and manufacturing practice must be made available to the Blood Transfusion Service involved, for submission as part of the supporting documentation to the SACBC.
Obtain SACBC listing of the component		
9. Investigators submit report and supporting data to the SACBC for consideration.	Investigators review outcomes and produce a report, which summarises findings and supports the case for a new blood component to be listed. The SACBC decides if: • the blood component is novel • the data support the ability to produce the blood component on a regular basis • the blood component is efficacious and safe.	Investigators who have been conducting speculative research with a manufacturer may enter the process at this point. This may also include data supplied by manufacturers, other Blood Services and published studies. Investigators should submit a draft specification for the component.
10. The SACBC decides whether the component may be recommended for inclusion in the Red Book guidelines.	If the SACBC decides that the blood component will be listed, it submits this recommendation to the Red Book JPAC. If the SACBC decides that the blood component will not be listed, it informs the submitting group and provides an explanation.	The SACBC may request further data in support of the submission prior to listing the blood component.

Table continues

Table 8.1 continued

Step	Details	Information
Joint Professional Advisory Committee		
11. Consider the recommendation that a new component should be listed.	Write to the SACBC notifying it of the decision. If not accepted, provide the SACBC with detailed reasons for the decision.	
SACBC		
12. Communicates the JPAC decision to appropriate parties.	If accepted inform investigators and request the SACIT to proceed with the provision of appropriate labels. Write to Medical Directors of the four UK Blood Transfusion Services. Provide copies of the data and report used to accept the new blood component. If not accepted inform investigators, with supporting reasons.	
SACIT		
13. Provides codes for the new blood component.	Code will be unique. ISBT 128/ABC Codabar will be supported.	
14. Provides a component label and updates the UKBTS Component Portfolio.	Label will be unique.	Label text will describe the key attributes of the component.
Blood Establishment		
15. Begin production of the new blood component.	Base procedures on those used during validation studies. Complete installation and process qualification.	Demonstrates without redoing the above validation that the blood component produced is equivalent to that defined in the UK guidelines.
16. Produce the blood component routinely.	Confirm procedures.	Continue to monitor production to the Red Book specification.

8.2 Evaluation of new red cell components for transfusion

8.2.1 Introduction

In establishing any novel component, the development process is expected to involve three stages:

- **Investigation:** Initial intensive investigation of a range of parameters on a relatively small number of units to establish concepts. This should involve *in vitro* studies with serial sampling, and may also involve *in vivo* studies. Components produced during this phase should not be used for transfusion.

- **Validation:** Operational validation on a larger number of units (e.g. 50 to 100) to establish routine operation of the technique, normally testing for those parameters listed in the current edition of the Red Book. These tests may be supplemented by a limited set of assays selected from the investigational phase to allow setting of routine quality parameters. This may involve *in vivo* studies and normally would involve sampling at the times shown below for routine testing.

- **Routine:** Ongoing routine validation using a small set of parameters selected on the basis of the above studies. This will not normally involve *in vivo* studies. For clarity the guidance on which tests need to be performed is as shown in Table 8.2. Advice may be sought from SACBC on the validation requirements for red cells produced from automated processing of whole blood or other technologies that are not specified in Table 8.2.

Red cell components may be derived either from whole blood or collected by apheresis and, in either case, the standard requirements for donor selection and for mandatory donation microbiological testing should be fulfilled. When well prepared, there is no evidence that the clinical performance of any of these products is different, and the guidance provided below applies equally to the various approaches.

In vitro assays should be performed on samples representative of the pack contents taken by an aseptic technique that does not appreciably alter the gross volume of the pack contents (must be kept to a minimum but in any case no greater than 10%). Parallel testing of units prepared by a well-established method is recommended, and the use of a split-pool or crossover design will increase the power of such comparisons. If required, *in vivo* studies, preferably with parallel testing of 'standard' components, should be performed on the last day of the proposed storage period. The number of units studied should be determined by statistical analysis based on the difference between test and control units to be detected. A sample size of at least 12 tests or controls would be required to detect a 30% difference in ATP and potassium at Day 35 of storage using an unpaired study. Fewer units will be required if a pooled and split study design is used, but should not be less than four.

Red cell components will be stored for the recommended storage period or longer in the case of experimental additive solutions (AS) that are designed to extend the shelf life of red blood cells (RBC). Samples will be taken weekly (or minimally at Days 1, 21, 35 and at the end of storage if this is >35 days) for *in vitro* studies. If required, autologous *in vivo* recovery studies should be undertaken at the end of the storage period.

8.2.2 *In vitro* studies

The measurements described below and in Table 8.2 will be made at the time of component production (Day 0/Day 1) or other relevant stages of component preparation. An equal number of appropriate control components (e.g. standard AS RBC) should be tested in parallel. Greater consistency of information may be obtained if two or more group-compatible components are pooled and divided prior to processing for *in vitro* studies only. The number of units to be studied should be based on the study objectives and design.

8.2.3 On the day of component production/collection

Weight, volume, haematocrit (L/L), haemoglobin (Hb, g/unit), platelets (x 10^9/unit), red cell loss* (%), platelet loss* (%), leucocyte depletion (given as residual WBC × 10^6/unit) and log depletion*. These results should be obtained by validated test procedures and be within the limits defined by the preliminary component specification.

* Relevant to procedures involving integral filtration or other methods that are likely to result in loss of cellular components during production. Validated techniques using flow cytometry or cell counting chambers should be used to count leucodepleted components and would currently be expected to exhibit a sensitivity of less than or equal to 1 leucocyte per microlitre.

Table 8.2 Evaluation of new red cell components for transfusion: recommended tests

New characteristic parameter	New pack	Leuco-depletion	New centrifugation/ component extractor (e.g. Optipress, Compomat etc.)	Novel anti-coagulant	Novel apheresis system	Novel additive solution	Irradiation	Pathogen reduction
Unit volume (mL)	✓	✓	✓	✓	✓	✓	✓	✓
Haematocrit (L/L)	✓	✓	✓	✓	✓	✓	✓	✓
Haemoglobin (g/unit)	✓	✓	✓	✓	✓	✓	✓	✓
MCV	✓	✓	✓	✓	✓	✓	✓	✓
WBC (x 10^6/unit) (post-leucodepletion)		✓						
Leucocyte subsets (%) (post-leucodepletion)		✓						
Residual platelets (x 10^9/unit)			✓	✓				
Hb loss (g) (post-filter)		✓	✓					
K^+ (mmol/L)	✓	✓	✓	✓	✓	✓	✓	✓
Haemolysis (%)	✓	✓	✓	✓	✓	✓	✓	✓
pH				✓		✓	✓	✓
Lactate (mmol/L)				✓		✓	✓	✓
Glucose (mmol/L)				✓		✓	✓	✓
ATP (µmol/g Hb)	✓	✓		✓		✓	✓	✓
2,3-DPG (µmol/g Hb)				✓		✓	✓	✓
Na^+ (mmol/L)				✓		✓	✓	✓
pCO_2 (kPa)				✓		✓	✓	✓
pO_2 (kPa)				✓		✓	✓	✓
Pathogen reduction*								
Prion protein (PrP^c) and microvesicles		?						?
24-hour recovery (%)				?		?	?	✓

Some components may need to be tested for a combination of parameters, e.g. apheresis red cells in a novel/ experimental additive solution (AS) that are also leucodepleted. In this case the sampling requirement includes that of a leucodepleted red cell component and that of an experimental AS component.

Key: ✓ = recommended; ? = optional; other tests are not excluded. * = normally undertaken by the manufacturer.

At the end of the storage period components should be checked for sterility and a representative sample labelled with ^{51}Cr (single label method) or ^{51}Cr plus ^{131}I-albumin (dual label method), washed, reinjected and blood samples taken at 5, 7, 10, 12.5, 15 minutes and 24 hours to calculate the 24-hour recovery. Results will be considered acceptable if the mean 24-hour recovery is >75% with a standard deviation of <9%. Alternative methods to ^{51}Cr labelling may be used if shown to yield equivalent results.

8.2.4 During storage

Parameters to be studied during storage of red cells include: haemoglobin, haematocrit, MCV, ATP, 2,3-DPG, glucose, lactate, potassium, haemolysis (soluble haemoglobin as a percentage of total haemoglobin per mL of whole product), pH, pO_2, pCO_2, cytokines. These may include interleukin-1α, IL-1β, IL-6, IL-8, TNF-α and TGF-β. Measurements should, wherever possible, be by bioassay (seek advice from SACBC). Cytokine measurements are complex and may be considered optional. As red cell components are leucocyte depleted, measurement of leucocyte-derived cytokines is probably not informative. Advice should be taken from SACBC on the selection of cytokine tests.

These results should be obtained by validated test procedures. Where manipulation of components during processing might increase the risk of bacterial contamination, microbiological sterility testing should be performed at the end of storage.

8.2.5 Autologous *in vivo* studies

See Table 8.2 for details of testing. An equal number of appropriate control components obtained from healthy volunteer donors with ethical approval (e.g. standard AS RBC) should be tested in parallel. The number of components transfused should be justified based on the study objectives and design.

8.3 Evaluation of new platelet components for transfusion

8.3.1 Introduction

In establishing any novel component, the development process is expected to involve three stages:

- **Investigation:** Initial intensive investigation of a range of parameters on a relatively small number of units to establish concepts. This should involve *in vitro* studies with serial sampling, and may also involve *in vivo* studies. Components produced during this phase should not be used for transfusion.

- **Validation:** Operational validation on a larger number of units (e.g. 50 to 100) to establish routine operation of the technique, normally testing for those parameters listed in the current edition of the Red Book. These tests may be supplemented by a limited set of assays selected from the investigational phase to allow setting of routine quality parameters. This may involve *in vivo* studies and normally would involve sampling at the times shown below for routine testing.

- **Routine:** Ongoing routine validation using a small set of parameters selected on the basis of the above studies. This will not normally involve *in vivo* studies. For clarity the guidance on which tests need to be performed is as shown in Tables 8.3 and 8.4. Advice may be sought from SACBC on the validation requirements for platelets produced from automated processing of whole blood or buffy coats or other technology that is not specified in Tables 8.3 and 8.4.

Platelet components may be derived from whole blood using platelet-rich plasma or buffy coat methods of preparation, or by plateletpheresis and, in either case, the standard requirements for donor selection and for mandatory donation microbiological testing should be fulfilled. For components prepared in a closed system, storage in specifically designed plastic bags is currently undertaken with gentle agitation for up to 7 days at 22 ±2°C. Platelet components may be subjected to leucodepletion, storage in platelet additive solutions in place of plasma and, in the case of whole blood derived components, pooling of four to six units to form an adult equivalent dose. When well prepared, there is no evidence that the clinical performance of any of these products is different, and the guidance provided below applies equally to the various approaches.

In vitro assays should be performed on samples representative of the pack contents taken by an aseptic technique that does not appreciably alter the gross volume of the pack contents (must be kept to a minimum but in any case no greater than 10%) on Days 1, 3, 5 and 7 (and further samples if an extension of shelf life is proposed or for components that have a shorter shelf life). For studies investigating an extension to shelf life, consideration should be given to testing the component 1 day after the proposed limit of shelf life (e.g. Day 8 for a 7-day shelf life). Parallel testing of units prepared by a well-established method is recommended, and the use of a split-pool or crossover design will increase the power of such comparisons. *In vivo* studies, preferably with parallel testing of 'standard' components, should be performed on the last day of the proposed storage period. The number of units to be studied should be based on the study objectives and design and determined by statistical analysis based on the difference between test and control units to be detected. A sample size of ten tests or controls would be required to detect a 30% difference in pH and CD62P at Day 7 of storage using an unpaired study. Fewer units will be required if a pooled and split study design is used.

8.3.2 Investigational phase

8.3.2.1 Guidance

Table 8.3 recommends an assessment format for different kinds of novel development that may be expected for platelet components. While these are listed against the recommended assays above, this is not intended to be restrictive and comparable alternatives may be employed. It is recommended that any protocol for the evaluation of a novel blood component or production method be discussed with the Chair of the SACBC before finalisation.

For leucodepleted components, leucocyte enumeration should involve validated techniques and would currently be expected to exhibit a sensitivity of less than or equal to 1 leucocyte per microlitre.

8.3.3 *In vitro* assessment

8.3.3.1 Background

In vitro assessments essentially use surrogate assays that are hoped to be indicative of the *in vivo* performance of platelets, as measured by haemostatic effect, *in vivo* recovery and survival and corrected count increment following transfusion. While a large number of *in vitro* assays have been proposed, only a few of these have been shown to correlate with post-transfusion indices. This area has been reviewed by the BEST group[1] and can be summarised in Table 8.3 (* = correlates with *in vivo* viability).

Any platelet production system that may be considered as having the potential for an increased risk of bacterial contamination or growth should include an assessment of sterility as part of the initial validation phase. It is recommended that at least 50 apheresis units or pools (each sufficient for a standard adult dose) should be assessed for sterility by a validated technique prior to *in vivo* assessment and routine introduction of the component into clinical use.

8.3.4 *In vivo* assessment

If *in vivo* assessment is required local ethical committee approval should be obtained prior to commencing the *in vivo* assessment.

Additional measurements at 4–6 and/or 24 hours post-transfusion may give some indication of platelet survival.

Table 8.3 *In vitro* assessment

		Recommended	Alternatives (may be used if validated against parameters that correlate with *in vivo* viability)
(a)		Product content Volume Platelet content Leucocyte content Plasma content (for additive developments only)	
(b)		Platelet morphology (proportion of discs) Determination of swirling Morphology index (phase microscopy)* Extent of shape change by ADP*	
(c)		Platelet metabolism ATP* Hypotonic shock response* pO_2/pCO_2 pH Glucose consumption Lactate production	
(d)		Extent of platelet activation P-selectin (CD62P) on platelet surface and in supernatant Beta thromboglobulin release	Surface GPIb/IX (CD42a/42b) Surface GPIIb/IIIa (CD41/CD61) Platelet fibrinogen binding Serotonin content or release Glycocalicin or PF4 release Annexin V binding (to phospholipid)
(e)		Extent of platelet lysis Supernatant lactate dehydrogenase	Soluble annexin V
(f)		Measurements reflecting *in vitro* function Aggregation in response to paired antagonists (e.g. 80 μM ADP and 8 μg/mL collagen)	*In vitro* bleeding time (in development) Platelet adhesion (e.g. Baumgartner)
(g)		Assays indicative of possible side effects Cytokines/chemokines, particularly platelet-derived (IL-6, IL-8, RANTES, TNF-α, TGF-β): optional, (if performed bioassay is preferable to immunoassay) FXIIa formation (particularly for novel plastics or filters) Bacterial contamination (at end of shelf life only) Pathogen reduction (for these processes only)	

Any *in vivo* assessments should be performed at the end of the proposed storage period, following generation of sufficiently reassuring data from *in vitro* studies. For studies investigating an extension to shelf life, consideration should be given to testing the component 1 day after the proposed limit of shelf life (e.g. Day 8 for a 7-day shelf life). Due to the inherent variability of patients, use of a crossover design or dual labelling technique in stable, afebrile thrombocytopenic patients without evidence of platelet consumption (or in volunteers) is strongly recommended so that each patient acts as their own control. The number of components transfused should be justified on the basis of the study objectives and design.

Platelet counts should be assessed immediately prior to infusion of an appropriate dose of ABO identical platelets and 1 hour post-infusion.

Two approaches are established:

- Use of radioisotope-labelled platelets in normal volunteers: This approach is not applicable to pooled products. ^{51}Cr, or preferably ^{111}In, are the recommended isotopes to determine platelet recovery and survival.[2] Alternative validated techniques may be used.

- Determination of recovery after transfusion: An appropriate adult dose (>240 × 10^9 platelets) of ABO identical platelets may be used to determine increments and therapeutic effect (bleeding time measurements are not recommended). Patients known or suspected to have lymphocytotoxic or human platelet antigen (HPA) antibodies should be excluded and should have no evidence of hypersplenism, sepsis, ongoing haemorrhage or other cause of increased platelet consumption.

Table 8.4 Evaluation of new platelet components for transfusion

Parameter	Leuco-depletion	Pathogen reduction	Extended storage	Sterile connection	New bag, additive or anticoagulant
Volume (d1)	✓	✓	✓	✓	✓
Platelet content	✓	✓	✓	✓	✓
Leucocyte content (d1)	✓	?	?		?
Leucocyte subsets (%)	?	?	?		?
Morphology, e.g. Swirl test	✓	✓	✓	✓	✓
Activation, e.g. beta thromboglobulin	✓	✓	✓		✓
Lysis, e.g. lactate dehydrogenase	✓	✓	✓		✓
Metabolic activity, e.g. ATP, pH	✓	✓	✓		✓
Function e.g. Aggregation	?	?	?	?	?
Cytokines/chemokines	✓	✓	✓		✓
FXIIa	?	?			?
Sterility	if dock on	✓	✓	✓	?
PrP^c and microvesicles	?				
Pathogen reduction*	?	✓			

Key: ✓ = recommended; ? = optional; other tests are not excluded. * = normally undertaken by the manufacturer. Planned studies may fall into more than one category in which case all indicated assays should be performed. d1 = Day 1.

8.4 Evaluation of new fresh frozen plasma/cryoprecipitate components for transfusion

8.4.1 Introduction

In establishing any novel component, the development process is expected to involve three stages:

- **Investigation:** Initial intensive investigation of a range of parameters on a relatively small number of units (e.g. 10) to establish concepts. This should involve *in vitro* studies with serial sampling, and may also involve *in vivo* studies. Components produced during this phase should not be used for transfusion.

- **Validation:** Operational validation on a larger number of units (e.g. 50 to 100) to establish routine operation of the technique, normally testing for those parameters listed in the current edition of the Red Book. These tests may be supplemented by a limited set of assays selected from the investigational phase to allow setting of routine quality parameters. This may involve *in vivo* studies and normally would involve sampling at the times shown below for routine testing.

- **Routine:** Ongoing routine validation using a small set of parameters selected on the basis of the above studies. This will not normally involve *in vivo* studies. For clarity the guidance on which tests need to be performed is as shown in Table 8.5.

8.4.2 *In vitro* evaluation of novel fresh frozen plasma

8.4.2.1 Suggested study design

Because of the wide normal range of some clotting factors and potential inter-batch variation of assays, it is suggested that novel units and controls be produced and assayed in parallel, with the novel technology being the only variable. A less costly alternative, if logistics permit, is to do a pooled paired comparison, where two units are pooled, and one half processed by the novel technique. This provides greater statistical power for fewer units assayed, and is particularly important for storage studies. Since levels of FVIII and von Willebrand factor are ABO group-dependent, investigators should consider an equal mix of group A and O donations in the experimental design. The number of units to be studied should be based on the study objectives and design, and determined by statistical analysis based on the difference between test and control units to be detected. A sample size of at least 16 test or controls would be required to detect a 30% difference in FVIII levels using an unpaired study. Fewer units will be required if a pooled and split study design is used.

For leucocyte depleted or pathogen reduction systems it is recommended that assays are performed on samples collected before and after the process under investigation. Ideally provision should be made for storing and testing aliquots from each pack at every time point, as thawing out three or four different packs at each time point introduces excessive variation. However, a pre-validation should be done to ensure that the behaviour of the aliquotted component during storage is the same as that in the main pack.

8.4.2.2 Assays required

The extent of any evaluation depends in part on the degree of novelty of the component. The list of assays below need not be applied in every setting. Table 8.5 gives a summary of which assays are recommended in different situations. Advice may be sought from SACBC on the validation requirements for plasma components produced from automated processing of whole blood or other technology that is not specified in Table 8.5.

All evaluations must include the routine quality control parameters such as FVIII:C.

Before freezing:

- volume, platelet count, WBC*, RBC, total protein
- prothrombin time (PT), activated partial thromboplastin time (APTT)
- factors I (fibrinogen), II, V, VII, VIII, IX, X, XI, XIII, von Willebrand factor (vWf):Ag, vWf:RiCof, which measures the functional activity or an assay validated as yielding equivalent results, vWf multimeric analysis, vWF cleaving protease
- inhibitors of coagulation – antithrombin, protein C, protein S, α2-antiplasmin
- markers of unwanted activation of coagulation* – prothrombin fragment 1.2, fibrinopeptide A, factor XIIa, thrombin-antithrombin (TAT) complexes.

*Particularly relevant to plasma which has been collected by any filtration technique, in which case the assays should be performed before and after filtration or to packs made of novel materials.

During storage:

- Consideration should be given to performing storage studies at ≥20°C in addition to those at ≤30°C to reflect hospital storage conditions. Samples should be taken at 12 and 24 months. Ideally, all clotting factors should be assayed at each time point, if only in a few packs. FVIII should be assayed at each time point as a minimum in addition to the proteins most severely affected by the initial process.
- Storage parameters may be assayed after the date of implementation of routine production, provided data 'keep ahead' of the age of any clinical product which might be issued.

8.4.3 *In vitro* evaluation of novel cryoprecipitate

It is assumed that this will be produced from a 'novel' start plasma so that investigators will be aware of any specific losses of clotting factors which should be particularly considered.

Assays to be performed before and after production, and during storage: fibrinogen, FVIII:C.

8.4.4 Cryosupernatant

The only clinical indication for this component is for plasma exchange procedures for patients with thrombotic thrombocytopenic purpura. Analysis of vWf multimers and cleaving protease is therefore appropriate. vWf multimeric and cleaving protease analysis should be performed in a laboratory recognised to be proficient in this technique and which is performing the assay regularly.

Table 8.5 Evaluation of novel plasma components

	Fresh frozen plasma						Cryo-precipitate	Cryo-supernatant
	Novel filter	New centrifuge/ component extractor	Novel anticoagulant	Novel apheresis system	Novel apheresis + anticoagulant	Pathogen reduction		
Volume	✓	✓	✓	✓	✓	✓	✓	✓
Leucocyte content	✓	✓	✓	✓	✓			
FVIII:C	✓	✓	✓	✓	✓	✓	✓	
Platelets	✓	✓	✓	✓	✓	✓	–	–
PT ratio	✓	–	✓	–	✓	✓	–	–
APTT ratio	✓	–	✓	–	✓	✓	–	–
Fibrinogen	✓	–	✓	–	✓	✓	✓	
II, V, VII, IX, X, XI, XIII	✓	–	✓	–	✓	✓	–	–
vWf:Ag	✓	–	✓	–	✓	✓		
vWf:RiCof	✓	–	✓	–	✓	✓		
AT III, Prot C, Prot S	✓	–	✓	–	✓	✓	–	–
TAT/Frag1.2/ FPA + FXIIa	✓	–	✓	✓	✓	✓	Omit if not elevated in source plasma	
C1 inhibitor	✓	–	✓	–	✓	✓		
vWf multimers	✓	–	✓	–	✓	✓		✓
vWF cleaving protease	✓	–	✓	–	✓	✓		✓
alpha-2 anti-plasmin	✓	–	✓	–	✓	✓		
Pathogen reduction*						✓		
PrP^c/ microvesicles	?	–						
Clinical trial	–	–	#	#	#	✓ *	#	#

Key: ✓ = recommended; – = not needed; # = consider individually. * = normally undertaken by the manufacturer.

8.4.5 *In vivo* studies

Whether or not *in vivo* studies are needed depends on the degree of novelty of the component, e.g. this may not be necessary for plasma which has been leucocyte depleted in the course of producing leucocyte-depleted red cells, but would certainly apply in the case of a novel pathogen reduced plasma which had been exposed to chemicals. Unlike red cells and platelets, administration to normal volunteers has not been traditional. Suitable patient groups to consider would be:

For fresh frozen plasma:

- correction of prolonged international normalised ratio (INR) prior to liver biopsy
- liver transplant recipients

- plasma exchange for thrombotic thrombocytopenic purpura (TTP)
- disseminated intravascular coagulation (DIC).

It is difficult to get permission to study neonates and usually considerable experience has to have been gained with the product in adults.

A randomised design is preferred, with standard fresh frozen plasma as control.

For cryoprecipitate:

- DIC
- liver disease/transplant
- congenital hypofibrinogenaemia, if maintained on cryoprecipitate.

8.5 Generic protocol for the evaluation of apheresis equipment

This protocol sets out the minimum requirements for new apheresis equipment and, in a generic form, the mechanism for assessing acceptability of the equipment hardware, the software and the associated apheresis sets. The specific validation or trial of apheresis collections from new equipment is covered in section 8.6. Novel components, as defined in section 8.1, produced as a result of new equipment will be assessed as detailed in other sections of this chapter.

8.5.1 Minimum requirements

8.5.1.1 General

Equipment should be CE marked or the Blood Service should participate to facilitate CE marking.

Manufacturers must comply with Good Automated Manufacturing Practice (GAMP).[3]

8.5.1.2 Equipment hardware

Equipment should contain the following:

- manual override system
- blood flow monitor
- in-line air detector
- integral blood filter
- anticoagulant flow indicator
- collection volume preset device
- visual audible alarm for procedure completion
- automatic standby mode for power failure
- power up self-check to include all critical safety and operational procedures.

8.5.1.3 Equipment software

Software should provide parameters:

- for accepted total blood volume calculation algorithm

- for accepted citrate reinfusion rate calculation algorithm
- for fixed upper limit citrate reinfusion (see Chapter 5)
- for programmable upper limit total collection volume
- must not exceed predetermined fluid reinfusion limits (e.g. citrate, saline)
- for alarm and prevent use of incorrect set (incongruent) for programmed procedure
- prevent procedure where predicted post-collection parameters fall outside programmable safety limits as defined in Chapter 5.

For other measures, see Chapter 5.

8.5.1.4 Apheresis sets

Apheresis sets should have:

- a closed system
- a visual system to minimise risk of transposition of fluid lines
- a microbial filter on 'spiked' lines
- a diversion line and pouch for sampling
- a means of preventing incorrect connections to the set for IV fluid (e.g. saline) and anticoagulant.

Consideration should be given to the incorporation of a pouch on the final pack to facilitate bacterial contamination testing.

For other measures, see Chapter 5.

The overall mechanism for equipment acceptance is given in Figure 8.1 for reference. Validation, installation qualification, operational qualification and performance qualification would be defined by the Blood Service, taking account of the advice within these guidelines.

8.6 Generic protocol for the evaluation of blood packs for whole blood donations and apheresis collections

8.6.1 Introduction

This protocol sets out in generic form the essential features of blood pack evaluations as required by the UK Blood Transfusion Services. National Services should exercise discretion in the extent to which the protocol should be applied. It may be appropriate to consider an abbreviated format, e.g. when the change to be evaluated represents the attachment of a filter to a pack assembly that is already in routine use, or where the change consists of a modified port access design.

The protocol is not intended for use with packs for stem cell collection and storage, although the principles outlined may be helpful. The principles of this section apply to components produced from whole blood donations as well as whole blood itself.

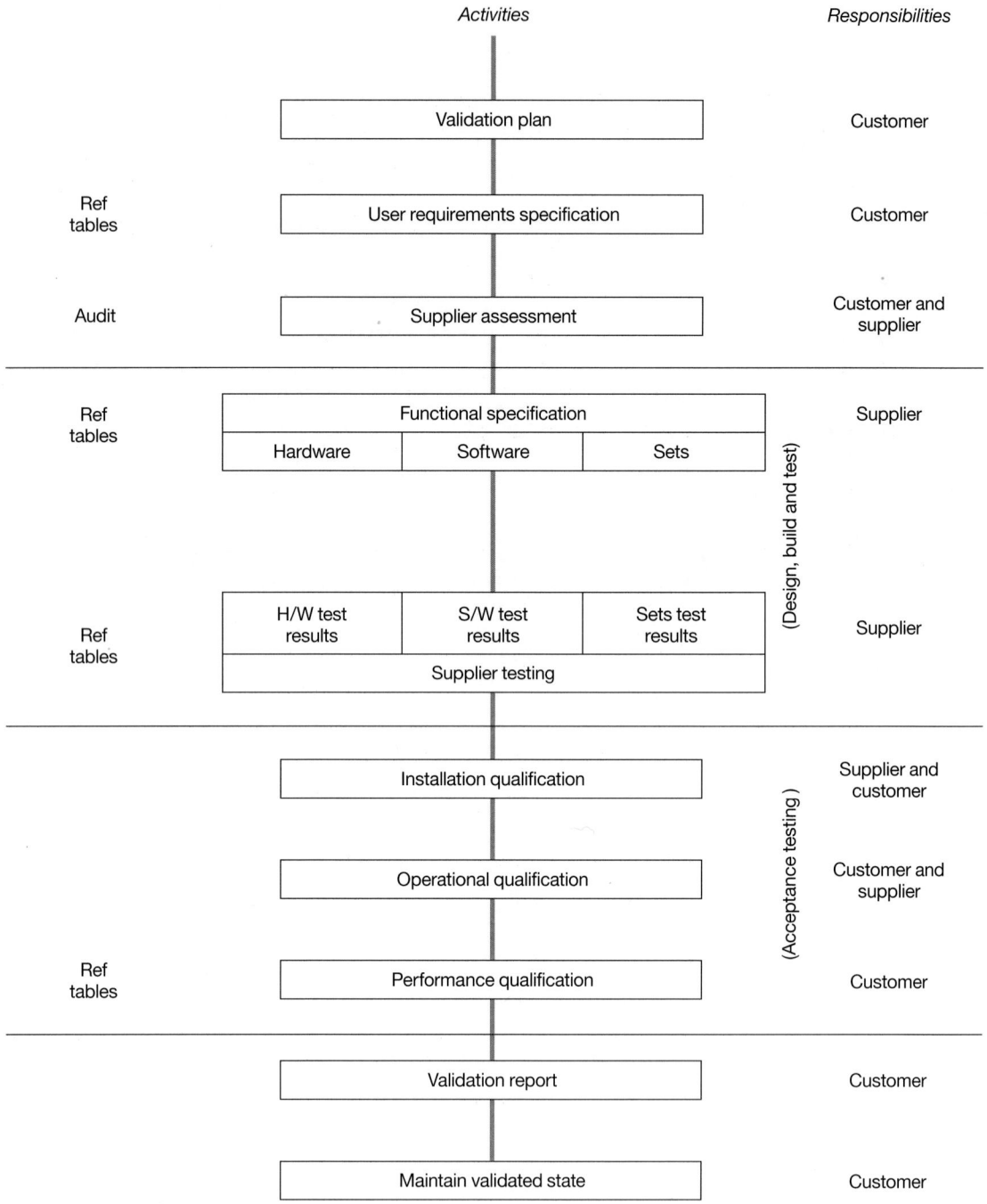

Figure 8.1 Generic flowchart of apheresis equipment acceptance

8.6.2 General principles

Each trial will be fully documented and will have a unique trial reference number. The key requirements are as follows:

- An evaluation outline: What type of pack is being investigated, where, when and the standards against which the assessment will be based.

- The evaluation objective: To demonstrate the packs are and remain free from defects and are suitable for the production and storage of components that meet current guidelines.

- Identification of any restrictions, e.g.:
  - situations where an evaluation would be required

- agreement on ownership and release of the evaluation report with the supplier/manufacturer
- limitations of the report and its distribution.

● How the trial will be controlled, e.g.:
  - the identity of the person/persons responsible for the trial and their reporting lines
  - sign-off procedures and authorities including concessionary changes
  - the trial protocol will be agreed with the supplier and any concessionary changes will require agreement in accordance with local procedures
  - trials will be conducted in three phases. Satisfactory performance and sign-off in Phase 0 is a prerequisite to progression to Phase 1 and satisfactory performance in Phase 1 is a prerequisite to progression to Phase 2
  - blood collected in Phase 0 will not be used for transfusion
  - all components prepared in Phase 1 will be subject to routine quality monitoring tests
  - a minimum of 1% of components prepared in Phase 2 will be subjected to routine quality monitoring tests
  - any testing that exceeds the minimum set out herein must be fully incorporated within the report.

● Confidentiality: Any data collected will normally be the property of the organisation performing the trial; blood pack suppliers/manufacturers who wish to release information arising from the trial will require confirmation in writing from the organisation performing the trial that they may do so.

● Quality monitoring: It is expected that packs evaluated under the trial protocol will be subject to routine quality monitoring and reporting procedures, e.g. pack faults, compliance with component specifications etc. It follows that any adverse findings during the trial would generate a corrective action.

Table 8.6 Summary of testing numbers required for evaluations and validations

Process	Testing	Phase 0	Phase 1	Phase 2	Local process qualification
Whole blood	Component evaluation	10–16 See Tables 8.2 to 8.5	None	None	None
	Quality monitoring	10–16 100% tested	125 100% tested	2000 from each of two batches Minimum 1% tested	125 100% tested
Apheresis collection	Component evaluation	10–16 See Tables 8.2 to 8.5	None	None	None
	Quality monitoring	10–16 100% tested	125 100% tested	300 100% tested	10 (each machine) 100% tested

A summary of the numbers to be tested for each evaluation or validation phase is given in Table 8.6. The numbers given are the minimum required. More detail is given in the relevant sections below. Deviations from this number must be agreed in accordance with local procedures.

8.6.3 Phase 0: Evaluation

After an initial familiarisation with novel bag/filters (pre-Phase 0) the purpose of Phase 0 studies is to:

- assess suitability to progress to Phase 1
- determine suitable quality monitoring parameters
- disclose any quality problems that might prevent components collected or prepared in these packs from being used for transfusion.

Processing conditions used in the Phase 0 evaluation should be the same as those applied to Phase 1 and 2 evaluations.

8.6.3.1 Component quality monitoring

Starting donations and all final components will be tested for compliance with relevant parameters listed in the component specifications in these guidelines. Where relevant, additional assays should be performed as specified in the Red Book generic evaluation protocols for new or novel blood components.

8.6.3.2 Goods inward inspection

- Check that appropriate storage information is shown on the packaging.
- Check the condition of packaging on receipt. Document damaged cartons and examine contents to assess the extent of any damage.

8.6.3.3 Quality assurance pack conformance inspection

Unless otherwise indicated, the following inspection will be performed and documented for all packs to be used in Phase 0 of the trial:

- pack batch number (eye-readable and machine-readable)
- pack type number (eye-readable and machine-readable)
- base label integrity and compliance with Chapter 26 of these guidelines for the uniform labelling of blood and blood components
- base label adherence (a sample of 20 at each temperature)
    - +22°C for 1 week
    - +4°C for 1 week
    - +4°C for 1 day, followed by −35°C for 1 week
- donation number, component type and blood group label adherence (a sample of 20 at each temperature)
    - +22°C for 1 week
    - +4°C for 1 week
    - +4°C for 1 day, followed by −35°C for 1 week

- seals, seams and welds satisfactory
  - absence of leaks
  - anticoagulant/additive free from turbidity, particulate matter and inclusions
- if the inspection requires removal of packs from their overwraps, either repackage and use according to the manufacturer's instructions or perform the examination immediately prior to donation
- check for acceptable handling and storage characteristics of unopened cartons of packs from receipt, through storage to use at sessions.

8.6.3.4 Checks to be performed by collection teams

Collection teams will follow routine procedures for recording pack faults, but additionally should comment on:

- ease of overwrap opening
- integrity of overwrap
- accuracy of instructions for use at time of collection
- acceptability of needle characteristics
- suitability of tubing (length and flexibility)
- general suitability.

8.6.3.5 Checks to be performed by processing team

The processing team will follow routine procedures for recording pack faults, but may additionally wish to comment on:

- breakage rates following freezing
- heat seal failures (in-house seals)
- suitability of tubing (length and flexibility)
- ease of cannula breakage
- ability to sterile dock (during secondary processing)
- integrity of join, following local, current, procedure
- compatibility with instructions for device for sterile connection
- assess packaging of frozen packs
- inspection of packs after overnight storage at 4°C.

When the minimum number of packs has been evaluated, the individual or group responsible for the trial will prepare and submit a Phase 0 report.

8.6.4 Phase 1: Validation

The purpose of this phase is to allow:

- staff to familiarise themselves with the packs and any associated equipment

- the generation of quality monitoring data
- the development of an appreciation of the suitability of the packs for routine use, i.e. progression to Phase 2 trial.

Phase 1 of the validation process normally will require not less than 125 packs to be tested at the centre undertaking the trial. Deviations from this number must be agreed in accordance with local procedures.

It is expected that a smaller number of packs will be used for familiarisation in other centres.

This phase will include the finalisation of standard operating procedures (SOPs) for use in Phase 2.

Blood components produced during Phase 1 may be used therapeutically where they comply with appropriate release criteria.

8.6.4.1 Component quality monitoring

Starting donations and all final components will be tested for compliance with relevant parameters listed in the component specifications in these guidelines.

8.6.4.2 Goods inward inspection

- Check that appropriate storage information is shown on the packaging.
- Check the condition of packaging on receipt. Document damaged cartons and examine contents to assess the extent of any damage.

8.6.4.3 Quality assurance pack conformance inspection

Unless otherwise indicated, the following inspection will be performed and documented for all packs to be used in Phase 1 of the trial:

- pack batch number (eye-readable and machine-readable)
- pack type number (eye-readable and machine-readable)
- base label integrity
- seals, seams and welds satisfactory
  - absence of leaks
  - anticoagulant/additive free from turbidity, particulate matter and inclusions
- if the inspection requires removal of packs from their overwraps, either repackage and use according to the manufacturer's instructions or discard
- check for acceptable handling and storage characteristics of unopened cartons of packs from receipt, through storage to use at sessions.

8.6.4.4 Checks to be performed by collection teams

Collection teams will follow routine procedures for recording pack faults, but additionally should comment on:

- ease of overwrap opening
- integrity of overwrap
- accuracy of instructions for use at time of collection

- acceptability of needle characteristics
- suitability of tubing (length and flexibility)
- general suitability.

8.6.4.5 Checks to be performed by processing team

The processing team will follow routine procedures for recording pack faults, but may additionally wish to comment on:

- breakage rates following freezing
- heat seal failures (in-house seals)
- suitability of tubing (length and flexibility)
- ease of cannula breakage
- ability to sterile dock (during secondary processing)
- integrity of join, following local, current, procedure
- compatibility with instructions for device for sterile connection
- assess packaging of frozen packs
- inspection of packs after overnight storage at 4°C.

8.6.4.6 End users

Set up a process by which users will feedback information on acceptability of the packs for use. This would involve blood bank and ward/theatre staff. Obtain details on:

Blood bank issues:

- acceptability to end users
- acceptability of number and condition of bleed line samples
- crossmatch/other label adherence
- leak and breakage rates.

Ward/theatre staff issues:

- general acceptability
- accessibility of ports for giving sets
- leak and breakage rates.

When the minimum number of packs has been evaluated, the individual or group responsible for the trial will prepare and submit a Phase 1 report.

8.6.5 Phase 2: Evaluation

A minimum of 2000 packs from each of two batches for whole blood collection processes or 300 sets for apheresis collection will be used in this phase to allow data on consistency of manufacture to be collected.

Relevant SOPs will be available before commencing Phase 2. Customer communication and any associated training will also have been done by this date.

Blood components produced during Phase 2 may be used therapeutically where they comply with the normal release criteria.

8.6.5.1 Goods inward inspection

- Check that appropriate storage information is shown on the packaging.
- Check the condition of packaging on receipt. Document damaged cartons and examine contents to assess the extent of any damage.

8.6.5.2 Quality assurance pack conformance inspection

Unless otherwise indicated, the following inspection will be performed and documented for packs to be used in Phase 2 of the trial:

- pack batch number (eye-readable and machine-readable)
- pack type number (eye-readable and machine-readable)
- base label integrity
- seals, seams and welds satisfactory
- absence of leaks
- anticoagulant/additive free from turbidity, particulate matter and inclusions.

8.6.5.3 Checks to be performed by collection teams

Collection teams will follow routine procedures for recording pack faults, but additionally should comment on:

- ease of overwrap opening
- integrity of overwrap
- accuracy of instructions for use at time of collection
- acceptability of needle characteristics
- suitability of tubing (length and flexibility)
- general suitability.

8.6.5.4 Checks to be performed by processing team

The processing team will follow routine procedures for recording pack faults, but may additionally wish to comment on:

- breakage rates following freezing
- heat seal failures (in-house seals)
- suitability of tubing (length and flexibility)
- ease of cannula breakage
- ability to sterile dock (during secondary processing)

- integrity of join, following local, current, procedure
- compatibility with instructions for device for sterile connection
- assess packaging of frozen packs
- inspection of packs after overnight storage at 4°C.

8.6.5.5 Component quality monitoring

A minimum of 1% of components (or as determined by statistical process monitoring) produced for whole blood collection processes or 300 of each component (one of each relevant component per procedure) for apheresis collection will be subjected to routine quality monitoring for parameters specified in this book.

8.6.5.6 End users

Set up a process by which users will feedback information on acceptability of the packs for use. This would involve blood bank and ward/theatre staff. Obtain details on:

Blood bank issues:

- acceptability to end users
- acceptability of number and condition of bleed line samples
- crossmatch/other label adherence
- leak and breakage rates.

Ward/theatre staff issues:

- general acceptability
- accessibility of ports for giving sets
- leak and breakage rates.

On completion, the individual or group responsible for the trial will prepare and submit a Phase 2 report on the suitability for use of the blood pack system within the service undertaking the trial.

8.7 References

1. Murphy S, Rebulla P, Bertolini F, Holme S, Moroff G, Snyder E, Stromberg R (1994). *In vitro* assessment of the quality of stored platelet concentrates. The Biomedical Excellence for Safer Transfusion (BEST) Task Force of the International Society of Blood Transfusion. *Transfusion Medicine Review*, 8(1), 29–36.

2. The Panel on Diagnostic Application of Radioisotopes in Hematology, International Committee for Standardization in Hematology (1977). Recommended methods for radioisotope platelet survival studies. *Blood*, 50(6), 1137–1144.

3. Good Automated Manufacturing Practice (GAMP) *Guide for Validation of Automated Systems in Pharmaceutical Manufacture*. Available at www.ispe.org.

Chapter 9
Microbiology tests for donors and donations: general specifications for laboratory test procedures

Blood donations make up the majority of donations collected and processed by the UK transfusion services, but tissue and stem cell donations are a growing part of their portfolio. While the screening requirements for blood, tissues and stem cells largely overlap, there are some important differences that should be acknowledged and incorporated into any guidelines.

For the purpose of these guidelines, tissue donations include all of the types of tissue normally retrieved from living or deceased donors, and stem cell donations include haemopoietic progenitor cells (HPC) and therapeutic cells (TP). These guidelines therefore specify the screening requirements for blood, tissue and stem cell donations managed by the UK transfusion services.

9.1 General requirements

All screening must be performed within Blood Safety and Quality Regulations (BSQR)[1] compliant laboratories and meet any other appropriate regulatory requirements.

Secure and effective procedures must be in place to ensure that:

- all donations, any subsequent components/products and their laboratory samples are correctly identified by barcoded and eye-readable numbers
- donations can be linked to their donor
- information about previous test results which would preclude issue of a subsequent donation cannot be automatically overridden by a subsequent negative test result
- donor samples are suitably stored under appropriate conditions of temperature and time to preserve the targets for which they will be screened
- the screening assays used are properly evaluated and validated
- tests are appropriately performed and controlled, and the results properly and accurately recorded, using validated procedures
- test results and other relevant test information are retained for the appropriate period, as set out in the BSQR[1] or equivalent
- appropriate confirmatory testing is available to investigate screen reactivity
- relevant data relating to screening and confirmatory test results are reported to a centralised surveillance system, allowing the monitoring of trends in screening test reactivity and confirmed positive results.

9.1.1 Test reagents, kits and equipment

All assays used must be CE marked and must have been assessed (in respect of sensitivity and specificity) and deemed suitable by the UK Blood Transfusion Services kit evaluation groups (NHSBT KEG or SNBTS/NIBTS MTEG) for the detection of the required markers in the donation types being screened. Unless specifically validated for alternative use/performance, test kits and reagents must be stored and used according to the manufacturer's instructions.

Each new manufacturer's lot of each assay should be assessed prior to being accepted and put into use.

Additionally, all testing laboratories must ensure that the expected standard of performance of the assays used is being achieved, by using appropriate assay batch pre-acceptance testing, delivery acceptance testing and statistical monitoring of test results on defined quality control samples.

All test procedures must be documented and an inventory maintained of kits and reagents in stock, including supplier, batch number, expiry date, date of receipt, version number of product insert and record of pre-acceptance testing.

Procedures must ensure the traceability of the batch number and manufacturer of kits and reagents and the serial number of equipment used to test every donation.

Equipment must be validated, calibrated and maintained. Appropriate records for these activities must be made and retained as defined in extant regulations (currently 30 years).

Appropriate reactivity with manufacturers' and any external control samples must be demonstrated with every series of tests.

A series/batch of tests is defined as the number of tests set up at the same time, under the same conditions and processed in a similar manner:

- Where the microplate format is used each plate constitutes a series of tests even if only a few wells are used.

- Where a closed system is used the size of a series/batch of tests must be determined by each individual Service through an appropriate risk assessment.

9.1.2 Recording and reporting of results

The laboratory final output should indicate the result of every test performed, using a system that provides positive sample identification. Each test result should be recorded by a system that does not require transcription. If manual completion of screening is performed it must be thoroughly documented and controlled and the results handled electronically following the same basic principles applied to fully automated testing.

9.1.3 Release of tested components/products

Standard procedures must ensure that no donations, or components/products prepared from them, can be released for issue until all the required laboratory tests (mandatory and additional) have been completed, documented and approved within a validated system of work. Compliance with this requirement can only be achieved by the use of a validated computerised system that requires the input of valid and acceptable test results for all the mandatory and required laboratory tests to permit the release of each individual donation.

Table 9.1 Screening required for blood donations

Infectious agent	Minimum requirement	Comments
HIV 1+2	anti-HIV 1+2 or HIV 1+2 Ag/Ab (M) HIV RNA*	RNA screening in pools of a maximum of 48 donations**
HCV	anti-HCV (M) HCV RNA (M)	RNA screening in pools of a maximum of 48 donations**
HBV	HBsAg (M) HBV DNA* anti-HBc [+ anti-HBs] (A)	DNA screening in pools of a maximum of 48 donations** Donations that are anti-HBc reactive and have anti-HBs >100 mIU/mL are considered suitable for release
Syphilis	anti-treponemal Ab (M)	
HTLV I/II	anti-HTLV I/II (M)***	Screening in pools of a maximum of 48 donations**
HCMV	anti-HCMV (A)	Ideally both IgG and IgM, but IgG alone is considered sufficient
Plasmodium sp.	anti-*P. falciparum/vivax* (A)	
Trypanosoma cruzi	anti-*T. cruzi* (A)	
West Nile Virus (WNV)	WNV RNA (A)	RNA screening in pools of a maximum of 16 donations****

(M) – mandatory (release criteria) for the purpose of these guidelines

(A) – additional due to specifically identifiable risk

* Although neither are mandatory for blood donations in most of the UK, HIV RNA and HBV DNA are included in the nucleic acid amplification techniques (NAT) screen as the commercial systems available are now triplex assays. HIV RNA is mandated within Scotland.

** The minimum sensitivity of the molecular screening is dependent upon pool size. The maximum validated pool size for use for blood screening within the UK Blood Transfusion Services is 48 donations.

*** anti-HTLV screening is not required for frozen plasma components if they are sourced independently from cellular components (Department of Health instruction 2010).

**** The maximum validated pool size for WNV NAT screening is 16 donations.

9.2 Microbiology screening

Note: The meanings of certain terms used in this section are defined in section 9.2.6.

9.2.1 Screening of donations/donors

Donation/donor screening can be broadly divided into two main categories:

- Mandatory: Absolute requirement prior to the release of components. There are, however, different reasons for a test to be defined as 'mandatory'. These include a European Union requirement, a specific instruction from the Department of Health, including its Advisory Committees, and an Act of Parliament.

- Additional (also known as Discretionary): Performed because of specific additional and identifiable donor or recipient risk.

Importantly, the mandatory requirements for blood donation and for tissue and stem cell donations are different, with some tests that are defined as 'Additional' for blood donations being 'Mandatory' for non-blood donations (Tables 9.1 and 9.2). Although not required for all donations, where

Table 9.2 Screening required for tissue and stem cell donations*

Infectious agent	Minimum requirement	Comments
HIV 1+2	anti-HIV 1+2 or HIV 1+2 Ag/Ab (M) HIV RNA (O)	Maximum pool size of 24 donations**
HCV	anti-HCV (M) HCV Ag and/or HCV Ag/Ab (O) HCV RNA (O)	Maximum pool size of 24 donations**
HBV	HBsAg (M) anti-HBc [+ anti-HBs] (M) HBV DNA** (O)	Donations that are anti-HBc reactive and have anti-HBs >100 mIU/mL are considered suitable for release
Syphilis	anti-treponemal Ab (M)	
HTLV I/II	anti-HTLV I/II***	Maximum pool size of 24 donations**
HCMV	anti-HCMV (A)	
Plasmodium sp.	anti-*P. falciparum/vivax* (A)	
Trypanosoma cruzi	anti-*T. cruzi* (A)	
West Nile Virus (WNV)	WNV RNA (A)	Maximum pool size of 16 donations****
(M) – mandatory		
(O) – optional, genomic screening for HIV, HCV and HBV is not mandated but can be performed on the original donation sample as an alternative to 180 days' quarantine and follow-up serological testing		
(A) – additional due to specifically identifiable risk		
* UK screening requirements. Other testing, e.g. Epstein-Barr virus, toxoplasmosis, may be required as additional tests depending upon specific additional risk and/or special requests for individual recipients. For certain product types that are exported there may be additional end user testing requirements.		
** All screening of deceased tissue donations is performed on individual samples. HCV and HIV RNA and anti-HTLV I/II screening of surgical tissues/stem cells can be performed using pools of a maximum of 24 samples. HBV DNA screening should be on individual samples.		
*** Not mandatory for avascular tissue donations but may be considered good practice.		
**** The maximum validated pool size for WNV RNA screening is 16 donations.		

additional tests are required, the results are an integral part of the criteria for the release of that donation/component/product. In addition, for certain donation types, there is the option of quarantine and follow-up serological testing before issue or the inclusion of genomic screening at donation.

Donations and any associated components/products must not be released to stock unless they have been tested and found negative for the mandatory, and any additional, microbiological screening required. In certain circumstances, for certain donation/component types, a reactive screen result may not preclude release of the donations/component.

9.2.2 Deceased neonatal and infant tissue donors

- Full microbiology screening of a maternal sample is always required.

- For still births and neonates less than 48 hours after birth, no microbiology screening of the neonate is required.

- For neonates between 48 hours and 28 days after birth, a neonatal sample is only required when there are identifiable risks of possible viral transmission. In this scenario only nucleic acid amplification techniques (NAT) testing of the sample is required.

- For infants more than 28 days after birth, full microbiology screening of an infant's sample is required.

9.2.3 Serology screening algorithms

9.2.3.1 Blood donations

- No sample which tests initially reactive for the first time in the routine screening assay can be released for clinical use unless subsequently shown to have a negative result on both tests in duplicate repeat testing using the same assay.

- Blood donations that are reactive on one or both of the repeat tests are unsuitable for use and must be labelled as biological hazard/not for transfusion.

- Samples which test initially reactive in the routine screening assay, but which originate from donors who have been previously investigated in a reference laboratory and have been shown to be demonstrating non-specific reactivity, may be tested on a second (alternative) screening assay of at least equal sensitivity to the primary screening assay, and can be considered suitable for clinical use if the reaction in the alternative screening assay is negative.

See flowchart for screening of blood donations provided in Figure 9.1.

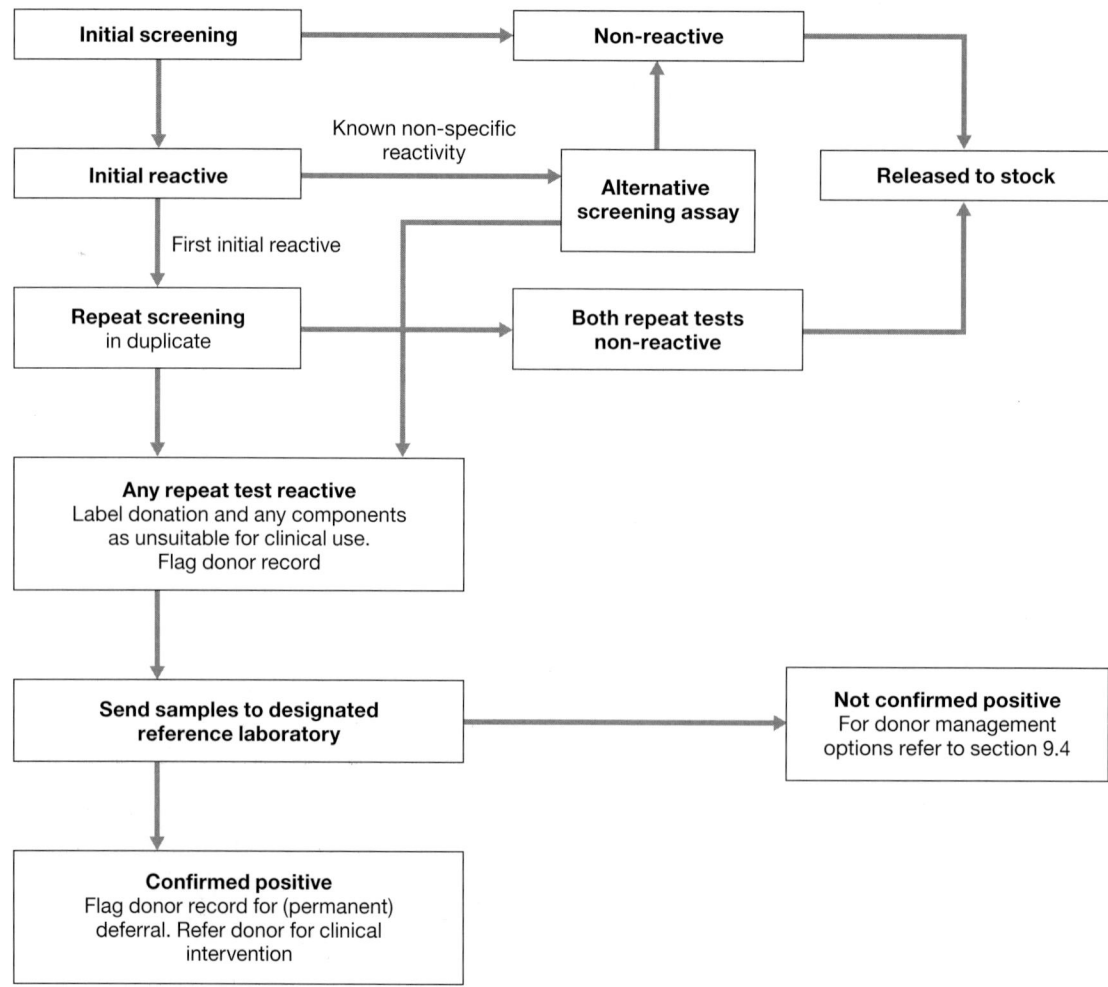

Figure 9.1 Serology screening: blood donations

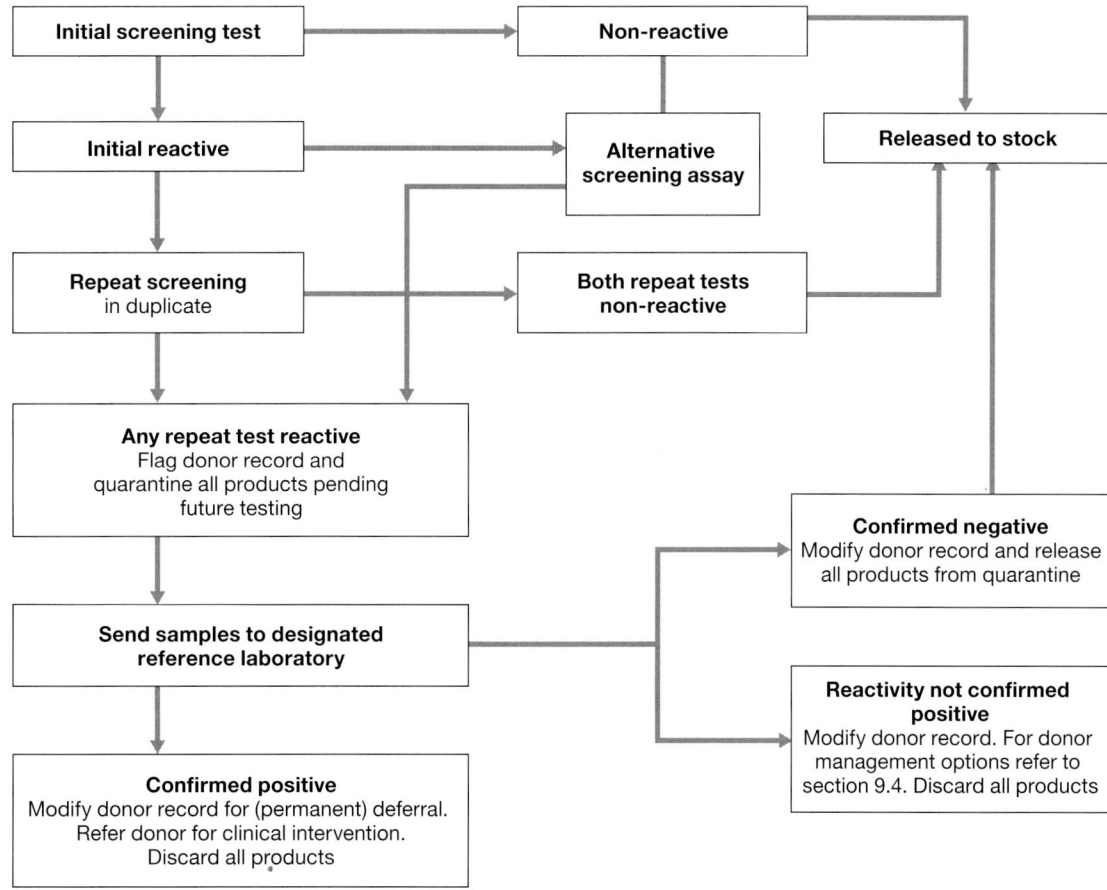

Figure 9.2 Serology screening and stem cell donations

9.2.3.2 Tissue and stem cell donations

- All initially reactive samples (see Figure 9.2) must be re-tested in duplicate using either the same assay or using an alternative assay that has been specifically evaluated to have at least equal sensitivity and ideally is based on different antigens and/or antibodies, and/or principles.

- Donations that are non-reactive on both of the repeat tests can be considered suitable for clinical use.

- Donations that are reactive on one or both of the repeat tests may in some clinical circumstances, and depending on the confirmatory results, be considered suitable for use (SaBTO Guidelines 2011[2]).

9.2.4 Molecular screening algorithm

- All initially reactive pool samples (see Figures 9.3 and 9.4) must be resolved to an individual (or more) reactive donation. All other non-reactive donations can be considered suitable for clinical use.

- Individual reactive donations are unsuitable for clinical use and must be labelled as biological hazard/not for transfusion.

- Stem cell donations from known infected individuals that are reactive on screening may in some clinical circumstances be considered suitable for use (SaBTO Guidelines 2011[2]).

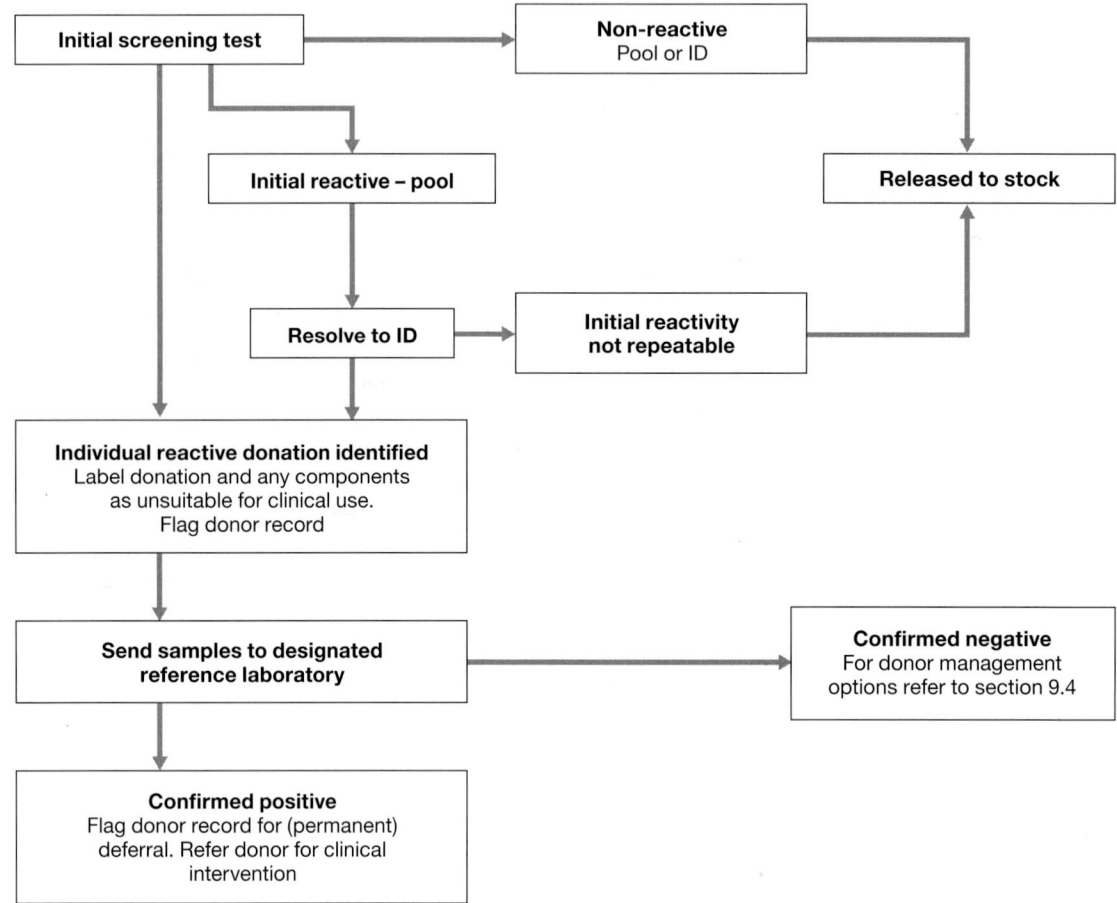

Figure 9.3 Molecular screening: blood donations

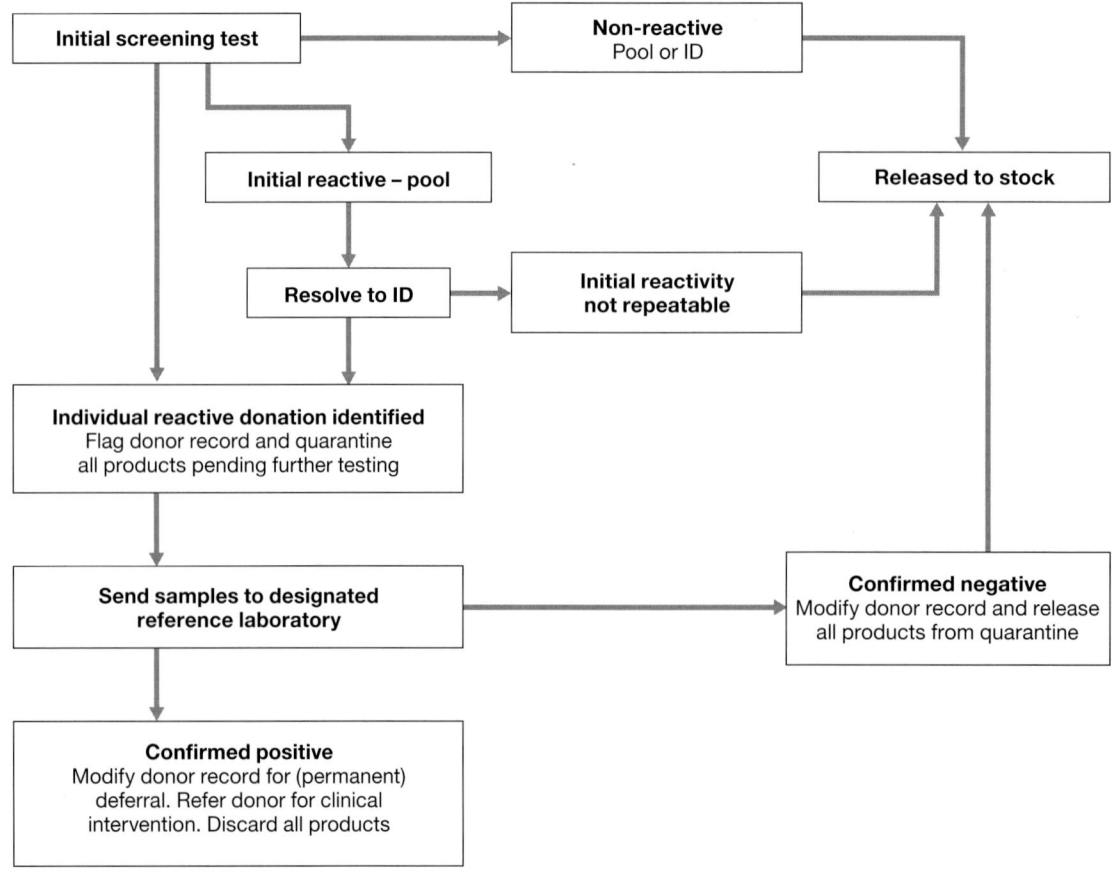

Figure 9.4 Molecular screening for tissue and cell donors

9.2.5 Confirmatory testing

When a donation is screen reactive for any of the serological or molecular mandatory or additional microbiology tests described above (except for anti-HCMV and anti-HBc, where anti-HBs is present at a level ≥100 mIU/mL), samples from the donor/donation must undergo confirmatory testing at a designated reference laboratory.

- If a positive result is confirmed, the donor record must be flagged as 'permanent exclusion risk – not to be used for clinical use' or equivalent. Arrangements should be made, as appropriate, to inform the donor and to ensure that the donor is referred for clinical intervention.

Note: Autologous stem cell donations may be collected from individuals who are known to be infected with one or more of the infectious agents for which donations are routinely screened. Such individuals are not generally classified as donors for the purposes of these guidelines.

- If a negative, inconclusive or indeterminate result is reported following confirmatory testing, and the initial reactivity is determined by the reference laboratory to be non-specific, use of further donations or the same donation (tissue and stem cell donors only) may be possible, as covered in section 9.4.

9.2.5.1 Specific requirements for HBsAg confirmation

The designated reference laboratory should, where appropriate, perform specific neutralisation tests for HBsAg to ensure that donors with low-level HBsAg reactivity are not incorrectly described as non-specifically reactive.

9.2.6 Definitions

Term	Definition
Non-reactive (NR)	A sample whose reactivity when first tested falls inside the assay cut-off as defined by the manufacturer's instructions. May also be referred to as a 'Negative' test result
Initial reactive (IR)	Any sample whose reactivity when first tested falls outside the cut-off as defined by the manufacturer's instructions
Repeat reactive (RR)	Any sample reactive on two or more occasions either in the same screening test (duplicate) or in two or more screening tests that are used in combination sequentially, to determine the suitability of a donation for release for clinical use
Alternative assay testing	When a test of similar modality and sensitivity is used sequentially to screen a sample which is either IR or RR in a first screening assay
Confirmatory testing	Further testing of a repeat reactive sample using a number of different assays in a reference laboratory to define whether the reactivity is specific to the microbe being screened for and indicative of potential infectivity
Positive	A sample whose reactivity in confirmatory testing meets pre-defined criteria. This may indicate current or past infection depending on the markers and microbe concerned
Inconclusive	A sample whose reactivity in confirmatory testing is not sufficient and/or specific enough to determine whether it reflects infection with the microbe being screened for
Negative	A sample which is either non-reactive in confirmatory testing or whose reactivity in confirmatory testing is deemed not to reflect infection

9.3 Specific assays

9.3.1 HBsAg

- The UK specification for the minimum level of sensitivity for the performance of HBsAg screening is 0.2 IU/mL. A UK HBsAg working standard (07/288 or equivalent) containing 0.2 IU/mL HBsAg is available from the National Institute for Biological Standards and Control (NIBSC). Laboratories using an assay of high analytical or dilutional sensitivity where the working standard reacts too strongly are advised to utilise the NIBSC HBsAg monitoring standard (07/286 or equivalent) set at 0.05 IU/mL in place of the working standard.

- In addition to the assay manufacturer's controls, the UK working standard must be included at least once in each series of tests to demonstrate acceptable sensitivity of the test method.

- No series of tests should be considered acceptable unless the result of the assay manufacturer's and the additional quality control samples have satisfied the criteria laid down.

- Each manufacturer's batch/lot of HBsAg test kits must be shown to conform with nationally established minimum criteria for specificity and sensitivity prior to being accepted for use for screening.

9.3.2 anti-HIV 1+2 or HIV 1+2 Ag/Ab combination

- The HIV 1+2 Ag/Ab combination assay is recommended for use within the UK Blood Services as the serological screening assay of choice.

- The UK requirement for the minimum level of sensitivity for the performance of HIV 1+2 serological screening is that a positive result should be obtained with the UK anti-HIV 1 working standard, available from NIBSC (99/750 or equivalent). Laboratories using an assay of higher analytical or dilutional sensitivity where the working standard reacts too strongly are advised to utilise the NIBSC HIV working standard 1/5 dilution (99/710 or equivalent) in place of the working standard. There is no specific requirement to demonstrate individual anti-HIV 2 or HIV p24 Ag reactivity.

- In addition to the assay manufacturer's controls, the UK working standard must be included at least once in each series of tests to demonstrate acceptable sensitivity of the test method.

- No series of tests should be considered acceptable unless the result of the assay manufacturer's and the additional quality control samples have satisfied the criteria laid down.

- Each manufacturer's batch/lot of HIV test kits must be shown to conform with nationally established minimum criteria for specificity and sensitivity prior to being accepted for use for screening, including demonstrating specific anti-HIV 2 reactivity and, as appropriate specific HIV p24 Ag reactivity.

9.3.3 anti-HCV

- The UK requirement for the minimum level of sensitivity for the performance of anti-HCV screening is that a positive result should be obtained with the UK anti-HCV working standard (06/188 or equivalent), available from NIBSC. Laboratories using an assay of higher analytical or dilutional sensitivity where the working standard reacts too strongly are advised to utilise the NIBSC HCV working standard 1/8 dilution (06/190 or equivalent) in place of the working standard.

- In addition to the assay manufacturer's controls, the UK working standard must be included at least once in each series of tests to demonstrate acceptable sensitivity of the test method.

- No series of tests should be considered acceptable unless the result of the assay manufacturer's and the additional quality control samples have satisfied the criteria laid down.

- Each manufacturer's batch/lot of anti-HCV test kits must be shown to conform with nationally established minimum criteria for specificity and sensitivity prior to being accepted for use for screening.

9.3.4 anti-HTLV I/II

- The UK requirement for the minimum level of sensitivity for the performance of anti-HTLV I/II screening is that a positive result should be obtained with the UK anti-HTLV working standard, available from NIBSC (03/104 or equivalent).

- In addition to the assay manufacturer's controls, the UK working standard must be included at least once in each series of tests to demonstrate acceptable sensitivity of the test method.

- No series of tests should be considered acceptable unless the result of the assay manufacturer's and the additional quality control samples have satisfied the criteria laid down.

- Each manufacturer's batch/lot of anti-HTLV I/II test kits must be shown to conform with nationally established minimum criteria for specificity and sensitivity prior to being accepted for use for screening.

9.3.5 Syphilis antibody

- The UK requirement for the minimum level of sensitivity for the performance of syphilis (specific treponemal antibody) screening is that, in the absence of a specifically defined UK working standard produced by NIBSC, a positive result should be obtained with the appropriate Health Protection Agency (HPA) syphilis quality control preparation.

- In addition to the assay manufacturer's controls, the HPA syphilis quality control preparation must be included at least once in each series of tests to demonstrate acceptable sensitivity of the test method.

- No series of tests should be considered acceptable unless the result of the assay manufacturer's and the additional quality control samples have satisfied the criteria laid down.

- Each manufacturer's batch/lot of anti-treponemal test kits must be shown to conform with nationally established minimum criteria for specificity and sensitivity prior to being accepted for use for screening.

9.3.6 Malarial antibody

The exclusion period for donors from malarial areas is given in the Joint UKBTS/HPA Professional Advisory Committee (JPAC) *Donor Selection Guidelines*.[3] These guidelines specify situations where donations may only be released if a test for malarial antibodies is negative.

- The UK requirement for the minimum level of sensitivity for the performance of malarial antibody (anti-*P. falciparum/vivax*) screening is that, in the absence of a specifically defined UK working standard produced by NIBSC, a positive result should be obtained with the HPA malaria antibody quality control preparation.

- In addition to the assay manufacturer's controls, the HPA malaria antibody quality control preparation must be included at least once in each series of tests to demonstrate acceptable sensitivity of the test method.

- No series of tests should be considered acceptable unless the result of the assay manufacturer's and the additional quality control samples have satisfied the criteria laid down.

- Each manufacturer's batch/lot of malarial antibody test kits must be shown to conform with nationally established minimum criteria for specificity and sensitivity prior to being accepted for use for screening.

9.3.7 anti-*T. cruzi*

The deferral criteria for donors from *T. cruzi* endemic areas are given in the JPAC *Donor Selection Guidelines*.[3] Donors at risk of *T. cruzi* must be tested for anti-*T. cruzi* and negative results obtained prior to the release of any donation for clinical use.

- The UK requirement for the minimum level of sensitivity for the performance of anti-*T. cruzi* screening is that, in the absence of a specifically defined UK working standard produced by NIBSC, a positive result should be obtained with a formally validated in-house anti-*T. cruzi* quality control preparation.

- In addition to the assay manufacturer's controls, the anti-*T. cruzi* quality control preparation must be included at least once in each series of tests to demonstrate acceptable sensitivity of the test method.

- No series of tests should be considered acceptable unless the result of the assay manufacturer's and the additional quality control samples have satisfied the criteria laid down.

- Each manufacturer's batch/lot of anti-*T. cruzi* test kits must be shown to conform with nationally established minimum criteria for specificity and sensitivity prior to being accepted for use for screening.

9.3.8 anti-HBc

The exclusion period for blood donors who have had body piercing, acupuncture etc. are given in the JPAC *Donor Selection Guidelines*.[3] Certain of these categories may require donations to be tested for anti-HBc and negative results obtained prior to release of any blood component for clinical use. Tissue and stem cells donations have anti-HBc screening as a mandatory requirement.

- The UK requirement for the minimum level of sensitivity for the performance of anti-HBc screening is that, in the absence of a specifically defined UK working standard produced by NIBSC, a positive result should be obtained with the HPA anti-HBc quality control preparation.

- In addition to the assay manufacturer's controls, the HPA anti-HBc quality control preparation must be included at least once in each series of tests to demonstrate acceptable sensitivity of the test method.

- No series of tests should be considered acceptable unless the result of the assay manufacturer's and the additional quality control samples have satisfied the criteria laid down.

- Each manufacturer's batch/lot of anti-HBc test kits must be shown to conform with nationally established minimum criteria for specificity and sensitivity prior to being accepted for use for screening.

- Donations found to be reactive for anti-HBc should be tested for anti-HBs (see section 9.3.10).

9.3.9 anti-HCMV

- The UK requirement for the minimum level of sensitivity for the performance of anti-HCMV screening is that, in the absence of a specifically defined UK working standard produced by NIBSC, a positive result should be obtained with the HPA anti-HCMV quality control preparation.

- In addition to the assay manufacturer's controls, the HPA anti-HCMV quality control preparation must be included at least once in each series of tests to demonstrate acceptable sensitivity of the test method.

- No series of tests should be considered acceptable unless the result of the assay manufacturer's and the additional quality control samples have satisfied the criteria laid down.

- Each manufacturer's batch/lot of anti-HCMV test kits must be shown to conform with nationally established minimum criteria for specificity and sensitivity prior to being accepted for use for screening.

9.3.10 anti-HBs

Donations found to be reactive for anti-HBc with levels of anti-HBs <100 mIU/mL are deemed unsuitable for release, whereas those with levels >100 mIU/mL can be considered suitable for release.

- The UK requirement for the minimum level of sensitivity for the performance of anti-HBs testing is that, in the absence of a specifically defined UK working standard produced by NIBSC, a positive result should be obtained with the HPA anti-HBs quality control preparation.

- In addition to the assay manufacturer's controls, the HPA anti-HBs quality control preparation must be included at least once in each series of tests to demonstrate acceptable sensitivity of the test method.

- No series of tests should be considered acceptable unless the result of the assay manufacturer's and the additional quality control samples have satisfied the criteria laid down.

9.3.11 Hepatitis C virus RNA (HCV NAT)

- The UK requirement for the minimum level of sensitivity for the performance of HCV NAT is 5000 IU/mL in an individual donation. An HCV international standard is available from the NIBSC.

- The assay must include a specific internal control for each sample tested.

- No series of tests should be considered acceptable unless the result of the assay manufacturer's and any additional quality control samples have satisfied the criteria laid down.

9.3.12 Hepatitis B virus DNA (HBV NAT)

- There is currently no specific UK requirement for the minimum level of sensitivity for the performance of HBV NAT. An HBV international standard is available from the NIBSC.

- The assay must include a specific internal control for each sample tested.

- No series of tests should be considered acceptable unless the result of the assay manufacturer's and any additional quality control samples have satisfied the criteria laid down.

9.3.13 Human immunodeficiency virus RNA (HIV NAT)

- There is currently no specific UK requirement for the minimum level of sensitivity for the performance of HIV NAT. An HIV international standard is available from the NIBSC.

- The assay must include a specific internal control for each sample tested.

- No series of tests should be considered acceptable unless the result of the assay manufacturer's and any additional quality control samples have satisfied the criteria laid down.

9.3.14 West Nile Virus (WNV)

The exclusion criteria for donors from a WNV risk area is given in the JPAC *Donor Selection Guidelines*.[3] These guidelines specify some situations where donations may only be released if a test for WNV RNA is negative. WNV RNA screening can be performed on donations provided by donors within the exclusion period and the donations released if WNV RNA negative.

- There is currently no specific UK requirement for the minimum level of sensitivity for the performance of WNV NAT.

- The assay must include a specific internal control for each sample tested.

- No series of tests should be considered acceptable unless the result of the assay manufacturer's and any additional quality control samples have satisfied the criteria laid down.

9.3.15 Other infectious agents

The JPAC *Donor Selection Guidelines*[3] may identify other infectious agents and specify some situations when screening may be applied in addition to donor deferral. In such situations any screening performed must:

- use assays specifically evaluated and validated for the screening of the donation type

- identify and utilise an independent quality control in each series of tests in addition to the manufacturer's assay controls

- ensure that the results of the assay manufacturer's and the additional quality control samples have satisfied the criteria laid down prior to release of the results

- require that each manufacturer's batch/lot of kits must be shown to conform with nationally established minimum criteria for specificity and sensitivity prior to being accepted for use for screening.

9.4 Reinstatement of blood donors

Where a blood donation sample is found to be repeatedly reactive on screening, the donation and any components must not be released for clinical use. The donor's record must be flagged in accordance with standard operating procedures to prevent the issue of subsequent donations while awaiting the results of confirmatory testing in the reference laboratory.

The screen repeat reactive sample must be sent to a designated reference laboratory for confirmatory testing.

If the donation sample is determined by the reference laboratory to be demonstrating non-specific reactivity, subsequent donations from the donor may be considered suitable for issue provided that the associated donation samples are negative in the primary or an alternative screening assay (Figure 9.5).

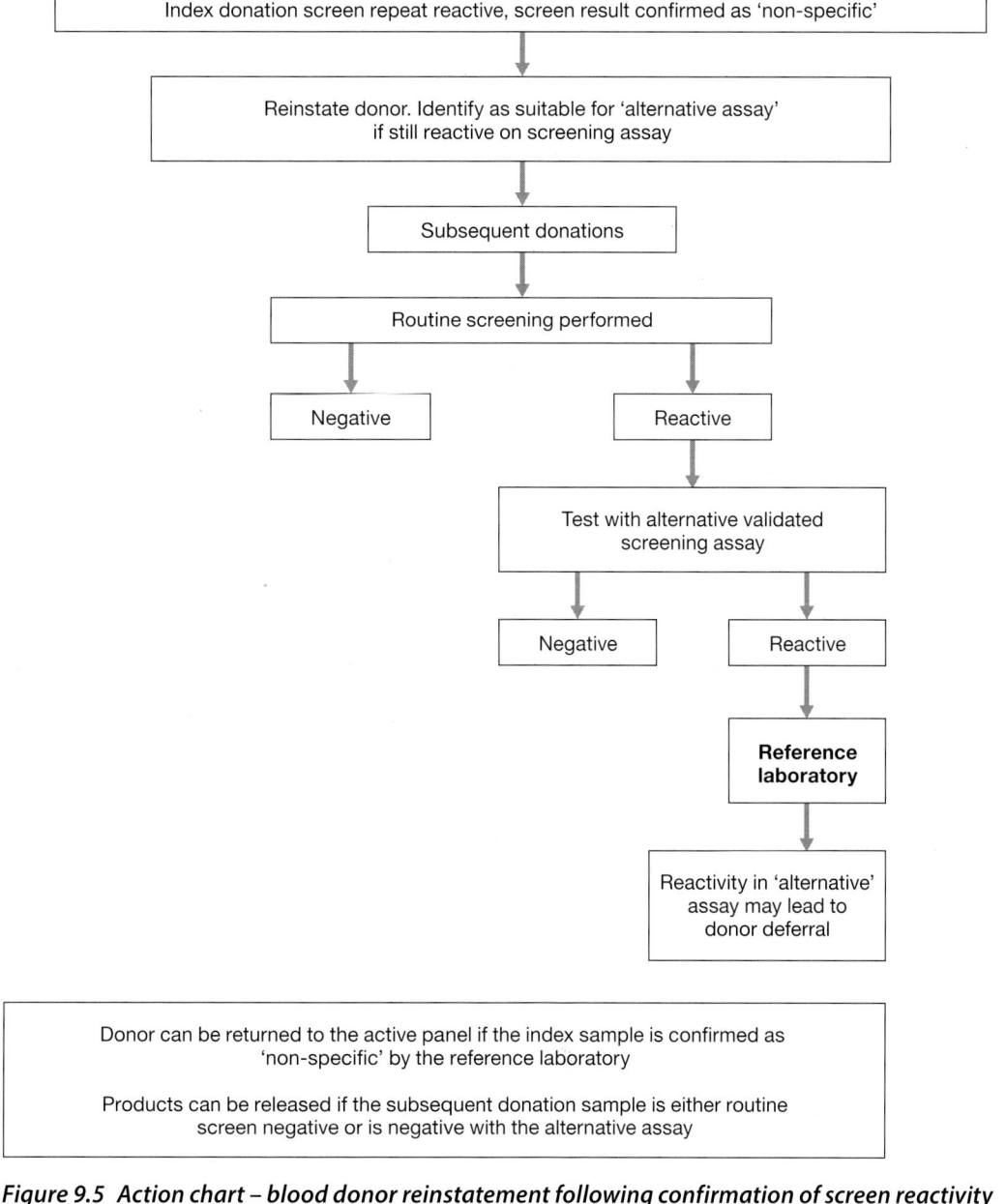

Figure 9.5 Action chart – blood donor reinstatement following confirmation of screen reactivity as non-specific

9.4.1 Process to reinstate a confirmed non-specific reacting blood donor

A donor with screen reactivity that is confirmed by the reference laboratory as 'non-specific' may be immediately returned to active status with no restrictions on any subsequent donations (see Figure 9.5).

However, in order to reinstate a donor whose sample remains reactive in the original screening assay, but confirmed by the reference laboratory to be demonstrating non-specific reactivity, the Blood Service must have the facilities to run appropriate alternative screening assays and to the same standard as primary screening. The following conditions must be met for this to be acceptable:

- The alternative assay must be of equivalent sensitivity to the original screening assay in which the index donation gave a repeatable non-specific reaction and conform to the UK requirements for microbiology screening tests.

- Donations taken subsequent to the return of the donor to the active panel may be used provided that the donation is non-reactive by the alternative assay.

- The donor's record must remain flagged with the information identifying previous non-specific reactivity for the marker.

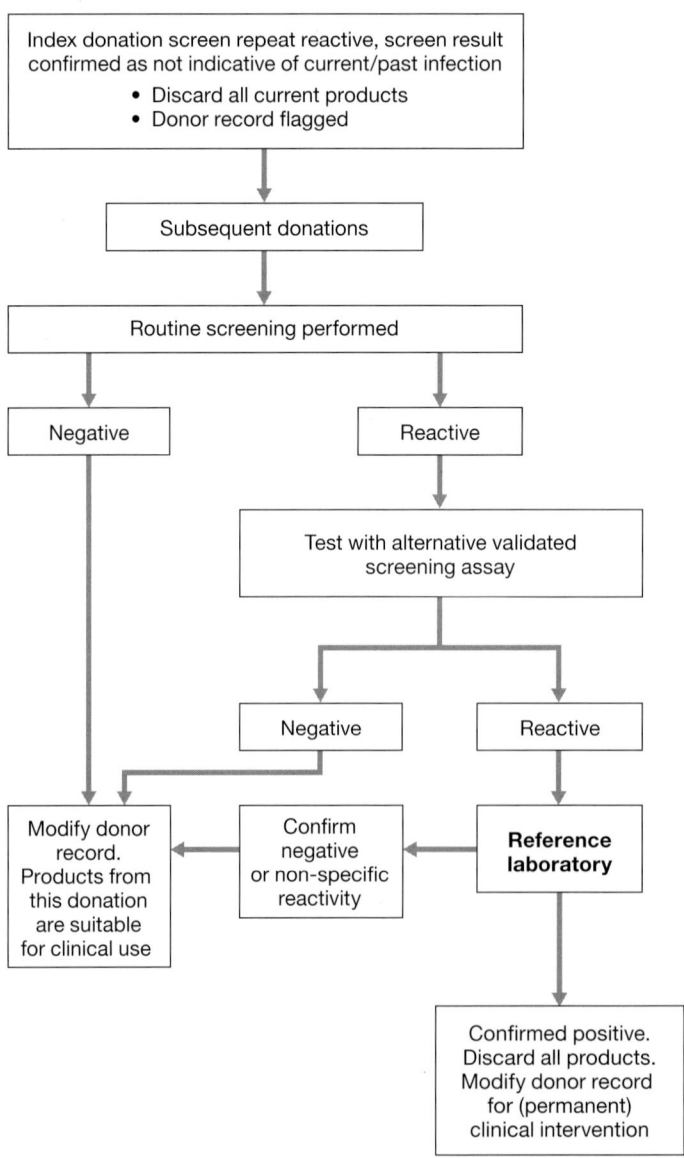

Figure 9.6 Action chart – tissue and cell donor reinstatement following confirmation that screen reactivity is not indicative of current or past infection

9.4.2 Process to reinstate a tissue/stem cell donor following confirmation that screen reactivity is not indicative of current/past infection

A tissue/stem cell donor with screen reactivity that is concluded by the reference laboratory as not indicative of current/past infection may be considered for return to active status on a subsequent donation, and products from the subsequent donation issued for clinical use, provided that:

- the subsequent sample tests negative with the primary screening assay OR
- the subsequent sample tests negative with an alternative validated screening assay OR
- the subsequent sample, reactive in both the primary screening assay and the alternative screening assay, is once again tested in the reference laboratory and is confirmed to be negative for evidence of the infection in question.

See Figure 9.6 for an action chart depicting tissue and cell donor reinstatement.

9.5 Recommended standards for the reduction of bacterial contamination of blood components

In recent years bacterial contamination of blood has been significantly reduced by the introduction of improved donor arm cleansing using 70% isopropyl alcohol/2% chlorhexidine gluconate applied as a single-step procedure, and diversion of the first 20–30 mL of the blood donation. The risk of bacterial contamination can be further reduced, but not eliminated, by screening of blood components.

9.5.1 Arm cleansing

There should be an effective, specified and validated method of arm cleansing, using an approved skin-cleansing system. 70% isopropyl alcohol/2% chlorhexidine gluconate is recommended by the National Evidence-Based Guidelines for Preventing Healthcare-Associated Infections in NHS Hospitals in England.[4] Adherence to the principles, protocols and practices relating to the correct use of the specified skin-cleansing system shall be regularly audited by periodic bacterial sampling and observation, and corrected if found to be lacking.

Periodic bacterial sampling of the skin of donors' arms may be carried out as an audit of correct use of the specified skin-cleansing system. If such sampling is performed, it will give an indication of how well staff are complying with the use of the system. In practice, it should be expected that bacterial sampling after skin cleansing with 70% isopropyl alcohol/2% chlorhexidine gluconate will reveal bacteria at a rate of no greater than 2 cfu per standard contact plate. Such levels may be difficult to achieve with other cleansing systems. Consistent finding of higher levels may require a review of compliance/re-education of relevant staff and further observational audits.

Periodic bacterial sampling may also take the form of anonymous sampling of staff fingertips after hand hygiene and after dealing with donors to assess levels of hand contamination and effectiveness of hand washing and decontamination in practice. Findings can then be fed back to staff as an educational tool.

9.5.2 Diversion of donation

A minimum of 20 mL of the first part of every blood donation should be diverted into a side-arm pouch, in order to minimise the level of bacterial skin contaminants in the collection bag. This diverted volume can be used as a source of blood samples for mandatory and other testing of the donation.

9.5.3 Screening of platelet components

There should be a means of detecting bacterial contamination of platelet components, using validated methods. The key requirements of a detection system are (i) effective sample size, (ii) a rapid test result or automated 24-hour readout with alarm notification and (iii) reliable detection of bacteria at a level indicating emerging risk to recipient.

Bacterial culture using an automated microbial detection system represents the most widely used and efficient method for screening of components. Its key feature is the continuous monitoring of incubation to allow immediate withdrawal of contaminated units.

The following protocols are considered to be optimal for single and two-test systems for the screening of platelets using an automated microbial detection system. Both require the use of a minimum 16 mL sample for aerobic and anaerobic culture and allow a 7-day shelf life. A two-test protocol is the ideal method for optimal performance, but this has significant operational issues. A single-test protocol with a minimum hold period of 36 hours before sampling will allow extension of shelf life of the product to 7 days providing incubation and monitoring is continued for the duration. Services may choose to initiate testing earlier than the 36-hour holding period (e.g. 18 hours), but these platelets will not qualify for a 7-day shelf life unless a second test is performed.

9.5.3.1 Single-test system

1. Platelet components are held for at least 36 hours after collection.

2. Minimum 8-mL samples are inoculated into each aerobic and anaerobic bottle.

3. If samples are negative after 12 hours of incubation, release product on a negative-to-date basis with 7-day shelf life and continue incubation and monitoring for the shelf life of the product.

4. A suitable protocol must be in place for confirmation of the presence of contamination.

5. Discard unused platelets on Day 8. (Time-expired units may be referred to the relevant bacteriology laboratory for surveillance testing.)

9.5.3.2 Two-test system

1. Platelet components are held for at least 18 hours after collection.

2. Minimum 8-mL samples are inoculated into each aerobic and anaerobic bottle.

3. If samples are negative after 24 hours of incubation, release product on a negative-to-date basis with 5-day shelf life and continue incubation and monitoring for the shelf life of the product.

4. A suitable protocol must be in place for confirmation of the presence of contamination.

5. Re-sample and test remaining stock at 4 days after collection and if negative at 24 hours release for use with a 7-day shelf life.

6. Discard unused platelets on Day 8. (Time-expired units may be referred to the relevant bacteriology laboratory for surveillance testing.)

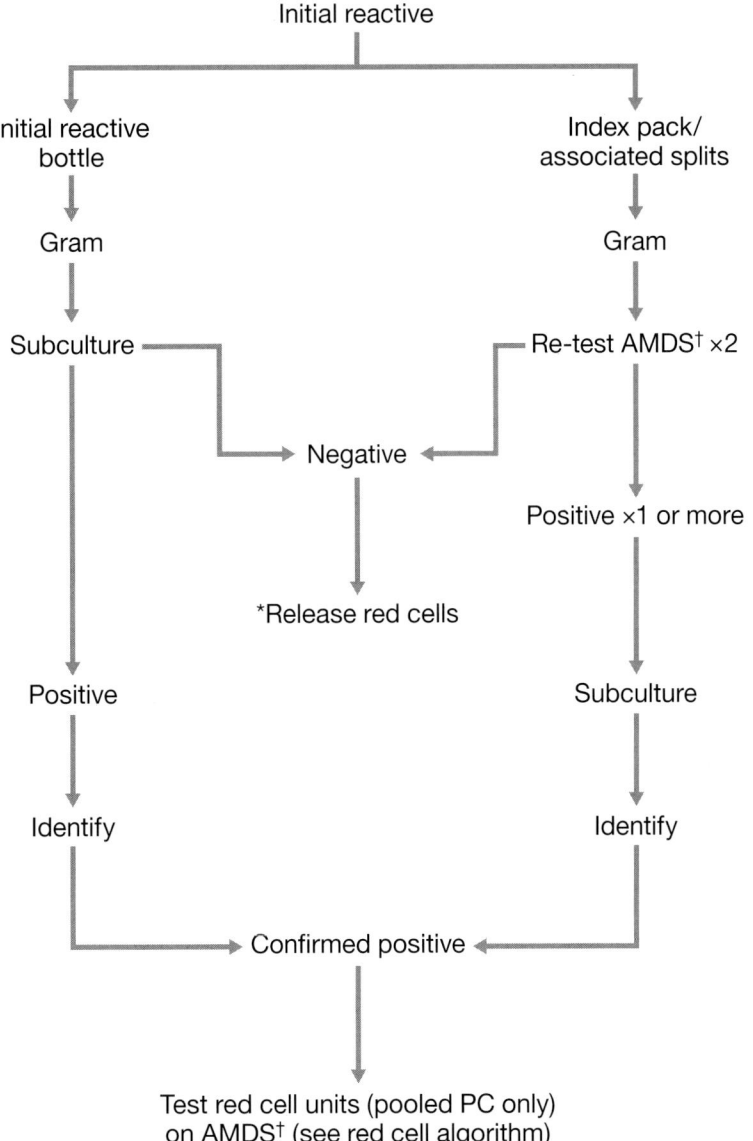

* Release of red cells requires a negative result from both the index culture bottles and testing of the platelet component.

† AMDS: Automated microbial detection system, re-test aerobic and anaerobic culture in duplicate.

Figure 9.7 Platelet components testing algorithm. If the index pooled platelet component is not available to re-test, the associated red cell unit should be tested.

The following definitions of screening test results are recommended.

Initial reactive: Positive bottle or bottles from which bacteria are isolated on initial screen.

Repeat reactive: Positive bottle or bottles from repeat testing of the index unit from which bacteria are isolated.

Confirmed positive: Bacteria detected from the initial and repeat tests which are of the same species.

Indeterminate: Bacteria detected in only the initial or repeat test, but not both, or bacteria detected in the initial or repeat reactives which cannot be matched at species level.

False positive: A positive signal is obtained for a culture bottle but no bacteria are detected on subculture.

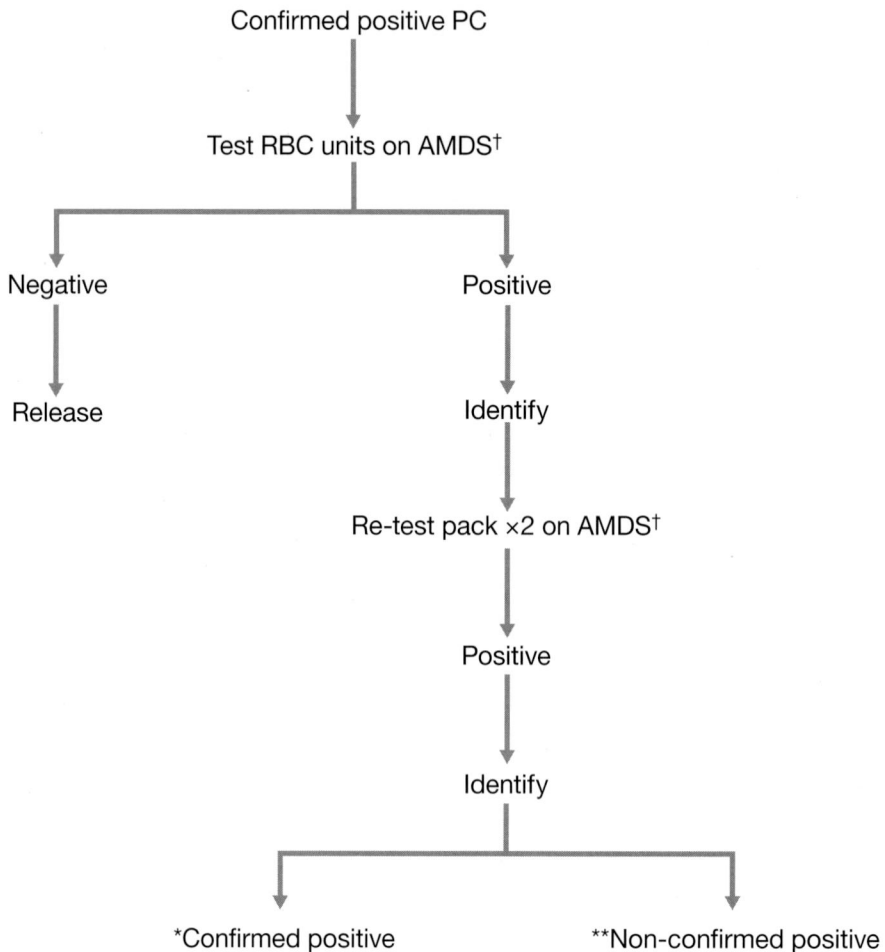

* Confirmed positive = a match at species level on the initial RBC test and re-test.
** Non-confirmed positive = negative repeat test and no match at species level with the PC confirmed positive result.
† AMDS: Automated microbial detection system, re-test aerobic and anaerobic culture in duplicate.

Figure 9.8 Red blood cell algorithm

False negative: Initial test negative but component associated with a post-transfusion reaction is subsequently positive on re-testing.

If the initial test is positive any components (plasma, red cells etc.) from the same donation must be quarantined pending the result of the repeat test and a recall procedure should be initiated for any platelet units or other components already issued.

The algorithms shown in Figures 9.7 and 9.8 are recommended for the confirmation of bacterial contamination of platelet components or red blood cells using an automated microbial detection system.

9.6 Recommended standards for microbiological screening

9.6.1 Tissues

All microbiological culture testing is subject to quality control tests in accordance with national accreditation standards and guidelines. This ensures that the risk of disease transmission is minimised and that tissue allografts are suitable for their intended use.

A written policy documenting the bacteriological acceptance criteria for specified tissues should be drawn up in consultation with a designated microbiologist.

Tissues must be screened for bacterial and fungal contamination by validated methods in accredited laboratories. Samples for bacterial screening (e.g. swab culture, bone chips etc.) should be obtained aseptically and placed in appropriate culture media at the time of retrieval or processing. Samples should be culture tested before and after exposure to decontaminating agents by enrichment liquid cultures to maximise the recovery of aerobic and anaerobic bacteria, and fungi. If pathogenic, highly virulent bacteria are recovered (e.g. *Clostridium* spp. *Streptococcus pyogenes*, *Staphylococcus aureus*, *Candida* spp.) the tissue should not be used for transplantation unless it is effectively sterilised by a process such as gamma irradiation. Cardiovascular tissues must be tested for the presence of *Mycobacterium* spp. Tissues contaminated with opportunist species of low virulence must be decontaminated by a validated process. Tissues which cannot be terminally sterilised (e.g. heart valves, amnion, menisci, osteochondrals) must be discarded if post-decontamination tests prove positive. An exception is cryopreserved skin allografts, which can be transplanted if non-pathogenic bacteria are present.

If no suitable sample is available for screening for bacterial and fungal contamination, then the products should be handled in the same way as those which have positive culture results for highly virulent bacteria: either discard or terminal sterilisation with a process such as gamma irradiation.

If a tissue fails culture testing, other tissues from the same donor should be discarded unless processed separately or an assessment of the risk shows otherwise.

9.6.2 Cord blood

Cord blood donations are subject to the NetCord-FACT International Standards for Cord Blood Collection, Processing and Release for Administration.[5] Cord blood collections must be screened for bacterial (aerobic and anaerobic) and fungal contamination using a system permissive for the growth of these microorganisms (European Pharmacopoeia 2.6.27). All donations positive for microbial growth should be discarded. Identification of any organism isolated needs to be undertaken and results reviewed by a microbiologist to identify potential sources of contamination. A trend analysis of contamination rates should be performed periodically to maintain quality.

9.6.3 Stem cells

Stem cell products (peripheral blood stem cells, bone marrow, whole blood and directed cords) are subject to the FACT-JACIE International Standards for Cellular Therapy Product Collection, Processing, and Administration.[6]

All products (fresh and cryopreserved) must be tested for microbial contamination (European Pharmacopoeia 2.6.27) unless the total sample volume is specifically requested by the transplant surgeon to optimise dose for the recipient. Microbial isolates recovered from products should be identified to species level and antimicrobial susceptibilities determined and stored in a cryobank. A trend analysis of data should be reviewed by a microbiologist to identify potential sources of contamination.

9.6.4 Autologous serum eye drops

Eye drops made from diluted autologous serum are used to treat ocular surface disorders. The serum is diluted with saline and bottled under aseptic conditions and bacteriologically tested (European Pharmacopoeia 2.6.27). It is recommended that 5% of batches should be tested for sterility by culture for aerobic and anaerobic bacteria. Identification of positive cultures needs to be performed and advice sought from a medical microbiologist regarding the suitability of a product for use via a quality concession.

9.7 Recommended standards for environmental monitoring of processing facilities

Environmental monitoring programmes must be in place for both uncontrolled and controlled processing facilities and must meet the requirements of appropriate regulatory bodies. They must form part of the quality management system ensuring that products are processed to the highest possible standards. Uncontrolled facilities include blood-processing laboratories and controlled facilities include cleanrooms used for the aseptic processing of tissues and stem cells.

The main aim of microbiological environmental monitoring is to provide a means of monitoring trends over time thereby ensuring that processing facilities continue to operate within acceptable bioburden levels. Individual test results, whether high or low counts, are rarely significant.

9.7.1 Key elements of an environmental monitoring programme

The monitoring programmes must define and document:

- The sites to be monitored and the rationale behind the selection of these sites.
- The types of samples to be taken and the techniques used.
- The monitoring frequency and the conditions under which the monitoring is to be performed, i.e. in the 'at rest' or 'in operation' states.
- Which personnel are authorised to perform environmental monitoring.
- The incubation regime for samples.
- The setting of limits (alert and action levels).
- The requirement for data and trend analysis.
- A procedure for the investigation of out-of-limit results including the identification of colony growth and the possible causes of the contamination.
- A procedure for corrective action in the event of out-of-limit results.

9.7.2 Monitoring techniques

Monitoring must be performed using standardised techniques and the main areas of sampling should include:

- Surface sampling using contact and swab plates with the latter being used in areas inappropriate for contact plates.
- Air sampling using settle plates and, in addition, in cleanroom environments, active air sampling and particle counting.
- Glove prints for assessing potential transfer of bacterial contamination to sterile product during aseptic processing (cleanrooms).

In controlled facilities, monitoring for fungal in addition to bacterial contamination must, as a minimum, be achieved through the use of settle plates with media specific for each type of contamination.

9.7.3 Culture media

Culture media used for environmental monitoring must be appropriate for the type of environment in which it is to be used, i.e. irradiated and triple wrapped media for use in cleanrooms, and for the range of organisms likely to be isolated. Media used for post-disinfection monitoring must contain agents, either individually or in combination, that will neutralise any residual surface disinfectant. Neutralising agents must be validated against the disinfectant(s) in use within the facility. Media storage must be in compliance with the manufacturer's recommendations and the monitored facility must be able to provide monitoring data to show that these storage requirements are met.

9.7.4 Alert and action levels

In cleanroom facilities, limits must be set for the results of both particulate and microbiological monitoring. These limits are specified in Annex 1 of the EC Guidelines to GMP (Manufacture of Sterile Medicinal Products[7]).

The action levels for microbiological monitoring in controlled rooms are taken as the limits given in the EU Guide. Alert levels must also be set in order to provide a warning of a possible deviation from normal operating conditions that may not require direct action but may need to be monitored more closely.

In uncontrolled facilities, action levels must be established using historical data. The monitoring programmes must define how the alert levels in controlled rooms and the action levels in uncontrolled rooms are to be determined.

9.7.5 Data and trend analysis

Monitoring results must be entered on a suitable database to allow data and trend analysis. The results must be reviewed by staff of the monitored facility on a regular basis with a formal documented review being held at a minimum of four times a year. This formal review must involve senior cleanroom/processing staff and representatives from the quality and microbiology departments.

9.7.6 Cleanroom gowning

Environmental monitoring programmes for controlled rooms also need to include procedures for:

- the qualification of staff with respect to cleanroom gowning for grade A and B environments
- the monitoring of staff upon leaving an aseptic area as a means of assessing operator bioburden levels.

Gowning qualification and exit suit monitoring should be performed for each cleanroom operator on a regular basis with the frequency, sampling method(s) used and monitoring sites clearly defined in the procedures.

9.7.7 Process simulations

Validation of aseptic processing should include a process simulation test using a nutrient medium. The process simulation test should imitate as closely as possible the routine process including all critical subsequent manufacturing steps. It should also take into account various interventions known to occur during the routine process as well as worst-case situations. Process simulation tests should be performed as initial validation with three consecutive satisfactory tests and repeated at defined intervals and after any significant modification to the heating, ventilation and air conditioning (HVAC) system, equipment or process.

Normally process simulation tests should be repeated twice a year (per shift and process). Alert and action levels should be defined and documented and any contamination investigated.

9.7.8 Cleaning and disinfection

Cleaning/disinfection validation should be performed in order to confirm the effectiveness of a cleaning/disinfection programme. As part of the validation, pre- and post-cleaning/disinfection environmental monitoring should be used to verify the acceptability of the frequency and efficiency of the programme in terms of microbiological contamination. Pre- and post-limits should be established and documented within the cleaning/disinfection programme. The monitoring results should be reviewed and, where limits have been exceeded, the contamination investigated and corrective action implemented.

Typically, three consecutive applications of the cleaning/disinfection procedure should be performed and shown to be successful in order to prove that the method is validated.

The cleaning and disinfection of controlled rooms is particularly important and should be performed in accordance with a written programme. Where disinfectants are used, more than one type should be employed on a rotational basis. Detergents and disinfectants should be monitored for microbial contamination and, when used in grade A and B areas, should be sterile prior to use.

9.8 Investigation of suspected bacterial contamination of blood components

Suspected cases of bacterial contamination of blood components may be notified by reports from the hospital of a significant transfusion reaction or, following a severe reaction, the identification of bacteria either within the pack or in a patient's blood culture.

A record of the original notification, clinical details and investigations carried out by the hospital must be made by the Blood Centre. The pack remains should be sealed and transported as soon as possible to a specialist bacteriology laboratory along with any bacterial isolates subsequently recovered from the patient's blood. If the patient has died without blood samples being obtained after the transfusion, it may be necessary for a post-mortem blood sample to be collected.

The contents of the pack, or if empty, a 20 mL saline wash out of the pack, should be sampled in the laboratory taking care to minimise the introduction of contaminants. A Gram stain may be informative but the sample should be cultured for bacteria (aerobic and anaerobic) and fungi using a system permissive for the growth of these microorganisms. If cultures prove negative no further action/investigation is necessary.

Where bacterial contamination is indicated, action must be taken to safeguard the safety of the blood supply by recalling all other components from the same donation(s) and these must be subjected to bacterial investigation. The possible source of a contamination needs to be investigated in consultation with a specialist microbiologist and appropriate swabs and other samples from the donor obtained for culture. If isolates of the same species are obtained from the pack and donor these must be submitted for molecular typing to establish the strain identity and possible route of transmission. Further decisions about the use of subsequent donations from the donor will depend on the circumstances and the type of contamination. An assessment should be carried out on a case-by-case basis to determine the risk of bacterial contamination through the use of further blood donations from the donor, and appropriate action taken.

9.9 References

1. Statutory Instrument 2005 No. 50. The Blood Safety and Quality Regulations 2005. Available at www.legislation.gov.uk.

2. SaBTO (2011). *Guidance on the Microbiological Safety of Human Organs, Tissues and Cells Used in Transplantation*. Available at www.dh.gov.uk/en/Publicationsandstatistics/Publications/PublicationsPolicyAndGuidance/DH_121497.

3. Joint UKBTS/HPA Professional Advisory Committee's (JPAC) *Donor Selection Guidelines*. Available at www.transfusionguidelines.org.uk.

4. Pratt RJ, Pellowe CM, Wilson JA, Loveday HP, Harper PJ, Jones SR, McDougall C, Wilcox MH. (2007). epic2: National Evidence-Based Guidelines for Preventing Healthcare-Associated Infections in NHS Hospitals in England. *Journal of Hospital Infection*, 65, S1–S64.

5. NetCord-FACT International Standards for Cord Blood Collection, Processing and Release for Administration, fourth edition 2010. Available at www.factwebsite.org.

6. FACT-JACIE International Standards for Cellular Therapy Product Collection, Processing, and Administration, fifth edition 2012. Available at www.jacie.org /Standards.

7. EC Guidelines to Good Manufacturing Practice Volume 4, Annex 1 (2008 revision): Manufacture of Sterile Medicinal Products. Available at http://ec.europa.eu/health/documents/eudralex/vol-4/index_en.htm

Chapter 10
Investigation of suspected transfusion-transmitted infection

10.1 General considerations

The guidelines in this section apply to reports of possible transfusion-transmitted infection (TTI) arising from blood or blood components supplied by the UK Blood Transfusion Services. Any suspected cases of TTI should be documented and fully assessed to determine whether further investigation of donors and/or donation samples is required or warranted. The guidance contained within this section covers the action to be taken at the Blood Centre in such cases.

Suspected cases of bacterial contamination of blood components may be notified by reports from the hospital of a significant transfusion reaction or, following a reaction, the identification of bacteria either within the pack or in a patient's blood culture. Reports will normally be received close to the time of transfusion of the blood component, when other components from the same blood donation may be in stock at either a Blood Centre or a hospital.

Because non-bacterial TTI may be asymptomatic, cases may not be recognised or detected until months or years after the transfusion. Many cases come to light through incidental screening of a patient who has received a blood component transfusion in the past or specific testing on development of late clinical features of the infection in question. Cases may therefore be notified by sources other than the hospital blood transfusion laboratory, but close liaison will be required with the reporting clinician and with the hospital blood transfusion laboratory that supplied the blood component for transfusion.

10.1.1 Documentation

Reports of possible TTI must be recorded and retained. Details of the notification should be confirmed in writing by the reporter.

For each report, confirmation of clinical and laboratory details will be required. Ideally, these should take the form of copies of the relevant recipient blood tests and computer printouts of transfusion records. Other forms of reporting of donation numbers (by letter, typed lists etc.) should be avoided in view of the risk of transcription errors.

10.2 Assessment of validity of the possible diagnosis of TTI

Clinical and laboratory details of the case should be reviewed to assess the validity of a diagnosis of possible TTI. Further information or test results may be required and requested at this stage.

Investigation of reported cases of TTI can be extremely time-consuming and impact on several different areas. In general, no investigation of archived samples or contact with involved donors should take place until all necessary information has been made available. However, in cases where complete details are not immediately available and a full assessment cannot be made, there should be consideration of the need to prevent issue of any further components from involved blood donors. Similarly, there should be consideration of the need to recall any in-date components from the same/recent donations to prevent their transfusion pending a decision about whether full investigation is necessary.

10.3 Non-bacterial TTI: identification of possible infectious donations

When a decision has been made to conduct an investigation into a reported non-bacterial TTI case, it may be possible to obtain sufficient information by reviewing results of testing of subsequent donations from the involved donor(s). If this is not the case, consideration should be given as to which donors require further investigation, and whether this can be satisfactorily carried out with samples already available at the Blood Centre from the index or any subsequent donation. This decision is dependent on the premise that subsequent samples may conclusively demonstrate the development of infectious markers (e.g. antibodies) in one of the implicated donors. It is expected that Blood Establishments will retain samples from each donation for a minimum period of 3 years in a suitable frozen archive. The retrieval of samples from this archive must be fully documented and be restricted mainly to such investigations.

If further investigation is required, and suitable blood samples are not available from the donor, then the decision may be made to contact the donor(s) and request further samples.

Decisions for each case and each donor will be on an individual basis depending upon the circumstances, timing, assessed likelihood of TTI and resources required. In cases of doubt, there should be a mechanism to ensure that there is a system for review and agreement on the way forward.

In instances where there is doubt whether a donor has been the source of a TTI, specialised molecular genotyping of both implicated donor and infected recipient may be necessary to prove conclusively whether TTI did indeed occur.

10.4 Investigation of possible bacterial TTI

Refer to section 9.8 for details of laboratory investigations.

10.5 Closing TTI investigations

Each investigation must be formally closed, with a conclusion and written notification to the reporter and any other interested party. In those cases where the recipient has been discharged from hospital, agreement should be reached as to who will notify the recipient: normally the general practitioner, or another clinician. It must be remembered that confidentiality of donor details is paramount and no information should be released which could lead, either directly or indirectly, to identification of the donor.

In cases of proven transmission, the recipient (or family, in the case of fatal cases) should be provided with an explanation of the cause of the transmission, and should be given the opportunity of a meeting with relevant staff, in keeping with NHS guidelines following a serious adverse event. Legal implications and the availability of any ex gratia payment schemes should be provided, as appropriate.

Each case investigated must be reported to the appropriate surveillance system: NHSBT/HPA transfusion-transmitted infection surveillance scheme for England and Wales, SNBTS National Microbiology Reference Unit for Scotland, Northern Irish Blood Transfusion Centre for Northern Ireland. These reports are collated and published in the annual report of the Serious Hazards of Transfusion (SHOT) scheme.

10.6 Look-back investigations

Look-back investigations are initiated on recognition that there may have been a risk of transmitting infection from a donor to a recipient. Such a situation may arise in the following circumstances:

- donors identified as infected through the introduction of a new screening test applied to all donations
- donors identified to be infected through seroconversion during their blood donation career
- donors identified to be infected and reported to the Blood Service from an outside source
- donors identified to be responsible for transmission of infection to a recipient.

10.6.1 General principles for look-back investigations

National look-back investigations, following introduction of a new screening test, should be managed through a generic system which incorporates the following steps:

- identification of potentially infectious donations
- identification of all blood components prepared from those donations
- documentation of the fate of the blood components
- notification of hospital transfusion laboratories in receipt of involved blood components
- identification of the fate of the component at the hospital, including details of any identified recipient
- for recipients not known to be dead, a procedure for notification, generally following notification of the general practitioner/hospital clinician
- a protocol for management of recipient notification and testing (if required)
- notification of recipient test results to recipient and other interested parties.

Look-back investigations following identification of a donor who has seroconverted and/or been responsible for transmission of infection and/or is identified through post-donation information should be carried out using the same principles.

Wherever possible, retrospective testing of stored samples should be carried out in order to identify those donations which must be included in the look-back. If samples can be tested, look-back should be performed to include the last seronegative donation, unless there is evidence about the timing of infection which would make such action unnecessary, e.g. a documented negative test result after the last negative blood donation, a clear history of risk exposure post-dating the last seronegative donation etc.

If retained samples are not available for testing, then case-by-case decisions on the number of donations to be included in the look-back will be influenced by the dates of donations and the availability of the particular hospital transfusion records.

10.6.2 Documentation and reporting

All cases of look-back should be documented in the same fashion as investigation of TTI. There should be a full audit trail of decisions made and actions taken.

Where look-back results in the identification of infected recipients, a report should be made to the surveillance system as appropriate, and cases included in the annual SHOT report.

Chapter 11
Reagent manufacture

11.1 Guidelines for reagent manufacture

11.1.1 Introduction

All reagents used to determine the group of human red cells and to detect red cell antibodies must comply with Directive 98/79/EC of the European Parliament and of the Council of 27 October 1998 on *in vitro* diagnostic medical devices[1] and all associated standards.

General guidelines for reagent manufacture are presented in this section. In other sections additional guidelines are given for particular reagents.

This document uses Fisher's notation to describe the presumed Rh genotype of red cell samples to be used. Where $R_z r$ or $r^y r$ red cells samples are to be used, the probable genotype should be confirmed, for example by extended Rh phenotyping.

Where specific reference to British Standard European Standard (BS EN) documents is given this is the most recent version. It is intended that these guidelines refer to the current requirements contained in the applicable documents so the phrase 'and subsequent revisions' should be assumed whenever a specific reference is given.

11.1.2 Reference preparations

The following reference preparations are available for use with these guidelines. Further details of these preparations can be found on the National Institute for Biological Standards and Control (NIBSC) website at www.nibsc.ac.uk:

- WHO International Standard for Minimum Potency of anti-A Blood Grouping Reagents
- WHO International Standard for Minimum Potency of anti-B Blood Grouping Reagents
- WHO International Standard for Minimum Potency of anti-D Blood Grouping Reagents
- ICSH/ISBT anti-Human Globulin Standard
- ICSH/ISBT Papain Reference Preparation
- ICSH/ISBT anti-D (for use with Papain Reference Preparation).

See section 11.3 for further information.

11.1.3 Definitions

Antibody identification is a test or combination of tests designed to determine the specificity of irregular antibodies.

Antibody screening is a test or combination of tests designed to detect irregular antibodies.

A **batch** of reagent is a defined quantity of material or of bulk, intermediate or finished product that is intended or purported to be uniform in character and quality, and which has been produced during a defined cycle of manufacture. A batch may be divided into sub-batches. A batch is sometimes described as a 'lot'.

A **batch of tests** is defined as a number of tests set up at the same time, under the same conditions and processed in a similar manner.

A **blood grouping kit** comprises a set of blood grouping components (reagents or materials) and 'instructions for use', packaged together, intended by the manufacturer to be used together for determining one or more blood groups.

A **blood grouping reagent** is a reagent, used alone or in combination with other materials, intended by the manufacturer for the determination of a blood group of an individual.

- A blood grouping reagent recommended by the manufacturer for the detection of A (i.e. subgroups A_1 and A_2) A_x and B should be named **anti-A,B blood grouping reagent**.

- A reagent recommended by the manufacturer for the detection of A (i.e. subgroups A_1 and A_2) and B but not of A_x, should be named **anti-A+B blood grouping reagent**.

A **blood grouping system** is an *in vitro* diagnostic medical device intended by the manufacturer to be used for determining one or more blood groups.

Clinically important or clinically significant antibody is a red cell antibody which will produce significantly accelerated red cell destruction when combined *in vivo* with its corresponding antigen.

Expiry date is the date beyond which performance of the reagent cannot be assured and is based upon the stability of the reagent.

Fresh serum for complement activity stored in the liquid state should be used within 8 hours of donation. When used after storage at −70°C or below, the 8-hour liquid storage period refers to the time both before and after frozen storage. Unless validated, the maximum period of frozen storage shall be 6 months at this temperature.

An **immediate container** is a medium adequate to protect the content(s) from contamination and/or physical damage. For example, a sealed vial, ampoule or bottle, a foiled pouch or a sealed plastic bag. The European Standard BS EN 375 requires a label on the immediate container and the outer container that is the material used in the packaging of the immediate container(s) of a product. It is a valid interpretation of that Standard that a microplate presented within a sealed pouch or foiled pouch does not require any label. It is considered by the Standing Advisory Committee for Immunohaematology that this interpretation will contribute to errors in identifying microplates in use within the laboratory. Therefore, in addition, the body of microplates presented in sealed bags or foiled pouches should be marked with a unique identifier to enable identification and traceability. Vials, ampoules, bottles and micro-well plates used as containers for a reagent for blood group serology should be transparent to permit visual inspection of the contents and consist of a material which does not cause deterioration of the reagent over the period recommended for use by the manufacturer.

Irregular blood group antibodies are those of specificity other than anti-A or anti-B.

The **manufacturer** is the natural or legal person with the responsibility for placing the device on the market under his or her own name, regardless of whether he or she has designed, manufactured, packaged, or labelled the device.

The name for a blood grouping reagent derived from monoclonal materials should include the word **monoclonal**.

A **monospecific blood grouping reagent** is one containing an antibody or blend of antibodies specific for one antigen, e.g. anti-A, anti-IgG.

A **polyspecific blood grouping reagent** is one containing a blend of antibodies specific for more than one antigen.

Polyspecific anti-human globulin reagent should be the name for a reagent which contains anti-human IgG and anti-human complement (C3d) activity, and is recommended by the manufacturer for use in both the direct and indirect anti-human globulin techniques, i.e. for the detection of red cell bound human IgG, and C3 complement in the form EiC3b and EC3d irrespective of the presence of other human immunoglobulin or human complement specificities.

Potency titre is a term used to describe the highest dilution of a reagent that effects a grade 2 endpoint reaction.

Prozone is the term used to denote the absence or weakening of agglutination with excess of antibody.

A **reagent control** is a reagent made to the same formulation as a blood grouping reagent but without the specific blood group antibody reactivity. If the reagent control contains serum or plasma, the reagent control should be shown to be free from specific blood group antibody reactivity.

A **reference preparation** is prepared nationally or locally and contains a known or agreed concentration of the activity being measured. It should be assayed to establish the sensitivity or calibration of a test procedure or reagent.

Sensitivity in relation to these guidelines is a term defining the limit of detectable specific reactions using reagents or test systems. These guidelines specify levels of sensitivity that should be achieved.

Shelf life is the period until expiry date.

Specificity in relation to these guidelines is a term defining the ability of a reagent or test system to react selectively. In particular terms, it represents the absence of unwanted or false-positive reactions.

Test monitors are a series of samples included as part of each batch of tests, which provide part of the release algorithm for a batch of tests.

Validation is the confirmation, through the provision of objective evidence, that the requirements for a specific or intended use have been fulfilled. Validation of a manufacturing method is to ensure that the product will be of the quality required for its intended use and that tests used in monitoring will accurately reflect the quality of the product.

Verification is the confirmation, through the provision of objective evidence, that specific requirements have been fulfilled.

Undiluted in these guidelines means the reagent as intended for use by the manufacturer. This term includes a diluted reagent if the reagent is supplied in a form requiring dilution by the user prior to use, as specified in the manufacturer's 'instructions for use'.

An **unequivocal** reaction in a test system is a reaction that is unambiguous. In the manual tube test, this is defined as a reaction of grade 3 or greater. In column tests this is defined as a 2+ reaction.

11.1.4 General manufacturing considerations

11.1.4.1 Good manufacturing practice

Reagents for blood group serology must be manufactured in accordance with Directive 98/79/EC of the European Parliament and of the Council of 27 October 1998 on *in vitro* diagnostic medical devices and all associated documents.

Guidance on the principles of good manufacturing practice can be obtained from *Rules and Guidance for Pharmaceutical Manufacturers and Distributors 2007*.[2]

- The method of manufacture should result in a product within an immediate container that is homogeneous and free of properties which adversely affect its intended use throughout its recommended shelf life. The reagent should have no precipitate, particles or fibrin gel.

- Each batch or sub-batch should be specifically identified by a distinctive combination of numbers and/or letters (batch reference) which permits its history to be traced.

- Reagents should be produced by a validated process that is shown to be suitable for the intended purpose, including any methods for preserving red cells prior to their preparation as reagent red cells.

- The manufacturer should monitor the batch-to-batch performance of the blood grouping reagent (e.g. by the reaction against some internal reference material) in order to provide consistency of performance. This is particularly important when the blood grouping reagent is provided as a test system, kit or kit component, when the performance may be dependent on the characteristics of other system variables or kit components.

11.1.4.2 Risk management

Risk management should be performed in accordance with:

- BS EN ISO 14971:2012 Medical Devices – Application of Risk Management to Medical Devices

- BS EN 13641:2002 Elimination or Reduction of Risk of Infection Related to *in vitro* Diagnostic Reagents.

11.1.4.3 Performance evaluation

Performance evaluation should be undertaken in accordance with:

- BS EN 13612:2002 Performance Evaluation of *in vitro* Diagnostic Medical Devices

- Reagents listed in Annex II, List A, of the EU *In Vitro* Diagnostic Medical Devices Directive must also comply with the Common Technical Specifications for *In Vitro* Diagnostic Medical Devices (2009/108/EC).

11.1.4.4 Stability data

Stability testing should be performed in accordance with:

- BS EN 13640:2002 Stability Testing of *in vitro* Diagnostic Reagents.

11.1.4.5 Date of manufacture

- For blood grouping reagents the date of manufacture is the date of commencement of the last potency test on the batch or sub-batch that indicates attainment of the required specification.

- For reagent red cells the date of manufacture is the date of collection from the donor. Where reagent red cells are prepared from more than one donor, the date of collection of the oldest donation should be recorded as the date of manufacture.

- Where a freezing process is used to preserve red cells before their preparation for issue as reagent red cells, the date of manufacture is the date of recovery from the frozen state.

11.1.4.6 Colour coding of reagents

No colouring agent should be added to reagents for blood group serology except that:

- Polyspecific anti-human globulin reagents may be coloured green, anti-A may be coloured blue, anti-B may be coloured yellow.

- The colorant should not interfere with the observation of the test result.

- 'Bespoke' antisera for use on automation may be coloured providing the information contained in the barcode on each bottle contains sufficient identifiers (specificity and lot number) to provide assurance that the intended test has been performed. The colours used for other specificities should not be coloured blue or yellow to avoid confusion with those for anti-A and anti-B reagents.

11.1.4.7 Freedom from microbial contaminants

- Reagents should be prepared using validated processes to produce a final product free from microbial contaminants that adversely affect the unopened product during storage at the recommended temperature. The manufacturer should routinely monitor the efficacy of the process used in the manufacture of the reagent.

- A preservative may be included in the reagent to minimise the effects of contamination during use if the preservative has been shown not to adversely affect the product during storage or use.

- Other than reagent red cells, all reagents for blood group serology recommended by the manufacturer for storage in the liquid state, should be filtered through a sterile filter of pore size not exceeding 0.22 µm. All reagents should be dispensed into the immediate container under aseptic conditions.

- Tests for contamination do not give absolute assurance of freedom from microbial contaminants. Bactericidal agents in common use for blood grouping reagents do not guarantee the absence of microbial agents after opening of the container.

11.1.4.8 Retained samples

- A minimum of 1% or three immediate containers, whichever is less, of each batch of reagents other than reagent red cells should be retained and stored as recommended by the manufacturer to enable analysis of reported defects. Such samples should be retained for at least 6 months beyond the expiry date.

- A minimum of two final containers of each batch of reagent red cells should be retained and stored as recommended by the manufacturer to enable analysis of reported defects. Such samples should be retained for at least 10 days beyond the expiry date.

11.1.4.9 Tests required

The manufacturer should test, as described in these guidelines, each lot of a reagent obtained from the immediate container to be supplied for use (see section 11.2.1).

11.1.4.10 Human source material

Existing procedures in the UK Blood Transfusion Services for consent to donate are sufficient to allow cellular and plasma materials collected as part of the donation process to be used as reagents without further explicit consent.

Samples/donations that are obtained specifically for reagent purposes will require additional consenting of the donor, and must have appropriate ethical approval. Donor materials that are obtained and retained for genomic or nucleic acid testing must comply with the regulations laid down by The Human Tissue Act 2004 (except Scotland).[3]

Residual samples retained from patient testing laboratories may be used without further explicit consent, if anonymised.[4] Additional samples taken from patients specifically for reagent use will require ethical approval and explicit consent. All patient samples acquired and retained must comply with the regulations laid down by the Human Tissue Act (2004).

Each individual donation or sample of human material in a reagent for blood group serology shall be tested and found negative for mandatory microbiological tests required by the UK Blood Transfusion Services for blood donations (see Chapter 9). A statement is required in the 'instructions for use' to this effect.

To ensure retrospective microbiological testing, an appropriate sample, collected at the same time as the donation used in the formulation of a particular reagent, should be archived until at least 6 months after the expiry date of the last batch of the reagent made from that material.

11.1.4.11 Label requirements

The label must conform to the requirements of:

- BS EN 18113:2011 Information Supplied by the Manufacturer with *in vitro* Diagnostic Reagents for Professional Use.

In addition, the instructions for use should meet the following criteria:

- The label fixed to the immediate container of a reagent should leave uncovered sufficient area of the full length or circumference of the container to allow ready visual inspection of the contents.

- The specificity of the reagent for blood group serology should be of a print size which is clearly legible. The print size of other information on the label should not exceed that used for the specificity of the reagent.

- The typeface used should clearly differentiate between antigens and related antibody specificities represented by upper and lower-case characters, e.g. C/c, S/s and K/k.

- For products needing to be prepared in the final form by the user following the instructions of the manufacturer and to be retained in the manufacturer's immediate container, a space should be available on the container label for the user to write the expiry date of the prepared product when stored as recommended by the manufacturer.

- The main panel of labels of enzyme-treated reagent red cells may be coloured pink in order to be distinguishable from non-enzyme-treated reagent red cells. Pantone colour reference 223 is recommended.

For other reagents, any colour appearing on the main panel of the label should comply with Food and Drug Administration regulations (21 CRF 660.28) as shown in Table 11.1.

Table 11.1 Label colour coding

Specificity	Colour	Code
anti-A	Blue	305C
anti-B	Yellow	102C
anti-C	Pink	204C
anti-D	Grey	429C
anti-E	Brown	465C
anti-CDE	Orange	151C
anti-c	Lavender	529C
anti-e	Green	577C

11.1.4.12 Instructions for use (package insert)

The instructions for use must conform to the requirements of:

- BS EN 18113:2011 Information Supplied by the Manufacturer with *in vitro* Diagnostic Reagents for Professional Use.

In addition:

- For blood grouping reagents containing monoclonal antibodies, the identity of the cell line(s) from which the monoclonal antibodies have been derived.

- For reagent red cells for antibody screening and for identification, the 'antigen profile' of the component cell samples is part of the instructions for use and should have the lot number and expiry date of the reagent to which it refers.

- A statement that loss of reactivity may occur during the stated shelf life of the red cells and that since this loss is partly determined by characteristics of individual blood donations or donors, which cannot be predicted or controlled, the conditions of storage and use recommended by the manufacturer should be rigidly applied.

- For enzyme-treated reagent red cells, information should be given concerning those antigens which are rendered inactive or less active by the enzyme treatment used.

11.2 Specifications, performance evaluation and quality control of blood grouping reagents

11.2.1 Blood typing antisera

11.2.1.1 General requirements

- It is essential that blood grouping reagents are prepared using reliable manufacturing procedures that are consistently capable of producing safe and efficacious products. The products must comply with requirements of the EU Directive (98/79/EC) on *in vitro* diagnostic medical devices and other relevant international standards detailed in section 11.3.

- The term weak D is used in these guidelines to indicate a weakened expression of a normal D antigen. The term partial D is used in these recommendations to indicate the expression of only a part of the normal D antigen. The reactivity of RhD blood grouping reagents against partial D red cells is determined by the nature of the D variant, the anti-D reagent and the technique used.

- The blood grouping reagent is satisfactory if an unequivocal positive result is obtained with all the red cell samples having the antigen corresponding to the blood grouping reagent being assessed, by all the methods recommended for use by the manufacturer.

- If reactivity is claimed by the manufacturer against weak variants or subgroups of a particular antigen, red cells from at least two confirmed/reference samples should be tested (see Table 11.3).

The grading system shown in Table 11.2 is used throughout these guidelines for manual tube/microplate serological testing.

Table 11.2 Grading system for serological tests

Reaction grade	Description
Grade 5	Cell button remains in one clump or dislodges into a few large clumps
Grade 4	Cell button dislodges into numerous large clumps
Grade 3	Cell button dislodges into many small clumps
Grade 2	Cell button dislodges into finely granular but definite, small clumps
Grade 1	Cell button dislodges into fine granules
Grade 0	Negative result
Unless otherwise stated, an unequivocal manual tube reaction is defined as a grade 3 or greater and for column tests as 2+ or greater	

11.2.1.2 Performance evaluation

Performance evaluation should be undertaken in accordance with:

- BS EN 13612:2002 Performance Evaluation of *In Vitro* Diagnostic Medical Devices.

- Reagents listed in Annex II, List A, of the EU *In Vitro* Diagnostic Medical Devices Directive must also comply with the Common Technical Specifications for *In Vitro* Diagnostic Medical Devices (2009/108/EC).

Stability testing should be performed in accordance with BS EN 13640:2002 Stability Testing of *In Vitro* Diagnostic Reagents.

Where appropriate, the following requirements should also be included in performance evaluation:

- In the case of polyclonal antibodies, contaminating antibodies to antigens having a prevalence of greater than 99% in the general population of the UK should be excluded by negative results in tests using samples of red cells from four different individuals who lack the antigen corresponding to the antibody specificity under test. Tests for the presence of contaminating ABO antibodies should be performed with red cells from a minimum of two individuals of group A1 and two of group B who lack the antigen corresponding to the antibody specificity under test.

- If tests using all methods recommended for use by the manufacturer do not exclude the presence of antibodies to the following antigens, these antibody specificities should be stated in the package insert[2] as not having been excluded in specificity testing:

    Xg^a, Do^a, Yt^a, Co^b, Wr^a and V^w.

- Blood grouping reagents which are chemically modified, and/or contain in their formulation a potentiator of agglutination, or require the user to add a potentiator, shall be tested, by all methods recommended by the manufacturer, with red cells lacking the antigen corresponding to the antibody specificity under test but sensitised with an IgG antibody to effect a grade 5 reaction in the anti-human globulin technique.

- Potentiated blood grouping reagents producing agglutination by those methods recommended by the manufacturer, should be supplied with a reagent control that has been shown to effect a degree of non-specific reaction with IgG-coated red cells similar to the corresponding blood grouping reagent.

- Blood grouping reagents recommended for use by a direct agglutination method should not contain antibodies reactive against red cells coated with IgG when used by direct agglutination methods recommended by the manufacturer.

11.2.1.3 Batch release testing requirements

Specificity tests

- The manufacturer should test the blood grouping reagent as a final product, by all methods recommended by the manufacturer for the specificity and reactivity claimed. Specificity should be determined by testing the reagent in accordance with the requirements outlined in Table 11.3.

- If a range of incubation times or incubation temperatures is recommended by the manufacturer, the range(s) should be used in these test procedures.

Requirements

- Blood grouping reagents should not produce a positive reaction when tested with red cells lacking the antigen corresponding to the antibody specificity under test, by any method recommended for use by the manufacturer. Should reactivity to a low-frequency antigen be observed with subsequent batches of a reagent, this fact should be brought to the attention of all primary consignees of that reagent.

- Rouleaux formation, prozone or haemolysis should not occur in tests using any of the methods recommended by the manufacturer.

Potency tests – tube or microplate methods

- Potency titrations should be performed in accordance with the manufacturer's recommended method of use using an appropriate diluent.

- Manufacturers should compare the potency titre of each batch of reagent with an appropriate reference preparation (see section 11.3).

- Potency titrations for each batch tested should equal or exceed any existing British or International reference preparations.

Table 11.3 Requirements for conventional blood typing reagents

Antibody specificity	Specification	Performance evaluation (as a minimum, two examples of the following reference cells should be included)*	Batch release testing — Specificity — Positive reactors Cell type	No.	Negative reactors Cell type	No.	Potency Cell type	No.
anti-A	Normally blue coloured. Should equal or exceed potency of reference preparation(s). Should detect variants and subgroups as detailed in the manufacturer's instructions for use	A_x, A_3	A_1	2	B	2	See insert of reference preparation(s)	
		A cord cells	A_2B	2	O	2		
			A_x*					
anti-B	Normally yellow coloured. Should equal or exceed potency of reference preparation(s). Should detect variants and subgroups as detailed in the manufacturer's instructions for use	B_x, B_3, B_v	B	2	A_1	2	See insert of reference preparation(s)	
		B cord cells	A_1B	2	O	2		
anti-A,B	Normally clear coloured. Should equal or exceed potency of reference preparation(s). Should detect variants and subgroups as detailed in the manufacturer's instructions for use	A_1, A_2, B, A_1B, A_2B	A_1	1	O	4	See insert of reference preparation(s)	
		$A_x\ A_3$	A_2	2				
		$B_x\ B_3$	B	2				
		A and B cord cells	A_x	2				
anti-A_1	Normally clear coloured. Should detect variants and subgroups as detailed in the manufacturer's instructions for use		A_1	2	A_2	2	A_1	2
			A_1B	2	A_2B	2		
					B	2		
					O	2		
anti-D	Normally clear coloured. Should equal or exceed potency of reference preparation(s). Should detect variants and subgroups as detailed in the manufacturer's instructions for use	Weak D (500 sites/cell)	R_1r	2	r'r	1	See insert of reference preparation(s)	
		C^w, C^x	R_2r	2	r''r	1		
		D^{VI} type 1, D^{VI} type 3, D^{IV}, D^V, D^{VII}, DFR, DBT, R_0^{HAR}	Weak D*	2	rr	1		

Table continues

Table 11.3 continued

Antibody specificity	Specification	Performance evaluation (as a minimum, two examples of the following reference cells should be included)*	Batch release testing					
			Specificity				Potency	
			Positive reactors		Negative reactors			
			Cell type	No.	Cell type	No.	Cell type	No.
anti-C	Normally clear coloured	C^w, Cx, r^{1S}	R_1r	1	R_2R_2	1	R_1r	2
	Potency titre greater than 4 vs by techniques detailed in manufacturer's instructions for use	R_2R_Z	R_1R_2 R_1R_Z	1 1	r''r	1		
			r'r	1	rr	1		
	Should detect variants and subgroups as detailed in the manufacturer's instructions for use							
anti-E	Normally clear coloured	R_1R_Z	R_2r	1	R_1R_1	1	R_2r	2
	Potency titre greater than 4 vs by techniques detailed in manufacturer's instructions for use	E^w	R_1R_2	2	r'r	1		
			r''r	1	rr	1		
	Should detect variants and subgroups as detailed in the manufacturer's instructions for use							
anti-c	Normally clear coloured	R_1R_Z, $R_1^wR_1$	R_1r	2	R_1R_1	3	R_1r	2
	Potency titre greater than 4 vs by techniques detailed in the manufacturer's instructions for use		R_1R_2	1				
			r'r	1				
	Should detect variants and subgroups as detailed in the manufacturer's instructions for use							
anti-e	Normally clear coloured	R_2R_Z	R_2r	2	R_2R_2	3	R_2r	2
	Potency titre greater than 4 vs by techniques detailed in the manufacturer's instructions for use		R_1R_2	1				
			r''r	1				
	Should detect variants and subgroups as detailed in the manufacturer's instructions for use							

11: REAGENT MANUFACTURE

Antibody specificity	Specification	Performance evaluation (as a minimum, two examples of the following reference cells should be included)*	Batch release testing					
			Specificity				**Potency**	
			Positive reactors		Negative reactors			
			Cell type	No.	Cell type	No.	Cell type	No.
anti-C^w	Normally clear coloured. Potency titre greater than 4 vs by techniques detailed in the manufacturer's instructions for use	$R_1^wR_1, r'^wr, R_1^wr$	R_1^wr or	2	R_1r	1	R_1^wr	2
			$R_1^wR_2$	2	R_1R_1	1		
			r'^wr	1	$r'r$	1		
anti-K	Normally clear coloured. Potency titre greater than 4 vs by techniques detailed in the manufacturer's instructions for use. Should detect variants and subgroups as detailed in the manufacturer's instructions for use	Kk Kp (a+b+)	Kk	4	kk	4	Kk	2
		Kk Kp (a−b+)						
anti-k	Normally clear coloured. Potency titre greater than 4 vs by techniques detailed in the manufacturer's instructions for use. Should detect variants and subgroups as detailed in the manufacturer's instructions for use	K+k+Kp(a+)	Kk	4	KK	4	Kk	2
			Kp(a+b+)	2				
			Kk Kp(a−)	2				
anti-Fy^a	Normally clear coloured. Potency titre greater than 4 vs by techniques detailed in the manufacturer's instructions for use. Should detect variants and subgroups as detailed in the manufacturer's instructions for use		Fy(a+b+)	4	Fy(a−)	4	Fy(a+b+)	2

Table continues

Table 11.3 continued

Antibody specificity	Specification	Performance evaluation (as a minimum, two examples of the following reference cells should be included)*	Batch release testing					
			Specificity				Potency	
			Positive reactors		Negative reactors			
			Cell type	No.	Cell type	No.	Cell type	No.
anti-Fy[b]	Normally clear coloured. Potency titre greater than 4 vs by techniques detailed in the manufacturer's instructions for use. Should detect variants and subgroups as detailed in the manufacturer's instructions for use	Fy^x	Fy(a+b+)	4	Fy(b−)	4	Fy(a+b+)	2
anti-Jk[a]	Normally clear coloured. Potency titre greater than 4 vs by techniques detailed in the manufacturer's instructions for use. Should detect variants and subgroups as detailed in the manufacturer's instructions for use		Jk(a+b+)	4	Jk(a−)	4	Jk(a+b+)	2
anti-Jk[b]	Normally clear coloured. Potency titre greater than 4 vs by techniques detailed in the manufacturer's instructions for use. Should detect variants and subgroups as detailed in the manufacturer's instructions for use		Jk(a+b+)	4	Jk(b−)	4	Jk(a+b+)	2
anti-S	Normally clear coloured. Potency titre greater than 4 vs by techniques detailed in the manufacturer's instructions for use. Should detect variants and subgroups as detailed in the manufacturer's instructions for use	SS, Ss, ss	Ss	4	ss	4	Ss	2

Antibody specificity	Specification	Performance evaluation (as a minimum, two examples of the following reference cells should be included)*	Batch release testing					
			Specificity				Potency	
			Positive reactors		Negative reactors			
			Cell type	No.	Cell type	No.	Cell type	No.
anti-s	Normally clear coloured Potency titre greater than 4 vs by techniques detailed in the manufacturer's instructions for use Should detect variants and subgroups as detailed in the manufacturer's instructions for use		Ss	4	SS	4	Ss	2
anti-M	Normally clear coloured Potency titre greater than 4 vs by techniques detailed in the manufacturer's instructions for use Should detect variants and subgroups as detailed in the manufacturer's instructions for use	NN He+	MN	4	NN	4	MN	2
anti-N	Normally clear coloured Potency titre greater than 4 vs by techniques detailed in the manufacturer's instructions for use Should detect variants and subgroups as detailed in the manufacturer's instructions for use		MN	4	MM	4	MN	2
anti-P_1	Normally clear coloured Potency titre greater than 4 vs by techniques detailed in the manufacturer's instructions for use Should detect variants and subgroups as detailed in the manufacturer's instructions for use		P_1 strong	4	$P_1(-)$	4	$P_1(+)$	2
			P_1 weak	4				

Table continues

Table 11.3 continued

Antibody specificity	Specification	Performance evaluation (as a minimum, two examples of the following reference cells should be included)*	Batch release testing					
			Specificity				Potency	
			Positive reactors		Negative reactors			
			Cell type	No.	Cell type	No.	Cell type	No.
anti-Le[a]	Normally clear coloured Potency titre greater than 4 vs by techniques detailed in the manufacturer's instructions for use Should detect variants and subgroups as detailed in the manufacturer's instructions for use		Le(a+b−)	4	Le(a−)	4	Le(a+)	2
anti-Le[b]	Normally clear coloured Potency titre greater than 4 vs by techniques detailed in the manufacturer's instructions for use Should detect variants and subgroups as detailed in the manufacturer's instructions for use	A1B Le(a−b+)	A1B Le(a−b+)	4	Le(b−)	4	Le(b+)	2

* For reagents where reactivity against the antigen is claimed

11.2.2 Anti-human globulin reagents

11.2.2.1 Introduction

Monoclonal antibodies have been developed which necessitate revision of the optimal composition of anti-human globulin reagents. For example, because of the limitations imposed by the presence of C3d on normal red cells, particularly in stored blood, conventional polyclonal anti-complement reagents rely on anti-C3c to detect *in vitro* bound complement and limited amounts of anti-C3d to detect *in vivo* bound complement. However, some monoclonal IgM anti-C3d reagents can be used at concentrations adequate to detect both *in vitro* and *in vivo* bound complement without causing unwanted positive reactions with normal red cells and fresh, inert, group-compatible serum in routine tests.

11.2.2.2 General requirements

- anti-IgG is the essential component since the majority of red cell alloantibodies are non-complement binding IgG.

- anti-complement should be present in reagents recommended for use with serum test samples.

- anti-light chain activity is desirable in reagents recommended for use with plasma test samples in order to detect IgM antibodies at levels unable to be detected in direct agglutination tests, especially with washed red cells.

- anti-C4d must be avoided. It is accepted that very low titres of anti-C4c may occur in reagents of animal origin.

- Reagents should be tested for the presence of heterospecific antibodies which can cause haemolysis or agglutination of unsensitised red cells in the indirect antiglobulin test and for the presence of unwanted positive reactions.

11.2.2.3 Performance evaluation

Performance evaluation should be undertaken in accordance with:

- BS EN 13612:2002 Performance Evaluation of *In Vitro* Diagnostic Medical Devices.

- Reagents listed in Annex II, List A, of the EU *In Vitro* Diagnostic Medical Devices Directive must also comply with the Common Technical Specifications for *In Vitro* Diagnostic Medical Devices (2009/108/EC).

Stability testing should be performed in accordance with:

- BS EN 13640:2002 Stability Testing of *In Vitro* Diagnostic Reagents.

11.2.2.4 Batch release testing requirements

Specificity testing

Tests for IgM or IgG red cell heterospecific antibodies

- Heterospecific antibodies can cause haemolysis or agglutination of unsensitised red cells in the indirect antiglobulin test. Details of tests for heterospecific antibodies are outlined in section 11.4.

Requirements

- The anti-human globulin reagent should not agglutinate or haemolyse washed unsensitised red cells from two individuals of group A_1 RhD positive, two individuals of group B RhD positive and two individuals of group O RhD positive, whether or not treated with proteolytic enzyme (e.g. papain, bromelin or ficin).

Tests for unwanted positive reactions

- These test for excess anti-C3d and anti-C3c, which can cause unwanted positive reactions in the indirect antiglobulin test, and for the presence of any undesirable antibodies in the reagent. Details of tests are outlined in section 11.4.

Requirements

- All reactions should be negative on macroscopic examination.

anti-IgG potency: polyspecific anti-human globulin and anti-IgG reagents for use in tube or microplate techniques

- The anti-human globulin reference reagent should be tested in parallel with the test reagent, each being titrated against red cells sensitised with potent IgG anti-D antibody.

Requirements

- The potency titre of the test anti-human globulin or anti-IgG reagent should be at least equal to that of the reference reagent.

Potency tests

anti-IgG potency by chequerboard titration studies with red cells sensitised with weak IgG antibodies (anti-D, anti-K and anti-Fy^a)

- Test anti-human globulin or anti-IgG reagents against a selection of weak antibodies to determine the optimum potency. Antibody preparations should not be diluted and the use of single-donor antibody preparations is preferred. Antibodies should include:

  - an IgG anti-D to give an anti-human globulin potency titre of 8–32 using a pool of group O R_1r red cells from four individuals
  - an IgG to give an anti-human globulin potency titre of 8–32 using Kk red cells
  - an IgG anti-Fy^a, to give an anti-human globulin potency titre of 8–32 using Fy(a+b+) red cells.

Details of tests are outlined in section 11.4.

Requirements

- The anti-human globulin reagent or anti-IgG reagent is satisfactory if the reaction grade at all dilutions attains or exceeds that of the reference reagent without significant prozone, against red cells sensitised with all dilutions of the anti-D, anti-K and anti-Fy^a. In this context, a significant prozone is more than one grade difference between the reaction of the anti-human globulin reagent undiluted and 1 in 2.

anti-complement potency; polyspecific anti-human globulin reagents for use in tube tests

- Test anti-human globulin or anti-complement reagents against a selection of complement-coated red cells to determine the optimum potency. C3 and C4 complement-coated red cells should be prepared as described in section 11.4. In addition, anti-complement activity may be evaluated by tests with complement-fixing antibodies, such as anti-Jk^a.

Requirements

- The anti-human globulin reagent should have an anti-C4c titre of 1 in 2 or less.
- The anti-human globulin reagent should not affect a macroscopic reaction with EC4d red cells.
- The reagent should attain the potency titre of the reference reagent.
- Conventional (polyclonal) anti-human globulin or anti-human globulin containing monoclonal IgG anti-C3d that attain adequate reactivity with an optimal incubation period different from that recommended for the detection of IgG antibody, should state in the instructions for use the appropriate incubation period required for the optimum detection of red cell bound C3c/d complement components.

Tests for unwanted positive reactions

- These test for excess anti-C3d and anti-C3c, which can cause unwanted positive reactions in the indirect antiglobulin test, and for the presence of any undesirable antibodies in the reagent. Details of tests are outlined in section 11.4.
- All test results should be negative as defined by the manufacturer in the 'instructions for use'.

Instructions for use

The instructions for use for anti-human globulin reagents used in tube and microplate tests should also include a statement that:

- Inadequate washing of red cells in the anti-human globulin test may result in neutralisation of the anti-human globulin reagent.

- Following completion of the wash phase in the anti-human globulin test, excess residual saline may dilute the anti-human globulin reagent, when added, beyond that in the manufacturer's assessment.

- No single test is capable of detecting all clinically significant antibodies.

- For each batch of antibody screening being undertaken by an anti-human globulin test, a positive and negative control should be included. The positive control should be a weak anti-D (not more than 0.1 IU/mL); the negative control an inert serum, tested against the antibody screening cells being used.

11.2.3 Reagent red cells

11.2.3.1 Introduction
Reagent red cells prepared from human blood are essential in ensuring safe transfusion practice. They are used in the determination of ABO blood groups, in the control of blood grouping reagents and of the anti-human globulin technique, and in the detection and identification of irregular red cell alloantibodies.

11.2.3.2 General guidelines for reagent red cell manufacture

- When testing reagent red cells, in order to confirm the presence or absence of antigens listed in the antigen profile, a sample from each individual should be tested whenever possible, with a minimum of two antisera for each specificity prepared from different donors/cell lines.

- Where such testing produces conflicting results, repeat and further testing with at least one additional example of the relevant antibody(ies) should be undertaken to confirm the antigenic status of that cell.

- Where such testing has been performed with only one example of any blood grouping reagent, this information should be stated in the antigen profile included within the package insert.

- Reagent red cells should be shown not to produce unwanted positive reactions by the methods recommended for use by the manufacturer.

- Except for IgG-sensitised and C3-sensitised red cells, reagent red cells should be negative in the direct anti-human globulin technique with anti-IgG, anti-complement and polyspecific anti-human globulin reagents.

- With the exception of umbilical cord blood, red cells used to test a patient's samples for irregular antibodies should not be pooled.

- Reagent red cells should be processed by a method and suspended in a medium that consistently ensures stability of the antigens specified in the antigen profile included within the package insert.

- All red cell reagents should be free of ABH-specific blood group substances and blood group antibodies, including anti-A and anti-B, demonstrable by the manufacturer's recommended methods of use.

- The method of manufacture should ensure that white cells are removed from donations of red cells before the white cells lyse and release enzymes, which may adversely affect the properties of the red cells.

11.2.3.3 Immediate container label and instructions for use sheet

The immediate container and instructions for use sheet for reagent red cells should also meet the following criteria:

- Include the statement 'pooled cells', if cells are prepared from pooled material.

- Where reagent red cells are intended for use in ABO grouping or control of ABO or D blood grouping reagents, only the ABO and D group need be stated.

- When the reagent red cells are a multi-container product such as a red cell panel, the label on the immediate containers and packaging should be assigned the same identifying batch reference and carry a number or symbol to distinguish one container from another. This number or symbol should also appear in the antigenic profile.

- The date of expiry of reagent red cells should be stated on the antigenic profile.

- Where reagent red cells are provided suspended in preservative medium, the components of the medium should be stated in the instructions for use.

- The concentration and limits of the red cell suspension (e.g. 3 ±0.2%) should be stated in the instructions for use.

- For enzyme-treated reagent red cells, information should be given in the instructions for use concerning those antigens which are rendered inactive or less active by the enzyme treatment used.

11.2.3.4 Reagent red cells for use in ABO and RhD grouping

- Reagent red cells should be groups A_1 and B. In addition, A_2, B or O red cells may be included.

- At least one of the set should be RhD positive and one RhD negative.

11.2.3.5 Reagent red cells for use in antibody screening

The detection of irregular antibodies in the serum of a patient is of greater clinical significance than if such antibodies are detected in blood donors. Reagent red cells of a lesser specification may be used when performing antibody screening tests on blood donor samples.

In general the following should apply:

- Reagent red cells for use in antibody screening should be confirmed as group O by an ABO blood grouping procedure that is capable of demonstrating the A_x phenotype.

- Where practicable, reagent red cells known to express antigens having a frequency of less than 1% in the general population of the UK should not be included in reagent red cells for antibody screening.

- Where practicable, red cells from individuals known consistently to effect troublesome reactions with HLA antibodies should not be used as reagent red cells for antibody screening.

11.2.3.6 Reagent red cells for use in antibody screening of patient samples

- As a minimum the following antigens should be expressed on the reagent red cells for antibody screening:

    C, c, D, E, e, K, k, Fy^a, Fy^b, Jk^a, Jk^b, S, s, M, N, P_1, Le^a and Le^b.

- As a minimum, reagent red cells from two individuals should be provided. These red cells should not be pooled. One reagent red cell should be R_2R_2; the other R_1R_1 (or $R_1^wR_1$).

- Apparent homozygous expression of the following antigens is desirable:

    Fy^a, Fy^b, Jk^a, Jk^b, S and s.

11.2.3.7 Reagent red cells for use in antibody screening of donor samples

- Reagent red cells may be:

    - provided unpooled from a minimum of two individuals OR
    - as a pool of red cells in equal proportions from no more than two donors OR
    - red cells from a single donor.

- Pooled reagent red cells for antibody screening should be used only for testing samples from blood donors, not samples from patients.

- As a minimum the following antigens should be expressed:

    D, C, c, E, e and K.

11.2.3.8 Reagent red cells for use in antibody identification

- Reagent red cells for use in the identification of irregular antibodies should be confirmed as group O by an ABO blood grouping procedure which is capable of demonstrating the A_x phenotype.

- Where practicable, red cells from individuals known consistently to effect troublesome reactions with HLA antibodies should not be used in reagent red cells for antibody identification.

- The antigen profile of reagent red cells for antibody identification should permit the identification of frequently encountered antibodies (e.g. anti-D, anti-E, anti-K and anti-Fya), and of commonly encountered alloantibody mixtures (e.g. anti-D+K).

- A red cell antibody identification panel comprises cells from eight or more individuals which should between them express the following antigens:

    C, C^w, c, D, E, e, K, k, Kp^a, Fy^a, Fy^b, Jk^a, Jk^b, S, s, Le^a, Le^b, M, N, P_1 and Lu^a.

- Red cells from one individual should be R_1R_1 and from another $R_1^wR_1$ and between them should express the antigens:

    K, k, Fy^a, Fy^b, Jk^a, Jk^b, S and s.

- Red cells from one individual should be R_2R_2, another r''r and those from another r'r.

- Red cells from a minimum of three individuals should lack the Rh antigens C, E and D. One of these three individuals should be K positive. Between them, red cells from these individuals should exhibit apparent homozygous expression of the antigens:

  c, k, Fy^a, Fy^b, Jk^a, Jk^b, S and s.

11.2.3.9 Reagent red cells (IgG-coated) for use in the control of the anti-human globulin technique

- To ensure that the anti-IgG activity in negative antiglobulin tests has not been fully or partially neutralised, control red cells 'sensitised' with IgG antibody are added to negative tests.

- Group O RhD positive red cells are sensitised with sufficient anti-D to render an indirect antiglobulin test negative when a volume of these sensitised red cells and a volume of serum diluted 1 in 1000 are added, but remains positive if a volume of saline instead of diluted serum is added.

11.2.3.10 Other reagent red cells

These reagent red cells should be manufactured in accordance with the relevant guidelines above.

11.2.4 Miscellaneous reagents

11.2.4.1 Fetal calf serum and bovine serum albumin

When used in the formulation of reagents, fetal calf serum and bovine serum albumin should be obtained from a closed herd in the female line since 1980, in which no animal has been clinically suspected of having bovine spongiform encephalopathy (BSE), and which has not been fed rations containing ruminant-derived protein during that period.

Bovine albumin, usually supplied as a 20% or 30% solution, can be used as a constituent of a diluent for use in automated blood grouping antibody detection machines, for antibody quantification or as a potentiator in antisera, monoclonal reagents and anti-human globulin. When diluted and used in the system prescribed it should not cause:

- red cells to become T/Tk etc. transformed

- inhibition of antigen:antibody reactions

- false-positive reactions or rouleaux.

11.2.4.2 Proteolytic enzyme preparations

The activity of each batch of proteolytic enzyme should be assessed to ensure batch-to-batch consistency using a biochemical assay (e.g. azo-albumin technique).[5]

For manual antibody detection techniques, red blood cells treated with the enzyme should achieve activity comparable to that of the reference enzyme preparation 92/658 and associated reference anti-D 91/562.

For automated antibody detection techniques for patient pre-transfusion samples red blood cells treated with the enzyme should readily detect a weak anti-D of no more than 0.1 IU/mL (e.g. NIBSC anti-D standard for assessing operator and test performance as described at www.nibsc.ac.uk).

For automated antibody detection techniques for donation testing the red blood cells treated with the enzyme should readily detect a weak anti-D of 0.5 IU/mL.

11.2.4.3 Water

The quality of water used in the production of a reagent should be adequate for that reagent. Ionic and non-ionic contaminants of water may interfere with components of reagents or may result in a conductivity or osmolality other than that intended. Water should have a conductivity of 1.0 µS/cm or less or a resistivity of 1.0 Mohm/cm or greater.

11.2.4.4 Saline

Saline is an isotonic solution containing 8.5 to 9.0 g/L NaCl (0.145–0.154 M) and should contain sufficient buffer to maintain pH 7.0 ±0.2 at 22 ±1°C during its shelf life.

11.2.4.5 Low ionic strength solution

The term low ionic strength solution (LISS) should not be used to denote a low ionic strength formulation other than that described by Moore and Mollison.[6] LISS should not be used in place of preparations designed for a particular technology. LISS has the following properties:

- pH 6.5–7.0 at 22 ±1°C
- conductivity 3.4–4.0 mS/cm
- osmolality 285–305 mOsmol/kg.

The reactions obtained by an indirect antiglobulin test (IAT) with a weak anti-D and D positive cells suspended in LISS should be equal to, or better than, those obtained with the same cells suspended in saline and incubated at 37°C for 15 minutes.

11.2.4.6 Weak antibodies for use as controls in antibody detection techniques

Weak antibodies, such as anti-D, -K, -Fy[a] can be used to control antibody detection techniques using indirect antiglobulin methods.

To act as a wash control the weak anti-D positive control could be diluted in serum or plasma. If the diluent is saline/bovine serum albumin, the control test could be positive, even though the cell washing was sub-optimal and this should be noted in the package insert.

These weak antibodies should:

- when used undiluted give a grade 2–4 reaction with red cells with homozygous antigen expression and have a mean IAT titre of 4 with the same cells.

For weak anti-D the antibody activity should be expressed in IU/mL.

11.3 Reference preparations

11.3.1 Introduction

One of the major components of the EU Directive (98/79/EC) on *In Vitro* Diagnostic Medical Devices is a requirement for traceability to reference materials of higher order. In the case of blood grouping reagents, which come under Annex II of the Directive, there are several national and international reference preparations already available to manufacturers to ensure adequate potency of anti-A, anti-B and anti-D grouping reagents and the potency and/or performance of a number of other serology reagents or procedures, for compliance with the Directive and the *Guidelines for the Blood Transfusion Services in the United Kingdom*.

As batch identifiers may change during the lifetime of these guidelines please refer to www.nibsc.ac.uk for guidance.

11.3.2 International Standards for minimum potency of anti-A and anti-B blood grouping reagents

These anti-A and anti-B preparations are the lyophilised residues of culture supernatants from murine monoclonal hybridomas BRIC 131 and ES4 respectively. The preparations, when reconstituted and diluted according to the supplied instructions, define the minimum acceptable potency of manufactured anti-A, anti-B, anti-A,B and anti-A+B blood grouping reagents, i.e. the titre of the grouping reagent should be at least equal to that of the appropriate minimum potency reference preparation.

11.3.3 International Standard for minimum potency of anti-D blood grouping reagents for use in direct tests

This preparation is the lyophilised residue of culture supernatant from a human-murine monoclonal heterohybridoma secreting an IgM anti-D (RUM-1). When reconstituted and diluted according to the supplied instructions, this material defines the minimum acceptable potency of anti-D grouping reagents in direct tube tests, i.e. the titre of the grouping reagent should be at least equal to that of the minimum potency reference preparation in tube tests using unmodified red cells and without additional agents.

11.3.4 International Council for Standardization in Hematology/International Society of Blood Transfusion (ICSH/ISBT) reference preparations for papain and anti-D

The intended use of these preparations is to ensure adequate sensitivity combined with freedom from false-positive reactions associated with some manufacturers' enzyme preparations and techniques. The recommended procedure is to test the papain reference material in conjunction with the anti-D 'for use with papain standard' using a titration series for sensitivity, and a series of inert sera for false-positive reactions, according to the specified two-stage reference method in the product insert and to compare the titration scores with those obtained from testing the manufacturer's enzyme preparation in its recommended technique with the anti-D reference preparation and the inert sera.

11.3.5 ICSH/ISBT standard for anti-human globulin

This preparation consists of lyophilised rabbit antisera against human IgG blended with murine monoclonal anti-C3d. This is intended for use in the evaluation of anti-human globulin reagents containing either of these components, or polyspecific reagents containing them both.

11.3.6 UKBTS/NIBSC anti-D reference preparation for assuring operator and test performance

The current preparation (07/304) consists of lyophilised human plasma with a reconstituted anti-D potency of 1.0 IU/mL. At 1 in 10 dilution, it is intended to be used to assure the efficacy of red cell washing prior to the addition of an antiglobulin reagent. At 1 in 20 dilution, it is intended to be used in intra-laboratory monitoring to assess test operator variability in the detection of weak, macroscopic agglutination in the spin-tube antiglobulin test.

11.4 Recommended serological techniques for reagent testing

11.4.1 Potency titrations

11.4.1.1 Introduction

The use of a semi-automatic pipette is recommended; one volume being in the order of 40 µL.

A separate pipette tip should be used for each reagent.

If the reagent is formulated with a medium to enhance its reactivity then the diluent for the determination of the potency titre should be a formulation identical to the reagent but with antibody protein replaced by non-antibody protein, e.g. fetal calf serum or bovine serum albumin. Otherwise, dilutions may be prepared in saline containing a final concentration of 20 g/L bovine serum albumin that has not been deliberately polymerised or otherwise potentiated.

Beginning with the undiluted blood grouping reagent, doubling dilutions (1 in 2, 1 in 4, 1 in 8 etc.) should be prepared. When preparing doubling dilutions, after the addition of the reagent or diluted reagent to an equal volume of the diluent, the tip of the pipette is emptied and blotted before the dilution is mixed and a volume transferred to prepare the subsequent dilution.

The potency titre is the reciprocal of the highest dilution of the reagent that effects a grade 2 reaction using the required technique.

The dilution caused by the addition of the cell suspension should not be considered in determining the potency titre.

11.4.1.2 Potency test methods for manual and microplate blood grouping reagents

Manual method – direct test

- Add one volume of each dilution of the reagent to a separate tube.
- Add one volume of 2–3% test red cell suspension to each tube.
- Mix thoroughly and incubate for the appropriate temperature and duration.
- Centrifuge and determine the reaction grade.

Manual method – indirect anti-human globulin test

- Add two volumes of each dilution of the reagent to a separate tube.
- Add one volume of 2–3% test red cell suspension in saline, or two volumes of 1.5–2% test red cell suspension in LISS.
- Mix thoroughly and incubate at 37°C for 45 minutes if the red cells are suspended in saline, or for 15 minutes if suspended in LISS.
- Wash the red cells four times.
- Add two volumes of anti-human globulin reagent to the button of test red cells. Mix. Centrifuge and determine the reaction grade.

Microplate method

Equipment

- Rigid polystyrene microplates with 'U'-shaped wells.

- Centrifuge with microplate carriers having a radius of at least 10 cm.
- Microplate shaker.
- Concave microplate reading mirror or automated plate reader.
- Red cells for microplate use, bromelin-treated if required.

Method

- Using a microplate, add one volume (25–50 µL) of each dilution of the reagent to one volume of 2–3% test red cells.
- Mix the contents of the wells using a microplate shaker. Incubate at 19–25°C for 15 minutes.
- Centrifuge the microplate at 100g for 40 seconds. Gently dislodge the red cells from the bottom of the wells using a microplate shaker.
- Determine the reaction grade using a concave mirror or automatic plate reader.

11.4.1.3 Avidity determination

- Mix over an oval area of approximately 20 mm × 40 mm on a glass slide, one volume of the undiluted reagent and one volume of a 30–45% red cell suspension in allogeneic serum or ABO group-compatible plasma.
- Maintain the slide at the recommended temperature for a slide test. If a range of incubation temperatures is given, for those blood grouping reagents where the antibody-antigen reaction is favoured by a colder temperature, the higher temperature should be used; for other blood grouping reagents, the lower temperature should be used.
- Determine the time from mixing at which macroscopic agglutination first appears and record the reaction grade at 1 minute.

11.4.1.4 Test used in performance evaluation and batch release testing of anti-human globulin

Tests for IgM and IgG red cell heterospecific antibodies

- These test for heterospecific antibodies which can cause haemolysis or agglutination of unsensitised red cells in the indirect antiglobulin test.

Method

- Divide 12 test tubes into two sets of six.
- Into each of the first set of tubes, add one volume of washed 2–3% untreated red cells in saline from two group A_1 RhD positive, two group B RhD positive and two group O RhD positive individuals.
- Into each of the second set of tubes add one volume of washed 2–3% enzyme-treated red cells (papain, bromelin or ficin) in saline from the same group A_1 RhD positive, group B RhD positive and group O RhD positive individuals.
- Add two volumes of the anti-human globulin reagent, as intended to be supplied for use, to each test tube. Mix thoroughly. Incubate the reactants for five minutes at 19–25°C.
- Centrifuge the tubes.
- Determine the reaction grade.

Control of enzyme treatment

Weak IgG anti-D known to be reactive with enzyme-treated red cells should effect a positive reaction with each washed, enzyme-treated, red cell sample by the following method:

- To separate tubes, add one volume of the weak IgG anti-D to one volume of each of the washed, 2–3% suspension of enzyme-treated, RhD positive red cell samples. Mix thoroughly. Incubate for five minutes at 37°C. Centrifuge the tubes. Determine the reaction grade.

- The weak anti-D used for this purpose must be absorbed to remove anti-A or anti-B.

- Each of the enzyme-treated RhD positive red cell samples should be agglutinated by the weak IgG anti-D.

Tests for unwanted positive reactions

These test for excess anti-C3d and anti-C3c, which can cause unwanted positive reactions in the indirect antiglobulin test, and for the presence of any undesirable antibodies in the reagent.

Method for preparation of the red cell suspensions from segmented bleed line samples

- Select integral segment lines from two packs of group A_1, two packs of group B and two packs of group O blood stored at 2–6°C for at least 10 days.

- Wash each of the red cell samples with saline sufficient to remove serologically reactive traces of plasma.

- Prepare suspensions of each red cell sample as 2–3% in saline and as 1.5–2% in LISS.

Incubation of red cells and fresh group-compatible serum

- Each of the six red cell samples described above is tested as a saline and a LISS suspension with a different, fresh, group-compatible serum.

- For each anti-human globulin reagent to be assessed, prepare two sets of six tubes.

- To the first tube of the first set of six tubes and the first tube of the second set of six tubes, add 1 mL of a fresh, single-donor group-compatible serum. Add 1 mL of a second fresh, single-donor group-compatible serum to the second tube of each set, and so on for the six different, fresh, group-compatible sera.

- To the first tube of the first set of six tubes, add 0.5 mL of a red cell sample as a 2–3% suspension in saline. Add 1 mL of the same red cell sample as a 1.5–2% suspension in LISS to the first tube of the second set of six tubes. Add 0.5 mL of the second red cell sample as a 2–3% suspension in saline to the second tube of the first set of tubes and 1 mL of the same red cell sample as a 1.5–2% suspension in LISS to the second tube of the second set of tubes, and so on for each of the six different, red cell samples.

- Incubate the first set of tubes (saline suspended red cell samples) for 45 minutes at 37°C. Incubate the second set of tubes (LISS suspended red cell samples) for 15 minutes at 37°C.

- Wash the red cell samples with saline sufficient to remove serologically reactive traces of serum. Resuspend the red cells to 2–3% in saline.

Tests with anti-human globulin reagents

- For each anti-human globulin reagent, prepare two sets of six tubes. To each of the first set of six tubes, add in sequence one volume of the 2–3% suspension of washed red cells from the saline test above.

- To each of the second set of six tubes, add in sequence one volume of the washed 2–3% suspension of washed red cells from the LISS tests above.
- Add two volumes of undiluted anti-human globulin, as supplied for use, to each of the 12 tubes. Mix thoroughly.
- Centrifuge the tubes.
- Determine the reaction grade.

anti-IgG potency: polyspecific anti-human globulin and anti-IgG reagents for use in tube or microplate techniques

The anti-IgG reference reagent (see section 11.3.5) should be tested in parallel with the test reagent, each being titrated against red cells sensitised with potent IgG anti-D antibody.

Method

Test cells

- A 2–3% suspension in saline of washed pooled group O R_1r red cells is prepared from four individuals.

anti-D

- anti-D suitable for use in this application should have a potency titre of greater than 512.
- To 4 mL of the potent IgG anti-D add 2 mL of the 2–3% suspension of pooled group O R_1r red cells.
- Mix and incubate at 37°C for 45 minutes.
- Wash the red cell sample with saline sufficient to remove serologically reactive traces of serum. Prepare suspensions of each red cell sample as 2–3% in saline.

Technique

- Prepare 1 mL volumes of twofold serial dilutions of the test anti-human globulin reagent and anti-IgG reference preparation from 1 in 8 to 1 in 4096 (ten tubes).
- Prepare a set of ten tubes for each anti-human globulin reagent to be assessed.
- Place two volumes of each dilution into each of the series of ten tubes.
- Add one volume of the 2–3% suspension of pooled sensitised R_1r red cells to each tube, mix and centrifuge.
- Determine the potency titre.

Controls

The washed, strongly sensitised 2–3% suspension of R_1r red cells gives a negative result when centrifuged and gives negative results using the direct anti-human globulin technique with anti-complement (anti-C3c, anti-C3d, anti-C4c and anti-C4d) reagents and with anti-human globulin diluent in place of the anti-human globulin reagent. (The anti-complement specificities may be present as mixtures in one or more reagents.)

Test for anti-IgG potency by chequerboard titration studies with red cells sensitised with weak IgG antibodies (anti-D, anti-K and anti-Fy^a)

Selection of weak IgG antibody preparations

Antibody preparations should not be diluted to attain the following potency requirements. The use of single-donor antibody preparations is preferred.

The following are selected:

- an IgG anti-D to give an anti-human globulin potency titre of 8–32 using a pool of group O R_1r red cells from four individuals

- an IgG anti-K containing a final concentration of 0.014M EDTA neutralised to pH 7, to give an anti-human globulin potency titre of 8–32 using Kk red cells

- an IgG anti-Fy^a containing a final concentration of 0.014M EDTA neutralised to pH 7, to give an anti-human globulin potency titre of 8–32 using Fy(a+b+) red cells.

Test cells

Prepare 10 mL of a 2–3% suspension of washed R_1r red cells pooled in equal proportions from four individuals. Similarly, prepare 10 mL of a 2–3% suspension of washed Kk red cells and 10 mL of a 2–3% suspension of washed Fy(a+b+) red cells.

Sensitisation of test cells

anti-D

- Using a set of five containers each of 20 mL to 25 mL volume, prepare 4 mL volumes of serial twofold dilutions of the anti-D from undiluted to 1 in 16.

- Add 2 mL of the 2–3% suspension of pooled R_1r red cells in saline to each container. Mix and incubate at 37°C for 45 minutes.

- Wash the red cells four times with 20 mL volumes of saline at each wash and remove the last supernatant.

- Add 2 mL of saline to the packed washed red cells to prepare the 2–3% suspensions of sensitised red cells.

anti-K

As above, but using the anti-K with the Kk red cells.

anti-Fy^a

As above, but using the anti-Fy^a, with the Fy(a+b+) red cells.

Preparation of anti-IgG and/or anti-human globulin dilutions

For each anti-IgG and/or anti-human globulin under test and the anti-IgG reference preparation, prepare 2 mL volumes of twofold serial dilutions from undiluted, that is as supplied for use, to 1 in 16.

Test method for anti-IgG or antiglobulin potency by chequerboard titration

anti-D sensitised red cells

- Prepare five sets of five tubes for each anti-human globulin reagent under test and the anti-IgG reference reagent.

- Place two volumes of the anti-human globulin reagent, undiluted to 1 in 16, in the appropriate tubes for each of the five sets of five tubes.

- Using the 2–3% suspension of red cells sensitised with the undiluted anti-D for the first set of five tubes, the 2–3% suspension of red cells sensitised with the anti-D diluted 1 in 2 for the second set of five tubes, and so on, finishing with the 2–3% suspension of red cells sensitised using the anti-D diluted 1 in 16 for the fifth set of five tubes, add one volume of the washed red cells to each of the sets of anti-human globulin dilutions (see Table 11.4).

- Mix thoroughly. Centrifuge the tubes, appropriately.

- Determine the reaction grade.

Table 11.4 Chequerboard test format

Set	anti-D used to coat red cells	Dilution of anti-human globulin reagent				
		N	2	4	8	16
1	Undiluted					
2	1 in 2					
3	1 in 4					
4	1 in 8					
5	1 in 16					

anti-K sensitised red cells

As above, but using the anti-K sensitised Kk cells.

anti-Fy^a sensitised red cells

As above, but using the anti-Fy^a sensitised Fy(a+b+) cells.

Controls

The unwashed 2–3% red cell suspensions sensitised with the undiluted anti-D, anti-K and anti-Fy^a give negative results in a spin-tube test. The washed sensitised cells should not react with the diluent or the anti-complement components of the anti-human globulin reagents.

Test for anti-complement potency; polyspecific anti-human globulin reagents for use in tube tests[7]

Preparation of the complement sensitised red cells

Various very low ionic strength medium techniques are used to prepare the iC3b, C4b, C3d and C4d sensitised red cells that are necessary for the assessment of anti-complement activity.

The C3 and C4 activation states produced on red cells by the various methods are shown in Table 11.5.

As a minimum, red cell samples from two individuals are to be prepared and tested as described below.

anti-C4b potency

Method

- Prepare a set of three tubes for each anti-human globulin reagent under test.

- Prepare doubling dilutions of the anti-human globulin reagent from undiluted to 1 in 4.
- Place two volumes of each anti-human globulin dilution in the appropriate tubes.
- Add one volume of 2–3% EC4b red cells to each tube. Mix thoroughly. Centrifuge the tubes.
- Determine the reaction grade.

Controls

The EC4b cells do not react with anti-C3c, anti-C3d, anti-IgG or saline or the inert anti-human globulin diluent using the direct anti-human globulin technique. They react with anti-C4c and anti-C4d reagents.

anti-C4d potency

Method

- Place two volumes of undiluted anti-human globulin in a tube.
- Add one volume of 2–3% EC4d red cells. Mix thoroughly. Incubate for 5 minutes at 19–25°C.
- Centrifuge the tubes. Determine the reaction grade.

Controls

The EC4d cells do not react with anti-C3c, anti-C3d, anti-C4c, anti-IgG or saline or the inert anti-human globulin diluent using the direct anti-human globulin technique. The undiluted anti-human globulin does not agglutinate unsensitised red cells that have been trypsin-treated, using the direct anti-human globulin technique.

anti-C3d potency

Method

- Prepare a set of seven tubes for each anti-human globulin under test and the anti-C3d reference reagent (see section 11.3.5) which is tested in parallel, at the dilution for the 'immediate test' stated in its accompanying instructions for use.
- Place two volumes of each anti-human globulin dilution in each of the tubes (undiluted, that is as intended to be supplied for use, to 1 in 64).
- Add one volume of the 2–3% EC3d/EC4d red cells to each tube. Mix thoroughly and centrifuge the tubes, appropriately.
- Determine the reaction grade.

Controls

The EC3d/EC4d cells do not react with anti-C3c, anti-C4c, anti-IgG, saline or anti-human globulin diluent using the direct anti-human globulin technique. They do react with anti-C3d.

Table 11.5 Complement C3 and C4 activation

Method of preparation	Initial state	State after trypsin treatment
Very low ionic strength medium* 37°C	iC3b/C4b	iC3d/C4d
Cold acquired haemolytic anaemia (alpha 2D, CHAD)	C3dg	C3d
Very low ionic strength medium* 37°C with EDTA	C4b	C4d
* These media are not to be confused with low ionic strength solution (LISS).		

11.5 References

1. Directive 98/79/EC of the European Parliament and of the Council of 27 October 1998 on *in vitro* diagnostic medical devices. *OJ*, L 331, 07.12.1998, p1.

2. Medicines and Healthcare products Regulatory Agency (2007). *Rules and Guidance for Pharmaceutical Manufacturers and Distributors 2007*. London: Pharmaceutical Press.

3. The Human Tissue Act 2004. Available at www.legislation.gov.uk.

4. The Working Party of the Royal College of Pathologists and the Institute of Biomedical Science (2005). *The Retention and Storage of Pathological Records and Archives*, third edition.

5. Phillips PK, Prior D, Dawes BA (1984). Modified azo-albumin technique for the assay of proteolytic enzymes for use in blood group serology. *Journal of Clinical Pathology*, 37, 329–331.

6. Moore HC, Mollison PL (1976). Use of low ionic strength medium in manual tests for antibody detection. *Transfusion*, 16, 291.

7. Lachmann PS, Voak D, Oldridge RG, Downie RM, Bevan PC (1983). Use of monoclonal anti-C3 antibodies to characterise the fragments of C3 that are found on erythrocytes. *Vox Sanguinis*, 45, 367–372.

Chapter 12
Donation testing (red cell immunohaematology)

12.1 Scope

These specifications provide guidance on the tests required for blood donations in the UK.

12.2 General requirements

Secure and effective procedures must be in place to ensure that:

- Specific procedures are written in the form of standard operating procedures.

- Blood donations, components and their laboratory samples are correctly identified by barcoded and eye-readable numbers.

- Donations can be linked to their donor.

- A donor's record is reviewed every time he or she donates.

12.3 Samples

Samples may be ethylenediamine tetra-acetic acid (EDTA) or clotted.

Where equipment/reagent manufacturers have defined protocols for storage and preparation, then these must be followed.

In the absence of protocols or recommendations from manufacturers, then validated protocols for sample storage and preparation must be defined.

Visual inspection to determine the suitability for testing must consider the following in relation to the equipment methods and samples used:

- haemolysis

- lipaemia

- clots

- volume

- cell:plasma (serum) ratio

- the buffy coat layer (note: a large buffy coat layer in the sample may give rise to erroneous results).

Labels should be examined for defective labelling.

Reconciliation of all samples to be tested should be completed prior to testing.

12.4 Reagents and test kits

Acceptance testing should be performed on each batch/delivery of reagents and test kits.

Reagents and test kits should be stored and used according to the manufacturer's instructions.

Reagents and test kits outwith these instructions must be validated.

Reagent antisera must be validated and assured for specificity and potency as per Table 11.3.

A system of inventory control must be in place that records, as a minimum, the reagent or test kit:

- lot number
- expiry date
- supplier
- stock levels.

Procedures should ensure the traceability of the batch number and manufacturer of reagents and kits and, if relevant, the serial number of equipment used to test every donation.

12.5 Equipment

Test equipment should be validated before being introduced into routine use and procedures must be in place to ensure that test systems and equipment are able to produce consistent and valid results.

Equipment must be used, cleaned, calibrated and maintained in accordance with the manufacturer's instructions and written procedures. It is recognised that during maintenance procedures equipment may be compromised and therefore a protocol for reinstatement of the equipment for routine use is required.

Any deviations from the manufacturer's instructions should be validated and documented.

An equipment log covering the following must be readily available for all equipment:

- service contract details
- downtime
- faults
- maintenance
- calibration.

These logs must be retained.

12.6 Test procedure

Test procedures must:

- be validated before being introduced into routine use
- be written in the form of standard operating procedures
- be performed in compliance with the standard operating procedures

- be monitored and reviewed
    - be performed by trained staff and the training records must be maintained
    - include the recording of test results.

12.7 Reporting of results

The report must indicate the result of each and every test, by a system that provides positive sample identification.

Reporting a series of tests by an 'assumed negative' procedure is potentially dangerous and not acceptable.

The acceptance and release of test results will be the responsibility of designated personnel of proven proficiency.

Information must be archived.

12.8 Release of tested components

Standard procedures must ensure that blood and blood components cannot be released for issue until all the required laboratory tests (mandatory and additional) have been completed, documented and approved within a validated system of work. Compliance with this requirement may be achieved by the use of a computer program, or suite of programs, which requires the input of valid and acceptable test results for all the mandatory and additional laboratory tests before permitting, or withholding, the release of each individual unit.

Where a computer-based system has failed, compliance may be achieved by the use of a system, which requires documented approval for the release of each unit, by a designated person.

12.9 Laboratory test categories

Laboratory tests include the following categories:

- Mandatory tests – required as part of the criteria for release of all blood donations and components for clinical use. Currently these are ABO and D blood grouping and irregular red cell antibody screening.

- Additional tests – undertaken in special circumstances:
    - increase the safety of transfusion for susceptible patients or clinical effectiveness of specific transfusions, e.g. by providing HbS screened red cells
    - while not required for all blood donations or components, when such tests are performed to meet a specific need the results are an essential part of the criteria for release of that component.

12.10 Mandatory testing of blood donations

Blood groups shall be determined using reagents that comply with Chapter 11 of these guidelines.

All mandatory tests must be performed using an automated test system in the first instance (see section 12.13). Any persistent failures may be resolved using manual methods (see section 12.14).

12.10.1 ABO blood grouping

- The ABO blood group must be determined on each blood donation.

- For a donor whose ABO blood group is unknown to the test centre (e.g. a first-time donor), the ABO blood group must be determined by testing the plasma/serum with group A_1 and B red cells. The red cells of the donation must be tested twice with anti-A and anti-B as a minimum. The ABO group can only be accepted if the results are in agreement.

- If the security of sampling analysis and data transfer is assured, it is sufficient to test the red cells from previously tested donors with anti-A and anti-B once. There is no requirement to test the plasma. The ABO blood group shall be accepted only if the results are in agreement with those of previous tests.

- Where an anti-A which detects A_x is deployed in the testing of all donations, anti-A,B is not required.

12.10.2 Quality control of ABO blood grouping

- Quality control procedures recommended by reagent and equipment manufacturers should be followed.

- The following minimum test monitors are required for each batch of ABO blood grouping tests:

  - anti-A, anti-B (and anti-A,B where used) must give appropriate reactions with A_1, B and O cells. A_2 and A_2B cells may also be used; however, where CE-marked reagents, validated as per guidelines in section 11.2 are used, they are not mandatory

  - reagent red cell samples must give appropriate reactions with anti-A, anti-B (and anti-A,B where used).

12.10.3 D grouping

- The D blood group must be determined on each donation of blood.

- In the testing of donors being grouped for the first time, two anti-D blood grouping reagents should be used capable of detecting between them D^{IV}, D^V and D^{VI} antigens. If two monoclonal anti-Ds are used, they should be from different clones.

- Donors whose blood gives an unequivocal positive reaction with both anti-D reagents should be regarded as D positive.

- Donors whose blood is unequivocally negative with both anti-D reagents should be regarded as D negative.

- If the results with the anti-D reagents are discordant or equivocal, the tests should be repeated. Where the D group is in doubt it is safer to classify such donors as D positive.

- For known (repeat) donors one anti-D reagent, or blended reagent, that detects weak D, D^{IV}, D^V and D^{VI} can be used.

12.10.4 Quality control of D grouping

- Quality control procedures recommended by reagent and equipment manufacturers should be followed.

- The following minimum test monitors are required for each batch of D grouping tests:
  - each series of D blood grouping tests must obtain appropriate reactions with R_1r red cells as a positive and with r'r or rr red cells as a negative
  - appropriate reactivity with red cell samples expressing weak D should also be assured as a minimum during validation as indicated in section 11.2.

12.10.5 Antibody screening

Blood and blood components with antibodies of probable clinical significance may be released, as shown in Table 12.1.

12.10.5.1 Routine antibody screen

- All donations must be tested for the presence of red cell antibodies. This is achieved by testing the donor's serum or plasma using a validated technique capable of detecting anti-D at 0.5 IU/mL or lower.

- Reagent red cells for routine antibody screening (see 11.2.3.7) may be:
  - provided from a minimum of two individual donations (not pooled); or
  - as a pool of red cells in equal proportions from no more than two donations; or
  - red cells from a single donation.

- As a minimum the following antigens should be expressed: D, C, c, E, e and K.

- Each batch of tests must include a test monitor of ≤0.5 IU/mL anti-D.

- Donations found to be reactive in the routine antibody screen should be further tested by an indirect antiglobulin test to determine the fate of the products as specified in Table 12.1.

12.10.5.2 Antibody screen for blood for neonates

- Blood for neonatal use must be screened and found negative for antibodies by an indirect antiglobulin test, performed using a two-cell panel expressing the following antigens as a minimum: C, c, D, E, e, K, k, Fy^a, Fy^b, Jk^a, Jk^b, S, s and M.

Table 12.1 Minimum release criteria for blood products with antibodies of probable clinical significance

Component	Antibody screen for blood for neonates	Donation plasma sample diluted 1 in 10	Donation plasma sample diluted 1 in 50
For neonatal use	Negative	Not applicable	Not applicable
Red cells in SAGM	Not applicable	Not applicable	Negative
All other components	Not applicable	Negative	Not applicable

12.11 Additional testing

12.11.1 Antibody identification

- Donations found to be reactive in the routine antibody screen may be further investigated for specificity.

12.11.2 Blood and blood components from group O donors with high titres of anti-A, anti-B and/or anti-A,B

- Red cells, platelets and fresh frozen plasma from group O donors with high titres of anti-A, anti-B and/or anti-A,B can result in haemolytic transfusion reactions (HTRs) when given to non-group O patients. Such group O donors are generally termed 'high-titre group O donors'.

- Reactions are more likely to occur when:
  - the serological titre of the anti-A, anti-B and/or anti-A,B in the component is high
  - the plasma volume of the transfused product is high
  - the blood volume of the recipient is small.

- Each Blood Establishment should have a testing and issuing policy to avoid the use of high-titre anti-A and/or anti-B in instances where a significant adverse clinical reaction is likely. The policy should cover the following components:
  - whole blood and red cells
  - fresh frozen plasma
  - apheresis platelet donations
  - pooled platelets containing plasma from a single 'high-titre' group O donor
  - blood/components for neonatal use.

- Where high-titre anti-A/B testing is deemed necessary, a saline agglutination test (performed as detailed in Chapter 11) should give a negative result, at a dilution of 1/128, or an equivalent dilution by other techniques.

- There should be a procedure in place to collect and review testing and patient outcome data and to implement changes in policy in the light of continuing clinical experience with the plasma-containing blood products issued.

- Components from group O donors with 'low titres' of anti-A, anti-B and/or anti-A,B can cause intravascular haemolysis in non-group O recipients if given in sufficiently large volumes.

- It is important to recognise that, although testing for high-titre ABO antibodies in blood donors may reduce the risk of HTR in 'out of group transfusion', it cannot be entirely eliminated through this route. Group O platelets can cause HTR even when tested and labelled negative for high-titre haemolysins. They should only be used for non-group O patients (particularly paediatric patients) as a last resort.

12.11.3 Additional phenotyping

- Red cell components should only be labelled with confirmed extended phenotypes.
- A confirmed phenotype is one where the typing has been carried out and results concur:

- in duplicate on the current donation, or
- once on the current donation and the result is in agreement with historical data from previous donations, or
- on two previous donations from that donor.

For labelling to be carried out under the last of these conditions, the security of the donor data, testing methodology used on each occasion and that of the historical test result data, **must** be assured through validation and risk assessment.

12.11.4 Quality control of additional phenotyping

- Quality control of procedures recommended by reagent and equipment manufacturers should be followed.
- The test monitors shown in Table 12.2 are required for each batch of tests.
- Within some test procedures reagent cross-contamination may occur. Test monitors should be selected in order to maximise the detection of such contamination.

Table 12.2 Test monitor red cell samples

Blood grouping reagent	Test monitor red cell samples	
	Positive	Negative
anti-C	R_1r	rr or R_2r
anti-E	R_2r or r″r	rr or R_1r
anti-c	R_1r or r′r	R_1R_1
anti-e	R_2r or r″r	R_2R_2
anti-K	K+k+	K–k+
Other specificities	Heterozygous positive	Antigen negative

12.11.5 HbS screening

Unless the Blood Centre recommends that screening of donations for HbS is unnecessary, each Blood Establishment should have a protocol in place which:

- Ensures the use of donations which are HbS screen negative for the manufacture of whole blood and red cell components for intrauterine transfusion, neonatal exchange transfusion and for the transfusion of children and adults with haemoglobinopathy. This protocol may be extended to further red cell products as deemed necessary by the Blood Establishment.

Note: Where the Laboratory Information Management System (LIMS) in use allows recording of the donor's HbS status, historical information may be used for the purposes described above, provided that the security of the donor data, testing methodology and that of the historical test result data, has been assured through validation and risk assessment.

- Ensures confirmatory testing for donors who are found to be HbS screen test positive.

12.12 Donations found to have a positive direct antiglobulin test

Direct antiglobulin test (DAT) positive donations may be identified incidentally by testing laboratories when:

- the autologous/reference control is positive in ABO/RhD blood grouping
- the antibody screen is positive
- anomalies are identified in extended phenotyping tests.

Non-red cell components may be prepared and issued from DAT positive red cell donations. Red cell units may be prepared and issued from DAT positive red cell donations provided that:

- the ABO and RhD groups are confirmed
- red cell antibodies have been excluded as per the mandatory antibody screening (see Table 12.1)

Donors who have been found incidentally to have a positive DAT at donation testing may remain as blood donors provided they continue to pass the health screening questionnaire and have a normal haemoglobin.

12.13 Automated testing

An automated system as a minimum must accomplish the following:

- positive sample identification, reading and interpretation of results
- matching of results to sample identification
- electronic transfer of results.

There should be documented contingency plans for the breakdown or total failure of automated testing systems. Protocol settings for automated systems must be documented and version controlled. Where possible, current versions of software and settings for automated systems should be backed up and readily available.

12.14 Manual testing

- A manual testing system is one in which the minimum automated testing criteria have not been met.
- Manual testing can be used to resolve anomalous results.
- Measures should be taken to minimise the testing batch size to avoid the potential for errors.
- Manual tests must be performed and controlled according to the manufacturer's instructions.
- Test results must be recorded.
- There must be a secure and validated method of entering results onto the host computer. Post result entry verification should be performed.

Chapter 13
Patient testing (red cell immunohaematology)

13.1 Scope

These specifications provide guidance on the tests required for investigations performed on patient samples in red cell immunohaematology (RCI) laboratories in UK Blood Transfusion Centres. These include pre-transfusion and compatibility testing, tests associated with supporting the prevention and treatment of Haemolytic Disease of the Fetus and Newborn (HDFN), assessment of fetomaternal haemorrhage, and titration studies supporting ABO mismatched transplant.

Extended testing of blood donors other than in the above contexts is covered in Chapter 12.

It is assumed that RCI laboratories comply with the following guidelines:

- *Guideline for Blood Grouping and Antibody Testing in Pregnancy* (British Committee for Standards in Haematology, BCSH).[1]

- *The Specification and Use of Information Technology (IT) Systems in Blood Transfusion Practice* (BCSH).[2]

- *Guidelines for Pre-transfusion Compatibility Procedures in Blood Transfusion Laboratories* (BCSH).[3]

- *The Estimation of Fetomaternal Haemorrhage* (BCSH).[4]

And also comply with:

- *The Clinical Pathology Accreditation (CPA-UK) Standard for Medical Laboratories.*[5]

- The Blood Safety and Quality Regulations 2005.[6]

This chapter is intended to cover practice in areas not included in published UK guidelines at the time of writing. Where practice differs either from published guidance or this chapter, laboratory managers should formally document the reasons for doing so and assess the associated risk.

13.2 Sample acceptance and labelling

Visual inspection to determine the suitability for testing should consider the following in relation to the equipment, methods and samples used:

- the presence of haemolysis
- the presence of lipaemia
- the presence of an atypically large buffy coat layer
- the presence of clots in an anticoagulated sample
- a low sample volume
- an unusually high or low cell:plasma (serum) ratio.

If any of the above is identified, then this should be documented and appropriate action taken.

Any systematic variation from BCSH guidelines must be covered by a risk assessment. Tests performed on individual samples not complying with guidelines are documented on an authorised concession.

All samples are labelled with both barcoded and eye-readable numbers.

Samples that are separated prior to referral to the laboratory (e.g. samples separated at 37°C for Paroxysmal Cold Haemoglobinuria investigations) should be clearly labelled and signed to indicate the person separating the samples. Accompanying documents should clearly state the nature of the samples, the person separating the samples, and the time and date of sample separation.

13.3 Pre-transfusion testing

13.3.1 Resolution of anomalous grouping

ABO grouping is the most important pre-transfusion serological test performed. Fully automated ABO and D grouping procedures have significantly improved the accuracy and security of results, and should be used wherever possible.

When anomalous ABO groups are encountered laboratory protocols should support investigation of the following findings.

Missing agglutinins in reverse grouping:

- obtain the patient's history, and review for information which may explain missing agglutinin (e.g. age, immunodeficiency)
- repeat the reverse group, increasing the sensitivity of the test, consider the use of tube techniques, lower incubation temperature, increased plasma:cell ratio and enzyme-treated red cells.

Unexpected additional reactions in the reverse group:

- investigate the presence of allo- or autoantibodies active at temperatures below 37°C
- consider repeating the reverse group at 37°C
- consider repeating the reverse group using cells negative for any identified alloantibody.

Unexpected reactions in the forward or D grouping, including positive diluent control:

- check for immunoglobulin coating of the patient's cells by performing a direct antiglobulin test (DAT)
- consider repeating tests using unpotentiated reagents in tube techniques
- consider techniques to remove or reduce immunoglobulin coating (e.g. warm wash to remove IgM) and repeat tests with appropriate controls.

Unexpectedly weak or mixed field reactions in forward or D group:

- obtain the patient's history, and review for information which may explain results (e.g. recent non-ABO identical transfusion, haemopoietic cell transplant)
- consider additional investigations which may include adsorption/elution, and flow cytometry

- panels of monoclonal anti-D reagents are commercially available for the investigation of partial and weak D phenotypes.

Genotyping is useful in resolving grouping problems, particularly weak and partial D types (see section 15.2). Genotyping alone must not be used to determine the ABO group for use in selection of blood for transfusion. Where the patient ABO group cannot confidently be assigned by serology, group O (high-titre negative) blood must be selected.

13.3.2 Antibody identification

In all cases of the investigation of alloantibodies laboratories should focus on:

- secure identification of alloantibodies detected
- exclusion of additional specificities to those identified
- selection of blood for transfusion (Daniels et al. 2002).[7]

When antibodies which cannot be identified have been detected, laboratories should consider referral to the International Blood Group Reference Laboratory (IBGRL).

When patients with rare phenotypes are encountered, laboratories should, when practicable, exchange material with other RCI departments via the UK Rare Red Cell Exchange to ensure continued supply of valuable materials.

Antibody identification techniques and protocols are described in BCSH guidelines and should be adhered to. More complex problems encountered by RCI laboratories and not covered by BCSH are considered below.

13.3.2.1 Complex antibody mixtures

When investigating complex antibody mixtures RCI laboratories should consider:

- extended phenotyping of the patient, e.g. C, c, D, E, e, K, M, N, S, s, P_1, Le^a, Le^b, Fy^a, Fy^b, Jk^a, Jk^b
- if this is impossible due to previous transfusion or heavy IgG sensitisation, genotyping offers an alternative source of information
- extending the range of techniques and incubation temperature to identify component antibodies
- using cells matching the patient's phenotype/genotype to confirm the presence of multiple antibodies rather than an antibody to a high-frequency antigen
- careful use of alloadsorption techniques to confirm the specificity of elements of the mixture.

13.3.2.2 Antibodies known as high-titre low-avidity (HTLA)

Antibodies traditionally known as HTLA include anti-Ch, –Rg, –Kn^a, McC^a, –Yk^a, –Cs^a and –Sl^a. Typically HTLA antibodies present as reacting with most panel cells by indirect autoglobulin test (IAT) with variable strength, with or without similar patterns using enzyme-treated cells. Experienced operators can recognise characteristic agglutination by microscopic examination of tube IAT, which have been described as 'loose', 'stringy' or 'gritty'. In investigating samples suspected to contain HTLA antibodies RCI laboratories should consider:

- Neutralising anti-Ch or -Rg specificities by incubating the patient's plasma with pooled group AB donor plasma before IAT is undertaken. Reactivity of these antibodies is usually abolished. A dilution control in which the patient's plasma is incubated with phosphate-buffered saline should be prepared and tested in parallel with the neutralised plasma.

- The use of a panel of cells lacking HTLA antigens.

13.3.2.3 Antibodies to high-frequency antigens (HFA)

Typically antibodies to HFA present with positive reactions of similar strength against all routine screen and identification panel cells. The most commonly encountered specificities include anti-k, $-Lu^b$, $-Kp^b$, $-Vel$, $-Co^a$, $-Yt^a$, $-Fy3$, $-U$ and $-In^b$. In investigating samples suspected to contain antibodies to HFA, RCI laboratories should consider:

- the ethnicity of the patient

- extended phenotyping as in section 13.3.2.1

- typing the patient's red cells with antibodies to HFA. Where possible, CE-marked reagents must be used, otherwise results must be considered in context of the reliability of the reagent in use, supported by adequate controls.

13.3.2.4 Antibodies to low-frequency antigens (LFA)

Typically antibodies to LFA present with negative antibody screen and are detected in crossmatch. The most commonly encountered specificities include anti-Kp^a, $-Wr^a$ and $-Co^b$. In investigating samples suspected to contain antibodies to LFA, RCI laboratories should consider:

- testing the patient's plasma with a panel of red cells expressing LFA

- phenotyping the incompatible unit(s) for LFA.

13.3.3 Autoantibodies

Autoantibodies are frequently encountered in pre-transfusion testing, and may be the cause of autoimmune red cell destruction, or may be clinically benign. In either case autoantibodies may interfere with pre-transfusion testing, either due to coating of patient's cells with immunoglobulin, or as pan-reactive antibody in patient's plasma. In providing safe transfusion in the presence of autoantibodies, RCI laboratories may adopt the following strategies.

13.3.3.1 ABO and Rh grouping in the presence of autoantibodies

Most modern test systems support routine, accurate grouping of the majority of patients whose cells are coated with immunoglobulin and who give a positive DAT. Cases which are problematic may present with reaction patterns that cannot be assigned to an ABO group, weak additional reactions and positive reagent controls. Such cases should be investigated as in section 13.3.1.

Laboratories should make a clear documented assessment, based on the recommendations of reagent and test system suppliers, how to manage cases with anomalous ABO and D groups. This is particularly important when potentiated reagents are included in test systems.

13.3.3.2 Alloantibody detection and identification in the presence of autoantibodies

In dealing with cross-reacting autoantibodies, which complicate the detection and identification of underlying alloantibodies, RCI laboratories should consider:

- The characteristics of available, validated IAT in testing patient plasma-containing pan-reacting autoantibodies. Some workers consider tube IAT to be less prone to interference by autoantibodies than column technologies.

- The use of the patient's own cells to adsorb autoantibody from the plasma, permitting detection and identification of alloantibodies.

- The use of cells from two or more selected donors to adsorb autoantibody. Typically these cells are enzyme treated to optimise removal of autoantibody.

13.3.4 Management of patients with autoantibodies

Consideration should be given to close matching of recipient and donor red cell types. This is to safeguard against the presence of alloantibodies undetected by tests on modified plasma, and to prevent further alloimmunisation. In patients who cannot be grouped by conventional serology, due to sensitisation of red cells or previous transfusion, genotyping offers a solution.

In patients with autoantibodies requiring regular transfusion, close matching of transfused red cells with the patient's own phenotype, to manage risk of transfusion reactions, may be used as a basis by scientists and clinicians to assess, and potentially reduce, the required frequency of testing. Such assessments should be fully documented and subject to planned review.

13.4 Antibody quantification and titration

Antibody quantification and titration is performed in RCI laboratories on patients' samples, to support the prediction and management of HDFN and ABO mismatched organ transplant.

13.4.1 Antibody quantification of anti-D, and anti-c for management of HDFN

In UK laboratories it is standard practice to quantify anti-D and anti-c by continuous flow analyser against standard anti-D and anti-c preparations. In doing so, laboratories must:

- procure and maintain fully validated and supported quantification equipment

- procure and maintain fully validated dilution equipment

- prepare calibration curves from standard antibodies

- ensure operation consistency by running archive samples in parallel with all alloimmune anti-D and all anti-c samples (the repeat archive test result value should be within 10% of its original reported value)

- participate in the NHSBT's Antibody Quantification Quality Assurance Scheme, regularly review the results and act on the findings.

13.4.2 Antibody titration of antibodies capable of causing HDFN

RCI laboratories undertake IAT titration to assess all antibodies capable of causing HDFN other than anti-D and anti-c. Protocols for these tests should focus on achieving reproducible results by:

- specifying the phenotype of red cells for use with each antibody specificity

- describing the dilution medium and method

- using calibrated pipettes for dilution and dispense of reagents

- using IAT for titration, typically column technology
- establishing means of consistently identifying the endpoint for titration
- using parallel titration of previous archive samples from the patient where available
- managing cases where there is a difference between the current and archive sample endpoints.

13.4.3 Antibody titration in ABO mismatched transplant

RCI laboratories undertake titration of ABO antibodies to allow clinical assessment of the feasibility of ABO mismatched transplant, and monitoring of treatment to reduce antibody titre in preparation for ABO mismatched transplant. Protocols for this procedure should consider all the previously listed elements of titration, and in addition:

- the use of the organ donor's cells for titration
- inactivation of the IgM component of ABO antibodies (e.g. dithiothreitol (DTT) treatment).

13.5 Post-examination

All patient records and test results should be maintained according to the requirements of the Caldicott Report (1997)[8] and Data Protection Act (1998).[9]

Authorising and reporting of routine test results should be the responsibility of designated laboratory personnel. Consultant grade staff should authorise non-routine and discrepant results, or designate other senior staff to do so.

Results reported by fax should be to a designated fax number. The sender should confirm the telephone number of the receiving fax machine and the designated member of staff to whom the report is to be addressed. The sender should indicate when the report will be sent and, following fax transmission of the report, confirmation that the fax has been received should be obtained from the intended recipient.

Where electronic data interchange is in place either direct to surgeries/hospitals or onto a web browser the system should be based on the principles of the Caldicott Report.[8] The system should be validated and password controlled with clearly defined access levels. Data should be encoded with an electronic signature to ensure that the information cannot be altered and can only be viewed by designated individuals.

13.6 References

1. *Guideline for Blood Grouping and Antibody Testing in Pregnancy.* Available at www.bcshguidelines.com/documents/antibody_testing_pregnancy_bcsh_07062006.pdf.

2. *The Specification and Use of Information Technology (IT) Systems in Blood Transfusion Practice.* Available at www.bcshguidelines.com/documents/IT_blood_testing_22052006.pdf.

3. *Guidelines for Pre-transfusion Compatibility Procedures in Blood Transfusion Laboratories.* Available at www.bcshguidelines.com/documents/Compat_Guideline_for_submission_to_TTF_011012.pdf.

4. *Guidelines for the Estimation of Fetomaternal Haemorrhage.* Available at www.bcshguidelines.com/documents/BCSH_FMH_bcsh_sept2009.pdf.

5. *The Clinical Pathology Accreditation (CPA-UK) Standard for Medical Laboratories.* Available at www.cpa-uk.co.uk.

6. The Blood Safety and Quality Regulations 2005. Available at www.legislation.gov.uk.

7. Daniels G, Poole J, de Silva M, Callaghan T, MacLennan S, Smith N (2002). The clinical significance of blood group antibodies. *Transfusion Medicine,* 12, 287–295.

8. Caldicott Report. Available at www.dh.gov.uk/prod_consum_dh/groups/dh_digitalassets/@dh/@en/documents/digitalasset/dh_4068404.pdf.

9. Data Protection Act 1998. Available at www.legislation.gov.uk/ukpga/1998/29/contents.

Chapter 14
Guidelines for the use of DNA/PCR techniques in Blood Establishments

14.1 Safety precautions

All human cells should be treated as potentially infectious. Materials should be handled and discarded according to in-house documented procedures for potentially infectious biological materials.

Operators working with ultraviolet (UV) light should wear opaque gloves and a UV protective visor, appropriate to the wavelength emitted. Exposure should be kept to a minimum.

Operators should wear nitrile gloves when handling ethidium bromide. Liquid preparations of ethidium bromide are available from commercial sources and are preferable to handling the powder form.

14.2 Avoidance of contamination

DNA should be purified by a standard method that has been reported to the scientific literature and validated in the laboratory. DNA should be suitably stored to protect the integrity of the material.

During the preparation of genomic DNA, great care should be taken to avoid contamination from any other source of DNA. Pre-polymerase chain reaction (PCR) and post-PCR procedures should be undertaken in separate areas and using separate laboratory coats in each area. The laboratory should have documented procedures which have been constructed to eliminate potential causes of contamination, including training of the operator. If contamination does occur, all procedures should be reviewed and appropriate corrective action taken. Proposed change to procedures should be validated prior to their introduction.

In order to avoid contamination, the use of separate working stations or clearly defined work areas is beneficial for each stage of the PCR process. For example:

- One to prepare reagents. This is particularly important to avoid contamination of primers.

- One dedicated to pre-PCR manipulation (e.g. DNA isolation). A Class II laminar flow cabinet should avoid contamination of the sample with DNA from the operator.

- One dedicated to setting up PCRs.

- One for manipulation of PCR-amplified DNA. PCR-amplified products should be kept away from areas used for pre-amplification manipulation and reagent preparation.

Each working station should be adequately and independently equipped. However, the use of such working stations should not absolve the laboratory from procedures constructed to eliminate contamination.

Examples of measures which will help to minimise contamination include:

- the use of new sterilised, disposable plastic tubes or glassware for handling DNA
- the use of freshly prepared and sterilised materials and reagents when making up solutions for DNA samples, particularly dH_2O and Tris buffers
- aliquotting reagents in small amounts to minimise the number of repeat samplings
- the change of gloves and coats when moving between the areas dedicated for pre- and post-PCR manipulations
- the use of positive displacement dedicated pipettes or plugged tips to carry out PCR preparations
- routine wipe-tests of pre-amplification work areas should be performed. If an amplified product is detected, the area must be cleaned to eliminate the contamination, re-tested and measures taken to prevent future contamination
- reagents used for amplification must not be exposed to post-amplification work areas.

14.3 Working practices

- DNA should be as intact as possible. Degraded DNA should be avoided.
- An archival record (e.g. photograph) of each electrophoretic run should be retained.
- The performance of probes and primers should be fully validated and characterised before they are put into use. Others should be used only for research purposes.
- Reagents (e.g. chemicals, enzymes) should be stored and utilised under conditions recommended by the manufacturer, including, for example, storage temperature, test temperature, shelf life, diluent buffer and concentration for use.
- Each lot of reagents must be tested before use in routine typing.
- For reagents and kits, the source, lot number, expiration date and storage conditions should be documented.
- Users should have procedures to ensure that periodic checks of probes and primers are carried out to detect their deteriorating performance or contamination.
- Thermal cyclers should be serviced at least annually according to the manufacturer's recommendations and a temperature calibration should be performed. A record of the service and calibration checks should be maintained.
- Laboratories should regularly check their primer sequences for newly discovered single nucleotide polymorphisms. This can be done by checking the National Genetic Reference Laboratory website at https://ngrl.manchester.ac.uk/SNPCheckV3/snpcheck.htm

Chapter 15
Molecular typing for red cell antigens

15.1 Introduction

Genes for all of the blood group systems have been isolated and the molecular bases for most of the clinically important blood group antigens are known. So it is now possible to predict, with a high level of accuracy, most blood group phenotypes from genomic DNA.

This technology is generally applied when:

- we need to know a blood group phenotype, but do not have a suitable red cell sample
- molecular testing will provide more or better information than serological testing
- molecular testing is more efficient or more cost-effective than serological testing.

15.2 Clinical applications of blood group molecular typing

Various clinical applications of blood group molecular typing are listed below:

- **Fetal typing:**[1] Typing of fetuses, usually for D, but also K, C, c or E, of alloimmunised women, to assess whether the fetus is at risk of haemolytic disease of the fetus and newborn (HDFN). The DNA source is cell-free fetal DNA in the mother's plasma. In the future this technology may be applied to all D negative pregnant women to determine their requirement for antenatal anti-D prophylaxis.

- **Transfused patients:** Typing of multiply transfused patients, where serological testing cannot be used because of the presence of transfused red cells.

- **Immunoglobulin-coated red cells:** Typing of red cells giving a positive direct antiglobulin test (DAT), usually in patients with autoimmune haemolytic anaemia, to help in the identification of underlying alloantibodies.

- **Determining Rh variants:** Molecular methods are used for identifying Rh variants, especially the weak and partial variants of D, to assist in the provision of the most suitable blood for transfusion.

- **Confirmation of D negative:** Detection of *RHD* in an apparently D negative donor could signal very weak D expression, which could immunise a D negative patient.

- ***RHD* zygosity:** Quantitative PCR can reveal whether a D positive person is homozygous or hemizygous for *RHD*. This cannot be done by serological methods. Testing fathers of fetuses at risk of HDFN provides limited information on the D type of the fetus.

- **Testing when suitable reagents are not available:** Molecular methods can replace serological methods when suitable serological reagents are unreliable or not available, e.g. Dombrock typing of donors.

- **Supporting the serological reference laboratory:** Molecular methods are valuable for supporting the serological reference laboratory in sorting out difficult problems.

15.2.1 Testing donors for multiple blood groups

It is probable that molecular methods will replace serology in the near future for testing donors for multiple blood groups. The new high-throughput molecular technology will be more accurate than serological methods and will probably be more cost-effective. Molecular tests could also be applied to screening for donors with rare blood group phenotypes such as S– s– U–, Lu(b–), k–, Js(b–), Yt(a–), or Co(a–), plus Vel– when the molecular basis has been elucidated.

For prediction of blood group phenotypes from DNA of donors, results should either be confirmed by serological testing or by testing twice by molecular methods. This does not apply to ABO and RhD, which are always determined by serological testing.

15.3 ABO typing by molecular genetics

Whereas ABO typing by serological means is straightforward and extremely accurate, the genetics of ABO is complex, rendering ABO molecular typing by available methods unreliable. This is particularly so in people of African origin, where hybrid *ABO* alleles are present. As it is never acceptable to obtain a false ABO typing, prediction of ABO phenotype by molecular methods is not currently recommended.

15.4 Methods available for molecular blood grouping

15.4.1 Fetal typing

The usual technology employed for fetal blood group typing, in which the mother lacks the antigen to be tested, is real-time quantitative PCR (RQ-PCR) on cell-free DNA isolated from the maternal plasma. For D, probes and primers are designed to detect two or three regions of *RHD*. Tests for fetal C, c, E and K involve RQ-PCR with allele-specific primers. A test for the housekeeping gene *CCR5* is also included to confirm that DNA is present and that there is not an excess of maternal DNA.

Three controls for fetal *RHD* are used: DNA from D negative pregnant women containing DNA from a D positive fetus, a D negative fetus, and from a D negative fetus with *RHD*Ψ. Positive and negative fetal DNA controls are used for C, c, E and K.

15.4.2 Typing from DNA obtained from peripheral blood

There is a large variety of platforms for detecting single nucleotide polymorphisms for the purpose of predicting blood group phenotypes of donors and patients from genomic DNA isolated from blood.[2,3] These include low-throughput methods involving allele-specific primers and gel electrophoresis, a very comprehensive DNA microarray platform that identifies many D variants, and higher throughput platforms such as allelic discrimination technology and platforms involving the application of fluorescent beads coated with oligonucleotide probes. Those platforms that offer the possibility of high-throughput testing do not include testing for ABO or D.

The usual tests for blood group polymorphisms that would be required for testing donors and patients would be D, C, c, E, e, M, N, S, s, K, k, Fy^a, Fy^b, Fy-null, Jk^a, Jk^b, Do^a and Do^b. Often some others are also included. See Table 15.1.

Homozygous positive, homozygous negative and heterozygous controls are used when available.

In addition, International Reference Reagents which can be purchased from the National Institute for Biological Standards and Control (see Annex 1 and www.nibsc.ac.uk) could be useful in the standardisation of blood group genotyping.

There are certain precautions that are required for all molecular testing and they are described in Chapter 14. In addition, there are certain tests in molecular blood grouping that must be carried out to ensure a reasonable level of accuracy. The hazards of ABO grouping are described above. There are numerous variants of D that could give rise to a false answer. Any test for D must reveal the D negative genes *RHDΨ* and *RHD-CE-D^S*, which are common in people of African origin. Testing for at least *RHD* exons 5 and 7, with the test for the former being designed to give a negative result with *RHDΨ*, is the minimum required. C typing should not depend on the *RHCE* nucleotide 48 polymorphism; testing for the *RHCE* intron 2 insert is more reliable. Duffy typing must include a test for the *GATA* mutation to detect the common silent allele.

15.5 External quality assurance

Although there is no National External Quality Assurance Scheme (NEQAS) for molecular blood grouping, it is important that any laboratory performing this testing for clinical purposes participates in some sort of external quality assurance scheme. The International Society of Blood Transfusion (ISBT) organises workshops every 2 years in which DNA samples from 'patients' and plasma from D negative pregnant women are distributed. In addition, it is possible to set up sample-exchange schemes with other laboratories carrying out similar work.

Table 15.1 Some blood group polymorphisms and associated gene sequence changes

System	Gene	Antigens	Molecular test
MNS	*GYPA*	M/N	59 C/T, 71 G/A
Rh	*RHD*	D	Presence/absence
	RHCE	C	Intron 2 insertion
		c	307 C
		E/e	676 G/C
Lutheran	*LU* or *BCAM*	Lu^a/Lu^b	230 A/G
Kell	*KEL*	K/k	578 T/C
		Kp^a/Kp^b	841 T/C
		Js^a/Js^b	1790 C/T
Duffy	*FY* or *DARC*	Fy^a/Fy^b	125 G/A
		Fy-null	−67t>c
Kidd	*JK* or *SLC14A1*	Jk^a/Jk^b	838G/A
Diego	*DI* or *SLC4A1*	Di^a/Di^b	2561 T/C
Yt	*YT* or *ACHE*	Yt^a/Yt^b	1057 C/A
Dombrock	*DO* or *ART4*	Do^a/Do^b	793 A/G
Colton	*CO* or *AQP1*	Co^a/Co^b	134 C/T

15.6 References

1. Daniels G, Finning K, Martin P, Massey E (2009). Non-invasive prenatal diagnosis of fetal blood group phenotypes: current practice and future prospects. *Prenatal Diagnosis*, 29, 101–107.

2. Anstee DJ (2009). Red cell genotyping and the future of pretransfusion testing. *Blood*, 114, 248–256.

3. Veldhuisen B, van der Schoot CE, de Haas M (2009). Blood group genotyping: from patient to high-throughput donor screening. *Vox Sanguinis*, 97, 198–206.

Chapter 16
HLA typing and HLA serology

16.1 Preamble

For the eighth edition we have made significant changes in both the structure and content to the previous version of this chapter concerning human leucocyte antigen (HLA) typing and antibody testing. This obviously reflects the continuing scientific and technical development in the field. DNA-based testing for HLA alleles now predominates over serological phenotyping and antibody detection/characterisation mostly involves non-cell-based methods. This HLA section is constructed of three main parts, concerning reagents (section 16.4), testing (sections 16.5, 16.6 and 16.7), and application to donor and patient investigations (section 16.8). For certain patient or donor investigations there is, of course, an overlap with the guidance given in this and the granulocyte or platelet immunology chapters (Chapters 17 and 18 respectively). This is particularly relevant to the laboratory investigations of platelet refractoriness and transfusion-related acute lung injury (TRALI), so diagrams are included (Figures 16.1 and 16.2) to indicate how the different guidelines relate to each other.

16.2 Introduction

The transfusion or transplantation of blood components bearing allogeneic HLA can stimulate clinically significant immunological responses. All cellular components except erythrocytes express HLA and any plasma-containing product may include HLA-specific antibodies which are potentially harmful to the recipient.

Prospective HLA typing of platelet donors is undertaken for transfusion of immune refractory patients and those with disorders of platelet function and structure. Potential haematopoietic progenitor cell (HPC) donors are HLA typed to be placed on one of the national donor registries.

HLA typing or antibody investigations may be undertaken for diagnostic purposes or to investigate harmful consequences of transfusion. Thus the diagnosis of immune refractoriness requires the demonstration of HLA-specific antibodies (or other platelet-specific antibodies) in the patient. As part of the investigation of TRALI, implicated donors are screened for HLA (and human neutrophil antigen, HNA)-specific antibodies and the patient is HLA typed if possible.

The European Federation for Immunogenetics (EFI) has established standards[1] (at the time of writing, version 5.7) for histocompatibility testing and where appropriate these guidelines will refer to the relevant EFI Standard, which will be stated in the text. In general, guidance for practice is indicated by the term 'should'. The use of the term 'must' is mostly limited to circumstances where an EFI Standard applies.

16.3 Terminology and nomenclature

All HLA assignments, irrespective of the method, must comply with the current WHO Nomenclature Committee for Factors of the HLA System Report[2] and Nomenclature for Factors of the HLA System, 2010[3] (and see EFI Standards D1.000–D1.320, inclusive). Examples of acceptable HLA assignments are as follows: HLA-B12, HLA-B44, HLA-B-44(12), HLA-B*44, HLA-B*44:09.

HLA may be serologically typed (to determine the phenotype) or typed by DNA molecular analysis. The term genotype is properly used to describe the genetic (DNA) constitution determined by the pattern of inheritance (EFI Standard D1.230).

HLA typing by DNA-based molecular techniques, which employ either DNA-based probes or primers, type for the presence or absence of sequence motifs. Kits using this technology are able to define the HLA alleles present in an individual to a variable level of resolution dependent on a number of factors. These include the number of probes or primers employed, the number of alleles defined for a given locus and the HLA alleles present in the individual. Although it is possible to achieve a high resolution or allele level typing using molecular methods, it is not a clinical requirement in transfusion practice. Therefore, patients and donors are typed to a low or medium level of resolution, and may present HLA typing results that include some ambiguity in interpretation.

Each serologically defined HLA antigenic specificity may be encoded by a number of different HLA alleles. Conversely many HLA alleles have no determined serologically defined antigen. Thus it is not always possible to assign a serological equivalent to each HLA allele.[4] One consequence of this is that it is not practical to subject serological and DNA-based typing to the same standard as this would need to be unacceptably low (i.e. the lowest common denominator). Both techniques are in general use, each having specific advantages and disadvantages, and under these circumstances professional judgement together with the following guidelines should be used to deliver an appropriate standard of HLA typing.

Caution should therefore be exercised if an HLA type assigned using DNA-based molecular techniques is converted into a serological equivalent and such conversion must always be avoided with alleles for which the phenotype has not been unequivocally defined.

16.4 Reagents

16.4.1 General guidelines

HLA reagents prepared from human source material should comply with the guidelines in section 11.1.4.10.

Exceptionally, reagents not tested at source as required in section 11.1.4.10, and for which no alternative exists, may be supplied for use with the expressed approval of the user and with the understanding that the reagent must be regarded as potentially infectious.

These reagents should be marked 'Potentially infectious – not tested at source for...', as appropriate, both on the immediate container label or multi-well tray or reservoir, and the outer packaging.

The instructions for use of these reagents should indicate that the reagent(s) has not been tested at source as required in section 11.1.4.10, and that the reagents are to be considered as potentially infectious. In addition, the package insert should give information on the safe disposal of the material and the container, multi-well tray or reservoir.

16.4.1.1 Immediate container label

HLA reagents issued separately: The label should conform to the requirements of EN ISO 18113:2009. In addition, the body of a container presented in sealed bags or foiled pouches should be marked with a unique identifier to enable identification and traceability.

Multi-component test systems: In addition to the label information required above, a test system comprising multiple components should be marked to ensure identification and traceability of all components, for example multi-well trays or reservoirs, strips and pre-prepared membranes.

The instructions for use should contain the information required by EN ISO 18113:2009, and should comply, where applicable, with the requirements of section 11.1.4.12.

16.4.2 Serological typing reagents

The following information must be provided for each individual serological HLA typing reagent or HLA typing set:

- The claimed HLA specificity(ies) of the reagent, the percentage of specific reactions giving a cytotoxicity score of 80% to 100% cell death, the values of the correlation coefficient r obtained by the pre-testing of the reagent against a well-characterised cell panel, and the reaction score.

- The manufacturer should provide information of the incidence of equivocal cytotoxicity scores within the package insert.

- HLA typing sets should include a representation of the multi-well tray or reservoir layout indicating the position, HLA specificity(ies) and batch (or sub-batch) reference of the HLA typing reagent contained in each well.

- Monoclonal antibodies should be identified as such.

- An instruction that thawing and refreezing of the HLA typing reagents should be kept to the absolute minimum from the date of manufacture to the date of use. HLA typing sera frozen in micro-well trays should be used within 1 hour of thawing. Sera supplied freeze-dried in micro-well trays should be used within 1 hour of their reconstitution; unused trays should not be refrozen for later use.

- When reagents are supplied as an HLA typing set for the detection of a single antigen, the instructions for use should indicate which controls are appropriate to demonstrate specificity and cross-reactivity.

- For HLA typing sets, a list should be provided of those specificities that cannot be adequately defined in the presence of other specified specificities.

- Each HLA typing set for Class I or Class II phenotyping should contain at least one positive control antibody preparation, previously shown to react with all target cells, and should include at least one negative control preparation, previously shown to lack antibody activity or be from a male with no history of blood transfusion.

16.4.2.1 Preservation

HLA typing reagents may be preserved in the liquid or in the dried state. Reagents should be stored as recommended by the manufacturer.

HLA typing reagents, after being thawed or reconstituted, should be transparent and should not contain any sediment, gel or particles visible on microscopy (x 200).

16.4.2.2 Stability and expiry date

Manufacturers should ensure that HLA typing reagents have a shelf life of at least 1 year, when stored as recommended.

Any extension by the user of the expiry date stated by the manufacturer should be supported by documented test data.

Manufacturers should notify all primary users if an HLA typing reagent or a constituent reagent of an HLA typing set stored as recommended fails to perform satisfactorily within the expiry date allotted by the manufacturer.

16.4.3 Requirements for phenotype assignment

HLA Class I and Class II serological typing must comply with EFI Standards E1.000 to E2.740 inclusive. HLA reagents and kits to be used for phenotyping lymphocytes by cytotoxicity should comply with the following:

- HLA typing reagents, when used by all methods recommended by the producer, should react with all lymphocyte samples with the corresponding antigen(s) when tested against a panel of lymphocyte samples bearing those antigen(s) collected from at least 25 individuals. HLA typing reagents should not react with any lymphocyte samples when tested against a panel of lymphocyte samples known not to bear the corresponding antigen(s) collected from at least 100 individuals. Reagents that conform to the requirements of this paragraph are termed operationally monospecific.

- Not more than half of the HLA typing reagents used together to detect an antigen should have the same extra claimed specificity.

- None of the HLA typing reagents used together should have been shown to react with more than 5% of the separate samples of a lymphocyte panel which do not express any of the antigen(s) that the reagent is claimed to detect.

- Manufacturers should indicate in the instructions for use those specificities whose detection does not comply with the requirements of any of the above.

16.4.4 Rabbit complement for use in HLA serology

16.4.4.1 General guidelines

Rabbit complement supplied for use in HLA serology should be stored as recommended by the manufacturer.

Manufacturers should be aware that highly active complement can cause unwanted specificities to become apparent in HLA typing reagents that have been characterised on less active but adequate complement.

16.4.4.2 Immediate container label

The label of the immediate container of rabbit complement for use in HLA serology should conform to the specifications in section 11.1.4.11.

16.4.4.3 Instructions for use

The instructions for use supplied with rabbit complement for use in HLA serology should conform to the specifications in section 11.1.4.12.

The instructions for use should offer guidance on the method of thawing. In addition, they should contain an instruction that the complement, once thawed from the immediate container or reconstituted from the freeze-dried state, should not be refrozen.

The instructions for use should state whether the rabbit complement has been tested and found suitable for use with monoclonal HLA typing reagents.

16.4.4.4 Potency tests on rabbit complement for use in HLA serology

Rabbit complement should be tested prior to use, in accordance with EFI Standards E2.700–E2.740.

16.4.5 DNA typing reagents

Methods available for HLA typing of DNA samples rely on identification of polymorphic HLA gene sequence motifs. In all widely used methods, the polymerase chain reaction (PCR) is utilised, either through the use of sequence-specific primers as in PCR-SSP, or to produce a locus-specific DNA template (e.g. HLA-A) which can subsequently be typed using a panel of sequence-specific oligonucleotide probes (PCR-SSOP). The locus-specific template may also be directly sequenced using locus or allele group-specific sequencing primers.

DNA can be prepared from various tissues by a variety of methods. The laboratory should prepare DNA by a standard method that has been reported in the scientific literature and validated in the laboratory for the HLA typing method to be used.

16.4.5.1 Instructions for use

In addition to section 11.1.4.12 of these guidelines, the instructions for use must adhere to the EFI Standards for Nucleic Acid Analysis (Section L) and should include the following:

- a statement explaining the test and intended application of the kit
- the principle of the procedure
- reagents and equipment required to perform the test
- detailed instructions for all components of the test
- the gene targeted as a PCR amplification control (PCR-SSP)
- the specificity and nucleotide sequence of all primers and probes used in the HLA typing kit
- a table or diagram indicating the location of the probes and/or primers utilised in the test
- a list of ambiguous combinations of alleles defined for each test kit – this may also be given as part of interpretative software
- the HLA alleles which are claimed to be detected by the HLA typing kit, further divided into the following groups:
  - those HLA alleles which have been detected in appropriately controlled validation tests
  - those HLA alleles which have not been directly detected in validation tests but where the reactivity of the allele is expected to be detected
  - those HLA alleles which have not been directly detected in validation tests and whose reactivity cannot be assumed to be detected by the kit
  - those HLA alleles that are known to produce weak or unreliable signals in the output systems

- the date and the source of the sequence information used in the kit design and a statement that new alleles described following the date of design may not be detected by the kit
- the control tests to be performed to check for contamination (negative control) of the test system
- the control DNA to be included to check for quality of sample DNA used
- the control test to be performed to generate a true positive signal
- acceptable limits of signal intensity should be specified for positive and negative results
- all computer software assisted interpretation of results should be validated on control DNA
- the chemical components of the kits should be listed and reference made to any toxic substances included in the kit with recommendations for their safe disposal. Reference to material safety data sheets should be given.

16.4.5.2 Requirements

Manufacturers should inform all primary users of a DNA-based HLA typing kit when any changes to a kit's ability to perform are detected. All users of DNA-based HLA typing kits should report any kit-related problems directly to the manufacturer and maintain records of such events.

16.5 Testing of HLA genes and gene products

DNA-based methods must identify all HLA alleles included in the most recent WHO Nomenclature Committee for Factors of the HLA System Report[2] and Nomenclature for Factors of the HLA System, 2010.[3] Alleles should be reported either as individual alleles or as allele groups with two digits (first field). Definitions of allelic, high, intermediate and low resolution molecular HLA typing are available through EFI.

The minimum level of resolution by serological typing is given in Table 16.1. Typing to the level of broad specificities is acceptable but the higher level to include the split specificities, as indicated, is recommended. HLA-C types Cw12 and Cw14 to Cw18 have not been formally designated as recognised antigens and may not be identified serologically.

16.6 Testing for HLA-specific antibodies

16.6.1 General guidance

HLA-specific antibody screening and characterisation must comply with EFI Standards Section F (Antibody Screening and Crossmatching) and Section M (Flow Cytometry).

All commercial HLA antibody test kits should be CE and *in vitro* device (IVD) marked and validated for use. Each batch of commercial test kit or in-house panel should be evaluated against a minimum of three sera of known HLA specificity from different cross-reacting groups.

Table 16.1 HLA antigens that are defined by serological typing (with broad specificities shown in brackets)

HLA-A	HLA-B	HLA-C	HLA-DR	HLA-DQ
A1	B7	Cw1	DR1	DQ5 (1)
A2	B8	Cw2	DR15 (2)	DQ6 (1)
A3	B13	Cw9 (3)	DR16 (2)	DQ2
A11	B18	Cw10 (3)	DR17 (3)	DQ7 (3)
A23 (A9)	B27	Cw4	DR18 (3)	DQ8 (3)
A24 (A9)	B35	Cw5	DR4	DQ9 (3)
A25 (A10)	B37	Cw6	DR11 (5)	DQ4
A26 (A10)	B38 (B16)	Cw7	DR12 (5)	
A29 (A19)	B39 (B16)	Cw8	DR13 (6)	
A30 (A19)	B41	Cw12#	DR14 (6)	
A31 (A19)	B42	Cw14#	DR7	
A32 (A19)	B45	Cw15#	DR8	
A33 (A19)	B44	Cw16#	DR9	
A34 (A10)	B46	Cw17#	DR10	
A36	B47	Cw18#	DR103	
A43	B48			
A66 (A10)	B49 (B21)		DR51	
A68 (A28)	B50 (B21)		DR52	
A69 (A28)	B51 (B5)		DR53	
A74 (A19)	B52 (B5)			
A80	B53			
	B54 (B22)			
	B55 (B22)			
	B56 (B22)			
	B57 (B17)			
	B58 (B17)			
	B59			
	B60 (B40)			
	B61 (B40)			
	B62 (B15)			
	B63 (B15)			
	B64 (B14)			
	B65 (B14)			
	B67			
	B71 (B70)			
	B72 (B70)			
	B73			
	B75 (B15)			
	B76 (B15)			
	B77 (B15)			
	B78			
	B81			
	Bw4			
	Bw6			

The products of the Cw12 and Cw14 to Cw18 genes have not been formally designated as recognised antigens and might not be identified serologically.

HLA-specific antibodies may be detected using reagent lymphocytes (or cell lines), solid-phase bound, purified HLA molecules, or particle bound, purified HLA molecules. If such techniques are used for screening (i.e. not characterisation of specificity) the following apply:

- There should be discrimination between HLA Class I and Class II-specific antibodies.

- Overall the target cells or molecules should cover either all the known HLA immunogenic epitopes or all HLA specificities (Class I, Class II, or both as appropriate) found in the population at over 0.5%.

16.6.2 Characterisation of antibody specificity

Sera containing HLA-specific antibodies may be interpreted in terms of specific antigens (i.e. whole gene products), cross-reactive groups, single epitopes, or any combination of these as long as standard and unequivocal nomenclature is used. Specificity characterisation may be helped by computer analysis but a final result must involve manual interpretation.

Panels of HLA typed cells or purified HLA molecules are used for identification. The composition of the panel should be sufficient to discriminate the specificities (Class I, Class II, or both as appropriate) given in Table 16.2. The full list of antigens comprising a panel should be supplied and typed to the higher level of resolution shown in Table 16.1.

There are many techniques available for the detection of HLA antibodies such as those developed for the detection and identification of HLA antibodies utilising Luminex microspheres. These assays are highly sensitive, leading to the detection of very low levels of HLA antibodies. Cut-off values for HLA antibody detection should be set in accordance with manufacturer's instructions and local clinical evaluation.

For DNA typed reagents the types should be supplied at the four-digit (second field) level (e.g. HLA-A*02:01) and null alleles identified.

16.6.2.1 HLA antibody characterisation by complement dependent cytotoxicity

Rabbit complement

Rabbit complement used for detection of HLA antibodies by complement dependent cytotoxicity should comply with guidelines in section 16.4.4.

Instructions for use

In addition to the information required in section 16.6.2, the instructions for use should include the following information on each individual preparation of HLA reagent lymphocytes or set of HLA reagent lymphocytes:

- the HLA phenotype of the reagent lymphocytes

- the nature of the HLA reagent lymphocytes (e.g. normal peripheral lymphocytes, separated peripheral B lymphocytes, separated peripheral T lymphocytes, chronic lymphocytic leukemia (CLL) cells, splenic lymphocytes, lymph node lymphocytes, lymphoblastoid cell line)

- the concentration of the lymphocyte suspension should be stated in the instructions for use for HLA reagent lymphocytes issued in individual immediate containers, or on the phenotype listing of batches issued as multi-immediate container products

- HLA reagent lymphocyte sets issued in multi-well trays should include a representation of the tray or reservoir layout indicating the location of the various HLA reagent lymphocytes in the wells of the tray

Table 16.2 Characterisation of HLA-specific antibodies

HLA-A broad specificities	Splits	HLA-B broad specificities	Splits	HLA-C broad specificities	Splits	HLA-DR broad specificities	Splits	HLA-DQ broad specificities	Splits
A1		B5	B51	Cw1		DR1		DQ1	DQ5
A2		B5	B52	Cw2		DR103		DQ1	DQ6
A3		B7		Cw3	Cw9	DR2	DR15	DQ2	
A9	A23	B8		Cw3	Cw10	DR2	DR16	DQ3	DQ7
A9	A24	B12	B44	Cw4		DR3	DR17	DQ3	DQ8
A10	A25	B12	B45	Cw5		DR3	DR18	DQ3	DQ9
A10	A26	B13		Cw6		DR4		DQ4	
A10	A34	B14	B64	Cw7		DR5	DR11		
A10	A66	B14	B65	Cw8		DR5	DR12		
A11		B15	B62	Cw12		DR6	DR13		
A19	A29	B15	B63	Cw14		DR6	DR14		
A19	A30	B15	B75	Cw15		DR7			
A19	A31	B15	B76	Cw16		DR8			
A19	A32	B15	B77	Cw17		DR9			
A19	A33	B16	B38	Cw18		DR10			
A19	A74	B16	B39						
A28	A68	B17	B57						
A28	A69	B17	B58			DR51			
A36		B18				DR52			
A43		B21	B49			DR53			
A80		B21	B50						
		B22	B54						
		B22	B55						
		B22	B56						
		B27							
		B35							
		B37							
		B40	B60						
		B40	B61						
		B41							
		B42							
		B46							
		B47							
		B48							
		B53							
		B59							
		B67							
		B70	B71						
		B70	B72						
		B73							
		B78							
		B81							
		Bw4							
		Bw6							

- for HLA reagent lymphocyte sets issued in multi-well trays or reservoirs the phenotype information may take the form of a listing of the phenotypes of each of the individual donations comprising the set

- the shelf life of the HLA reagent lymphocytes following recovery from long-term storage and subsequent storage in conditions recommended by the manufacturer should be stated in the instructions for use

- when HLA reagent lymphocytes are provided suspended in preservative or medium, the components of the preservative or the name of the medium should be stated in the instructions for use.

Reagent lymphocytes

Freshly isolated or previously frozen lymphocytes should have a viability of at least 80% and should contain less than 1% platelets or granulocytes.

Reagent B lymphocytes isolated for the identification of Class II antibodies should contain less than 10% of non-B cells.

The background incidence of spontaneous cell death, as assessed by a negative control serum, should be less than 30%.

Reagent lymphocytes supplied as previously frozen in test trays should contain 1000 to 2000 lymphocytes per well, after recovery following manufacturer's instructions.

The manufacturer should specify in the instructions for use those antigens known to be present or absent, and those for which no testing has been performed. HLA-A, HLA-B, HLA-C, HLA-DR and HLA-DQ serologically defined specificities should be included in this statement.

16.6.2.2 HLA antibody characterisation by solid-phase and particle bound methods

Purified HLA captured onto a microtitre well, nylon membrane or microparticles can be used as sensor molecules for characterising sera containing HLA-specific antibodies.

Antibody binding can be detected by ELISA or fluorescence. The detector reagent should be able to identify IgG and discriminate between IgG, IgA and IgM.

Human material

If a product is prepared from human source material then the guidance in section 11.1.4.10 must be followed.

Instructions for use

The instructions for use must comply with the requirements of EN ISO 18113:2009 and the information required in section 16.6.1. In addition, the instructions for use should include the following information on each individual preparation or component of a set of HLA screening product:

- the HLA antigens represented in each container

- the concentration of any cells or particles in suspension should be stated in the instructions for use of HLA screening product issued in individual immediate containers or on the antigen information table of batches issued as multi-immediate container products or multi-well trays or reservoirs

- HLA screening products issued in multi-well trays should include a representation of the tray or reservoir layout indicating the location of the HLA antigens in the wells of the tray

- the expiry life of the HLA screening product following reconstitution or preparation and subsequent storage in conditions recommended by the manufacturer should be stated

- when components of an HLA screening product contains preservatives the name of the chemical preservatives and the components which contain them should be stated.

Validation

Kits for the detection of HLA antibodies should be validated for sensitivity and specificity on a batch basis using a panel of clinically representative HLA antisera. A panel of sera shown to be inert for HNA and HLA antibodies should also be used.

16.7 Leucocyte crossmatching in blood transfusion

Crossmatching may be used in the diagnosis of TRALI and the treatment of HLA- or HNA-sensitised patients with granulocyte transfusions. Unusually it may also be used in the management of patients refractory to random donor platelet transfusion.

A patient's serum should be comprehensively screened for HLA-specific antibodies prior to the crossmatch being performed. The chosen crossmatch technique should be of similar or greater sensitivity than the screening technique.

The presence of HLA-specific antibodies in a current patient serum sample that gives rise to a positive crossmatch excludes that donor providing platelets or leucocytes for that particular patient.

16.7.1 Lymphocytotoxic crossmatch

Assessment of leucocyte crossmatches must comply with EFI Standards within F6.000 and the standards for serological investigation given above.

16.7.1.1 Cytotoxic crossmatch requirements

A policy to determine which sera should be crossmatched should be established and based on local clinical data, where possible, before a crossmatch service is provided.

A negative control serum derived from a pool of sera that has been previously shown not to react with lymphocytes by complement-dependent cytotoxicity (CDC) should be used.

At least one positive control serum reacting with all lymphocytes or a mixture of anti-HLA-Bw4 and anti-HLA-Bw6-specific reagents should be used to confirm the activity of complement and HLA expression on the cell surface.

The crossmatch should be performed with and without dithiothreitol (DTT) to distinguish between IgM and IgG antibodies. An IgM control reagent should be included in the crossmatch test as a control for DTT activity.

Each patient's serum should be tested in triplicate to control for unusual reactions in individual wells of the microplate.

16.7.2 Flow cytometric crossmatch

The flow cytometric crossmatch (FCXM) offers greater sensitivity than the microlymphocytoxicity test for the detection of HLA-specific antibodies in patients receiving blood products. The FCXM may be performed with platelets, lymphocytes and/or granulocytes from the donor.

A two- or three-colour FCXM should be used with one antibody directed against human IgG conjugated to a fluorochrome (e.g. fluorescein isothiocyanate (FITC)). Antibody conjugated to different fluorochromes (e.g. anti-CD3 (T cells) and phycoerythrin (PE) and anti-CD19 (B cells) and allophycocyanin (APC)), should be used to identify the cell lineage under investigation, unless a purified cell population is used, to distinguish between anti-HLA Class I and II reactivity. Testing must be in compliance with EFI Standards M4.000.

16.7.2.1 FCXM requirements

A policy to determine which sera should be crossmatched should be established and based on local clinical data, where possible, before a crossmatch service is provided.

A negative control serum derived from a pool of sera that has been previously shown not to react with lymphocytes by flow cytometry should be used.

At least one positive control serum reacting with all lymphocytes or a mixture of anti-HLA-Bw4 and anti-HLA-Bw6-specific reagents should be used to confirm the activity of complement and HLA expression on the cell surface.

Each patient's serum should be tested in duplicate to control for unusual reactions.

An additional weak positive control, which gives a fluorescent intensity just greater than the cut-off point between positive and negative, may also be included to evaluate assay performance.

16.8 Application of HLA/HPA testing to patients and donors

16.8.1 Donor and patient testing

The most common cause of immunological refractoriness to random donor platelet transfusion is the presence of HLA-specific antibodies in the patient receiving platelet transfusion. The management of this group of patients may involve the provision of HLA-compatible platelets and/or crossmatch-negative donors.

HLA Class I typed platelets should normally be provided for refractory patients with the aim of minimising exposure to mismatched Class I antigens. In the absence of a zero mismatched donor, a compatible donor can be selected on the basis of a lack of antigens or alleles corresponding to the antibody specificities identified in the patient. Where a patient's antibodies have not been characterised, a crossmatch can be performed; however, it is best practice to establish the patient's antibody specificities if long-term platelet support is envisaged.

There are several crossmatch techniques for the detection of donor reactive antibodies that may involve the use of donor lymphocytes or donor platelets. The basic principle is the same for most of the techniques in that serum or plasma from the patient is incubated with donor cells and reactivity is detected by flow cytometry or cytotoxicity. Platelets from donors negative in the crossmatch testing may be used for transfusion of the patient whose serum has been crossmatched.

HLA and/or granulocyte-specific antibodies present in donor plasma have been implicated in nearly 80% of TRALI cases (patient leucocyte antibody or inter-donor reactions in pooled products have also been reported as causes of TRALI). The identification of leucocyte-specific antibodies in implicated donors provides support for the diagnosis of TRALI.

16.8.2 Apheresis platelet donors

All potential plateletpheresis donors used for the provision of HLA selected platelets should be typed for HLA-A, HLA-B and HLA-C. If serological typing is used the minimum level of typing should be for the HLA Class I specificities listed in Table 16.1. For all donors HLA-Bw4 or HLA-Bw6 should be assigned.

If DNA-based typing is performed on donors a typing strategy should be employed that allows for HLA alleles to be defined to at least the two-digit (first field) level of resolution. Typing should also be capable of determining the presence of the Bw4 and Bw6 epitopes.

Each donor should be HLA typed twice using samples collected on separate occasions, such that only if the second test confirms the first should the donor provide platelets for clinical use.

16.8.3 Testing of donors/cord units for related haematopoietic stem cell transplant (EFI Standard I1.000)

DNA-based HLA typing, to at least the two-digit (first field) level of resolution, should be performed on donors. High-resolution typing may also be necessary as detailed below.

Initially, all potential related stem cell donors must be typed for at least HLA-A, HLA-B and/or HLA-DR to assess compatibility. Further testing must then be undertaken to establish a phenotypic match for HLA Class I and II loci, as described in local protocols. HLA types of the matched patient and donor must be confirmed on a second sample. If HLA haplotype inheritance can be established by typing family members, then high-resolution typing is not required to establish a genotypic match. However, if haplotype inheritance is not established, high-resolution typing of HLA Class I and/or Class II should be undertaken as required by the local transplant protocol. Intra-familial donors who are not HLA identical siblings require both Class I and Class II high-resolution typing as required by the local transplant protocol.

As a minimum related cord units must be typed at low resolution for HLA-A, -B and -DRB1. Extended typing must be undertaken if required by the transplant protocol.

Prior to cord unit transplant, confirmatory typing at low resolution must be performed for HLA-A, -B and -DRB1. Typing must be performed on a segment of the tubing integrally attached to the unit, on a satellite vial or on the content of the thawed unit.

16.8.4 Testing of donors/cord units for unrelated haematopoietic stem cell transplant (EFI Standard I2.000)

DNA-based HLA typing, to at least the two-digit (first field) level of resolution, should be performed on donors. High-resolution typing may also be necessary as detailed below.

As a minimum all potential unrelated donors should be typed for HLA-A, -B , -C and -DRB1. HLA types of patient and donor should be confirmed, although the original type from the unrelated donor registry is acceptable for this purpose. The need for high-resolution typing of HLA Class I and II will depend upon local transplant protocols.

As a minimum cord units must be typed at low resolution for HLA-A and -B and high resolution for -DRB1. Extended typing must be performed if required by the local transplant protocol. Prior to commencement of patient conditioning, a minimum low-resolution confirmatory type of at least HLA-A, -B and -DRB1 must be performed upon receipt of the shipped unit. Typing must be performed on a segment of the tubing integrally attached to the unit, on a satellite vial or on the content of the thawed unit.

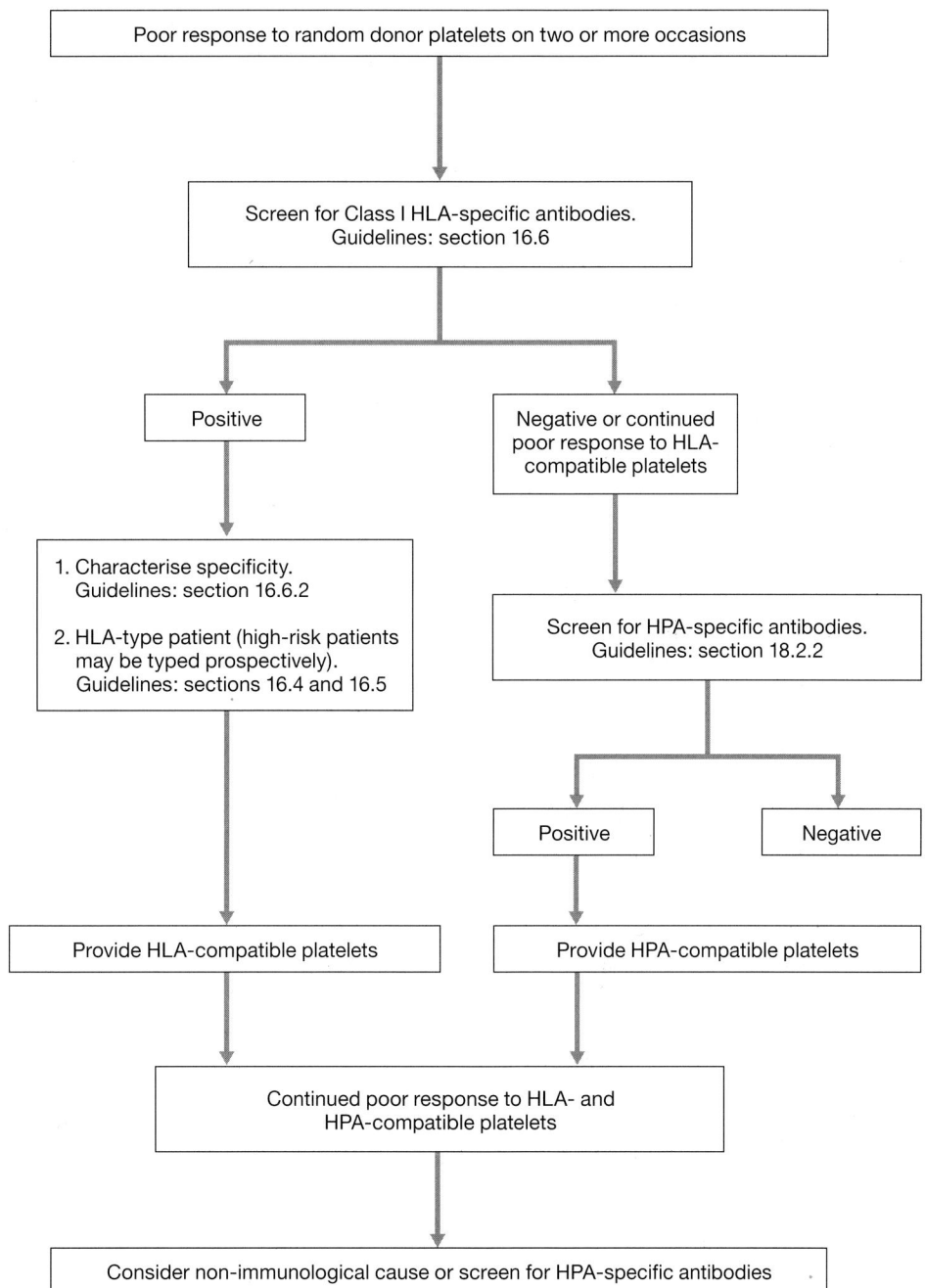

Figure 16.1 Algorithm for laboratory investigation of platelet refractoriness

16.8.5 Investigation of refractoriness

The investigation of refractoriness (see Figure 16.1) and the provision of selected platelets in such cases should comply with the British Committee for Standards in Haematology (BCSH) Guidelines for the Use of Platelet Transfusions.[5] Serological investigation of suspected immune refractoriness requires screening for HLA Class I-specific antibodies only, but the screening technique must detect HLA-A, HLA-B, and HLA-C-specific antibodies. Any screen-positive patient should be tested further for specificity to include all the Class I antigens listed in Table 16.2.

If a patient has HLA-specific antibodies that cannot be completely characterised, or a specificity corresponding to any of the donor's HLA Class I antigens cannot be excluded, then a crossmatch between donor and patient may be performed as described above.

16.8.6 Investigation of TRALI

Sera from all implicated donors must be screened for both HLA Class I and Class II-specific antibodies and HNA antibodies (see section 16.6.2).

Any screen-positive serum should be further characterised for HLA Class I and Class II to identify the antibody specificity.

If any of the implicated donors are shown to have HLA-specific antibodies the patient should be typed for HLA Class I and Class II to determine the presence of alleles/antigens corresponding to the antibody specificities found in the donor(s).

If a donor serum has HLA-specific antibodies that cannot be completely characterised, or a specificity corresponding to any of the patient's HLA antigens cannot be excluded, then a crossmatch between donor and patient should be performed.

See Figure 16.2 which gives an algorithm for laboratory investigation of TRALI.

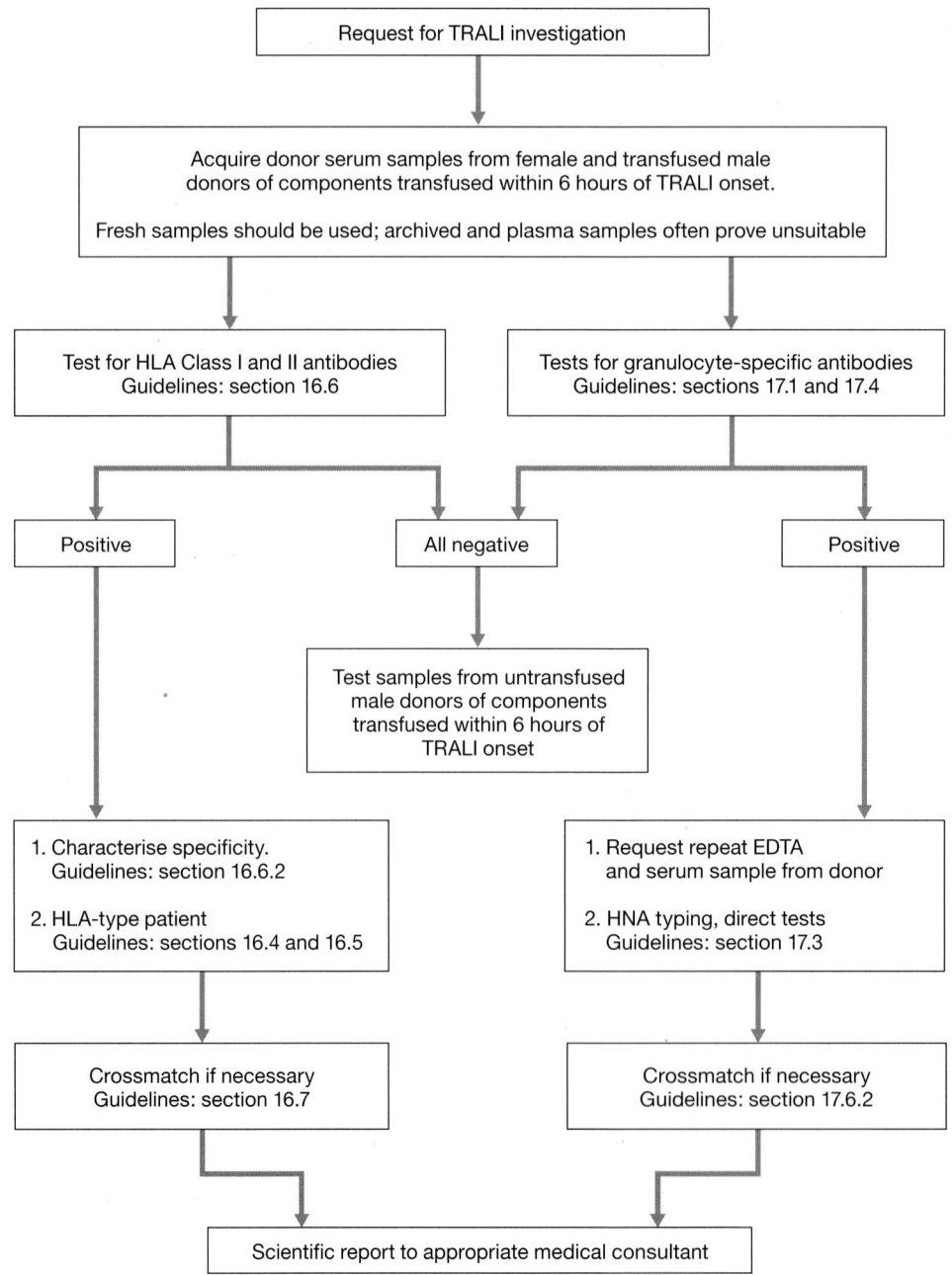

Figure 16.2 Algorithm for laboratory investigation and reporting of TRALI case

16.8.7 Investigation of febrile transfusion reactions

If an investigation is requested, sera from patients should be screened for both HLA Class I and Class II-specific antibodies. Any screen-positive serum should be further characterised for HLA Class I and Class II specificities to include all those listed in Table 16.2.

16.8.8 Investigation of female donors to reduce the incidence of TRALI

Many transfusion services have introduced screening for HLA or HLA and HNA antibodies to reduce the incidence of TRALI. An initial screen for HLA antibodies may be followed by a screen for HNA antibodies to further reduce the potential incidence of TRALI (see section 16.8.6). Female blood donors should be investigated for HLA antibodies following the guidelines set out in section 16.6. There is no requirement to determine the specificity of any HLA antibodies detected or type the donor for HLA.

16.9 References

1. The European Federation for Immunogenetics (EFI) Standards. Available at www.efiweb.eu.

2. WHO Nomenclature Committee for Factors of the HLA System Report. Available at www.anthonynolan.org.uk.

3. Marsh SGE (2010). Nomenclature for Factors of the HLA System. *Tissue Antigens*, 65, 291–455.

4. Holdsworth R *et al.* (2009). The HLA dictionary 2008: a summary of HLA-A, -B, -C, -DRB1/3/4/5, and -DQB1 alleles and their association with serologically defined HLA-A, -B, -C, -DR, and -DQ antigens. *Tissue Antigens*, 73, 95–170.

5. British Committee for Standards in Haematology (2003). Guidelines for the Use of Platelet Transfusions. *British Journal of Haematology*, 122, 10–23.

Chapter 17
Granulocyte immunology

17.1 Reagent manufacture/reference preparations/cell panels

17.1.1 HNA typing reagents

There are several human neutrophil antigen (HNA) genotyping and phenotyping techniques. The latter are generally based on the use of polyclonal HNA alloantibodies obtained from immunised donors or patients or monoclonal antibodies. HNA typing techniques that do not require polyclonal antibodies derived from donors or patients are the techniques of choice.

HNA typing reagents prepared from human source material should comply with the guidelines in section 11.1.4.10.

An 'Instructions for use' sheet (package insert) should be prepared and supplied with antibody typing reagents, see section 11.1.4.12. Information in the instructions for use sheet should further indicate the immunoglobulin class of the antibodies and the presence of any other contaminating antibodies reactive by the recommended methods.

HNA typing reagents used in genomic DNA and polymerase chain reaction (PCR)-based techniques should comply with the guidelines in Chapter 14.

17.1.2 Composition of granulocyte cell panel for HNA antibody detection

It is recommended that laboratories make all reasonable efforts to include cells in their panel that will aid the detection and identification of clinically significant HNA antibodies. The panel should consist of granulocytes typed for HNA-1a, 1b, 1c, 2, 3a, 3b, 4a, 4bw, 5a and 5bw by validated HNA typing techniques. Ideally, the panel should contain granulocytes that are homozygous for HNA-1a and HNA-1b and be from Group O donors. The panel can be expanded to include granulocytes homozygous for other HNA as indicated by the results of laboratory testing.

HNA typing of a granulocyte panel donor should be based on two concordant typings performed on samples obtained on different occasions. Wherever possible, both phenotyping and genotyping should be performed for the above antigens.

17.1.3 The preparation of granulocytes/lymphocytes

Granulocytes and lymphocytes for use in serological investigations should be prepared with regard to the following criteria:

- Granulocytes/lymphocytes should be prepared from donors/patients within 24 hours of venesection. Precautions must be taken to minimise activation of granulocytes during isolation.

- Granulocyte/lymphocyte preparations should be essentially free from red cells that would otherwise interfere with the technique or its reading.

- The viability of isolated granulocytes should be sufficient as to not interfere in the technique or its reading.

17.1.4 Selection of normal control sera

Normal control sera should be taken from untransfused male blood donors. The sera should be screened and found negative for granulocyte-reactive antibodies (e.g. clinically non-significant autoantibodies are occasionally detected in apheresis donors). An appropriate number of normal sera should be used, so that in any given assay a statistically relevant normal range can be determined.

17.1.5 Selection of positive control sera

At least one positive control should be included in each assay. The selection and number of positive control sera will depend on the technique and the HNA type of the granulocytes being used. In glycoprotein-specific assays, a positive control for each glycoprotein used should be included as a minimum. If different capture monoclonal antibodies are used, the positive control selected should be reactive with the monoclonal antibody selected.

17.1.6 Reference preparations

Sensitivity of techniques should be monitored on the basis of the inclusion of a 'weak positive' control. For anti-HNA-1a, the internal sensitivity control should be calibrated against the WHO International Reference Reagents for anti-HNA-1a (NIBSC code 09/284) when diluted as instructed by the manufacturer.

In-house sensitivity standards, with similar reaction strengths to the above reagent, should be prepared for other HNA antibodies.

17.1.7 Quality control schemes

Laboratories should take part in regular external quality control exercises such as the International Granulocyte Immunology Workshops for HNA antibody detection and for HNA genotyping. Effective mechanisms should be in place to correct poor performance in the quality scheme.

17.2 Nomenclature

The current nomenclature for HNA and corresponding antibodies must be used for recording granulocyte-specific alloantigen and alloantibody specificities[1] (see Table 17.1).

Table 17.1 Current nomenclature for HNA and corresponding antibodies

System	Antigen	Original name	Glycoprotein	CD
HNA-1	HNA-1a	NA1	$Fc_\gamma RIIIb$	CD16
	HNA-1b	NA2	$Fc_\gamma RIIIb$	CD16
	HNA-1c	SH	$Fc_\gamma RIIIb$	CD16
HNA-2	HNA-2	NB1	GP56-64kDa	CD177
HNA-3	HNA-3a	5b	CTL-2	
	HNA-3b	5a	CTL-2	
HNA-4	HNA-4a	MART[a]	CD11/18	CD11b
	HNA-4bw		CD11/18	CD11b
HNA-5	HNA-5a	OND[a]	CD11/18	CD11a
	HNA-5bw		CD11/18	CD11a

17.3 HNA typing methods

HNA types should be determined using antibody-based and DNA/PCR-based techniques that have been validated in the laboratory.

Polyclonal human anti-HNA antisera used in serological techniques should be well characterised. There is no requirement to use typing antisera that are ABO compatible with the granulocytes since the available evidence suggests that granulocytes either do not express Blood Group A or B antigens or do so very weakly.

17.4 HNA antibody detection methods

There are several techniques for the detection of HNA-reactive antibodies. These techniques can be divided into non-specific (where intact granulocytes are used, e.g. granulocyte immunofluorescence test, granulocyte agglutination test) and specific assays (where glycoprotein capture, or purified glycoproteins or recombinant antigens are used, e.g. monoclonal antibody immobilisation of granulocyte antigen test). Laboratories should use tests with adequate sensitivity for the detection and identification of HNA-reactive antibodies. It is recommended that more than one technique is used to detect HNA-specific antibodies.

The combination of chosen technique(s) and the composition of the cell panel cells (if applicable) must ensure:

- The detection of clinically significant HNA-reactive alloantibodies to the antigens of the HNA-1, HNA-2, HNA-3, HNA-4 and HNA-5 systems.

- The detection and identification of HNA-reactive antibodies in samples containing a mixture of both HNA and HLA-reactive antibodies, including antibodies to HNA-3 system antigens, which is expressed on both granulocytes and lymphocytes.

- The identification of the individual HNA specificities in samples containing mixtures of alloantibodies against several HNA antigens (e.g. masking of certain HNA specificities by composition of the panel).

- Techniques should be available to detect cytotoxic and non-cytotoxic anti-lymphocyte antibodies and thereby aid the distinction between granulocyte-specific, lymphocyte-reactive and HLA Class I and Class II antibodies.

Where granulocyte-specific antibodies are detected, which appear to have allo-specificity, but the specificity cannot be determined, the samples should be referred to a reference laboratory for further antibody specificity investigations. However, laboratories should make all reasonable efforts to screen against the widest possible range of HNA antigens.

17.4.1 Validation of laboratory kits

- Kits for the detection of HNA-reactive antibodies should be validated for sensitivity and specificity on a batch basis using a panel of clinically representative HNA antisera. It is recommended that the sensitivity of HNA antibody detection should be monitored using a panel of antisera containing 'weak' reactive HNA antibodies (not obtained by dilution of strongly reactive HNA typing sera). A panel of sera shown to be inert for HNA and HLA antibodies should also be used.

- Kits for HNA typing should be validated for specificity on a batch basis using nine donors (three donors homozygous for each HNA allele together with three heterozygotes).

17.5 Donor testing

17.5.1 HNA typing

HNA typing of donors whose granulocytes may be transfused to support HNA-immunised recipients should, wherever possible, be typed twice using samples collected on different occasions. However, it may be necessary to issue HNA-selected products on the basis of a single or 'unconfirmed' type.

17.5.2 Investigation of HNA antibodies

HNA antibody specificities should only be assigned when the sample investigated has been tested and a minimum of three positive and three negative reactions obtained with a single technique or a minimum of two positive and two negative reactions with two techniques. A report identifying the antibody can be issued at this stage. A donor with an HNA alloantibody should receive an HNA antibody card and an information leaflet, wherever this is available. However, before an HNA antibody card and information leaflet is issued, the donor should be typed (on one occasion but ideally by two methods) and found negative for that antigen.

17.5.3 Investigation of female donors to reduce the incidence of TRALI

Many transfusion services have introduced screening for HLA or HLA and HNA antibodies to reduce the incidence of transfusion-related acute lung injury (TRALI). An initial screen for HLA antibodies may be followed by a screen for HNA antibodies to further reduce the potential incidence of TRALI. Female blood donors should be investigated for HNA antibodies following the guidelines for donor investigation, except that there is only a requirement to test for IgG antibodies. The screening techniques used should enable detection of HNA-1a, -1b, -2 and -3a antibodies which are known to be implicated in causing TRALI.

HLA antibodies should be investigated using the guidelines set out in section 16.6.

17.6 Patient testing

17.6.1 HNA typing

Patients should be typed for HNA following the guidelines for donor HNA typing. A provisional type can be issued on the basis of a phenotype/genotype performed on one occasion. However, it is recommended that, if possible, a second typing technique be used on the first occasion of testing, especially where quality exercises or routine practice have revealed technical problems in typing for particular polymorphisms.

17.6.2 Investigation of HNA antibodies

Patients should be investigated for HNA antibodies following the guidelines for donor investigation. However, laboratories providing diagnostic tests for neonatal alloimmune neutropenia (NAIN) are advised to investigate cases with a clinical diagnosis of possible NAIN and a negative HNA antibody screen for antibodies against low-frequency or 'private' antigens. An effective approach is to use granulocytes from the child's father as an additional panel cell (paternal granulocytes should be HNA typed as a 'patient sample'). Alternatively, laboratories may refer such cases to a reference laboratory.

In the investigation of TRALI, implicated donor samples should be investigated for the presence of both HNA and HLA Class I and Class II antibodies (see also section 16.6). There is usually no requirement to investigate the patient's serum for HNA or HLA antibodies, but if this is necessary both pre- and post-transfusion samples (where available) should be investigated. Where antibody specificities are identified, the donor and patient should be typed to determine the presence or absence of the cognate antigen. If required, a crossmatch may be performed between the implicated donor serum samples and granulocytes/lymphocytes from the patient to determine the clinical relevance of any antibodies and the presence of any low-frequency antibodies. When 'pooled' platelet products are implicated in a case of TRALI, consideration should also be given to the possibility of the formation of inter-donor immune complexes. In such cases, all the donors who contributed to the pool should also be HNA and HLA typed. In a small proportion of TRALI cases, patient antibodies may react with infused donor cells/antigens and it may be necessary to incubate the patient's serum with granulocytes/lymphocytes from the donor.

Crossmatch studies in both suspected NAIN and TRALI cases require that the granulocytes/lymphocytes are isolated from the patient's blood samples within 24 hours of venesection.

A patient or donor with HNA alloantibodies should receive an HNA antibody card and an information leaflet wherever this is available.

17.6.3 Controls for direct tests for granulocyte bound immunoglobulins

Anticoagulated blood samples, less than 24 hours old, from a sufficient number of different normal donors to give a statistically valid normal range, should be used as control samples for the determination of granulocyte-bound immunoglobulins.

17.7 References

1. Bux J (1999). Nomenclature of granulocyte alloantigens. ISBT Working party on Platelet and Granulocyte Serology, Granulocyte Antigen Working Party. International Society of Blood Transfusion. *Transfusion*, 39(6), 662–663.

Chapter 18
Platelet immunology

18.1 Reagent manufacture/reference preparations

18.1.1 HPA typing reagents

- There are several human platelet antigen (HPA) genotyping and phenotyping techniques. The latter are generally based on the use of polyclonal HPA alloantibodies obtained from immunised donors or patients, or monoclonal antibodies. HPA typing techniques that do not require polyclonal antibodies derived from donors or patients are the techniques of choice.

- HPA typing reagents prepared from human source material should comply with the guidelines in section 11.1.4.10. An 'Instructions for use' sheet (package insert) should be prepared and supplied with antibody typing reagents. Information in the 'Instructions for use' should further indicate the immunoglobulin class of the antibodies and the presence of any other contaminating antibodies reactive by the recommended methods.

- HPA typing reagents used in genomic DNA and PCR-based techniques should comply with the guidelines in Chapter 14.

18.1.2 Composition of platelet cell panel for HPA antibody detection

- It is recommended that laboratories make all reasonable efforts to include cells in their panel that will aid the detection and identification of clinically significant HPA antibodies. The panel should consist of platelets typed at a minimum for HPA-1, -2, -3, -5 and -15 by validated HPA typing techniques. Ideally, the panel should contain platelets that are homozygous for HPA-1a, -1b, -2a, -2b, -3a, -3b, -5a, -5b, -15a and -15b and be from Group O donors.

- HPA typing of a platelet panel donor should be based on two concordant typings performed on samples obtained on different occasions. Wherever possible, phenotyping for the above antigens should also be performed on one occasion.

18.1.3 Selection of normal control sera

Normal control sera should be taken from non-transfused group AB male or ABO compatible blood donors. The sera should be screened and found negative for platelet-reactive-antibodies (e.g. clinically non-significant autoantibodies or EDTA-dependent antibodies are occasionally detected in apheresis donors). An appropriate number of normal sera should be used so that a statistically relevant normal range in a given assay can be determined.

18.1.4 Selection of positive control sera

At least one positive control should be included in each assay. The selection and number of positive control sera will depend on the technique and the HPA type of the platelets being used. In glycoprotein-specific assays a positive control for each glycoprotein used should be included as a minimum.

18.1.5 Reference preparations

- Sensitivity of techniques should be monitored on the basis of the inclusion of a 'weak positive' control. For anti-HPA-1a, -3a and -5b, the internal sensitivity control should be calibrated against the WHO International Reference Reagents for anti-HPA-1a (NIBSC code 05/106), anti-HPA-3a (NIBSC code 03/190) and anti-HPA-5b (NIBSC code 99/666) when diluted as instructed by the manufacturer.

- In-house sensitivity standards, with similar reaction strengths to the above reagents, should be prepared for anti-HPA-1, -3 and -5, and, if possible, for anti-HPA-2 and -15 antibodies.

Table 18.1 Current HPA nomenclature

System	Antigen	Original names	Glycoprotein	CD
HPA-1	HPA-1a	Zw^a, Pl^{A1}	GPIIIa	CD61
	HPA-1b	Zw^b, Pl^{A2}		
HPA-2	HPA-2a	Ko^b	GPIbalpha	CD42b
	HPA-2b	Ko^a, Sib^a		
HPA-3	HPA-3a	Bak^a, Lek^a	GPIIb	CD41
	HPA-3b	Bak^b		
HPA-4	HPA-4a	Yuk^b, Pen^a	GPIIIa	CD61
	HPA-4b	Yuk^a, Pen^b		
HPA-5	HPA-5a	Br^b, Zav^b	GPIa	CD49b
	HPA-5b	Br^a, Zav^a, Hc^a		
	HPA-6bw	Ca^a, Tu^a	GPIIIa	CD61
	HPA-7bw	Mo^a	GPIIIa	CD61
	HPA-8bw	Sr^a	GPIIIa	CD61
	HPA-9bw	Max^a	GPIIb	CD41
	HPA10bw	La^a	GPIIIa	CD61
	HPA11bw	Gro^a	GPIIIa	CD61
	HPA12bw	Iy^a	GPIbbeta	CD42c
	HPA13bw	Sit^a	GPIa	CD49b
	HPA14bw	Oe^a	GPIIIa	CD61
HPA-15	HPA-15a	Gov^b	CD109	CD109
	HPA-15b	Gov^a		
	HPA-16bw	Duv^a	GPIIIa	CD61
	HPA-17bw	Va^a	GPIIIa	CD61
	HPA-18bw	Cab^a	GPIa	CD49b
	HPA-19bw	Sta	GPIIIa	CD61
	HPA-20bw	Kno	GPIIb	CD41
	HPA-21bw	Nos	GPIIIa	CD61
	HPA-22bw	Sey	GPIIb	CD41
	HPA-23bw	Hug	GPIIIa	CD61
	HPA-24bw	$Cab2^{a+}$	GPIIb	CD41
	HPA-25bw	Swi^a	GPIa	CD49b
	HPA-26bw	Sec^a	GPIIIa	CD61
	HPA-27bw	Cab^{3a+}	GPIIb	CD41

18.1.6 Quality control schemes

Laboratories should take part in regular external quality control exercises such as the National Institute for Biological Standards and Control (NIBSC) Platelet Immunology Quality Scheme for HPA antibody detection and for HPA genotyping. Effective mechanisms should be in place to correct poor performance in the quality scheme.

18.1.7 Nomenclature

The current HPA nomenclature must be used for recording platelet-specific alloantigen and alloantibody specificities[1] (see Table 18.1). Any subsequent additions can be found in the Immuno Polymorphism Database (IPD) website (www.ebi.ac.uk/ipd/hpa/).

18.2 Methods

18.2.1 HPA typing methods

- HPA types should be determined using antibody-based and DNA/PCR-based techniques that have been validated in the laboratory.

- Polyclonal human anti-HPA antisera used in serological techniques should be well characterised. When used in techniques with 'intact' platelets the antisera should be ABO compatible with the platelets to be typed. Alternatively, anti-A and anti-B antibodies may be removed by absorption or neutralisation. This is not a requirement when using human antisera in glycoprotein capture assays, but reactivity against ABO incompatible platelets should be assessed. Sera shown to contain anti-A/B activity in these assays should be subject to the same requirements as those used in 'intact' platelet assays.

18.2.2 HPA antibody detection methods

- There are several techniques for the detection of HPA-reactive antibodies. These techniques can be divided into non-specific (where intact platelets are used, e.g. platelet immunofluorescence test, solid phase adherence assay) and specific assays (where glycoprotein capture, or purified glycoproteins or recombinant antigens are used, e.g. monoclonal antibody-specific immobilisation of platelet antigen assay). Laboratories should use tests with adequate sensitivity for the detection and identification of HPA-reactive antibodies.

- The combination of chosen technique(s) and the composition of the cell panel cells (if applicable) must ensure:

  - the detection of clinically significant HPA-reactive alloantibodies in the HPA-1, HPA-2, HPA-3, HPA-5 and HPA-15 systems

  - the identification of HPA-reactive antibodies and their specificity in samples containing a mixture of HPA and HLA-reactive antibodies

  - the identification of the specificities in samples containing mixtures of alloantibodies against several HPA antigens (i.e. avoiding the masking of certain HPA specificities by the composition of the panel).

- Where HPA-reactive antibodies are detected, but the specificity cannot be determined, the samples should be referred to a reference laboratory for antibody specificity investigations. However, all reasonable efforts should be made to screen against the widest possible range of HPA antigens.

18.2.3 Validation of laboratory kits

- Kits for the detection of HPA-reactive antibodies should be validated for sensitivity and specificity on a batch basis using a panel of clinically representative HPA antisera. It is recommended that for monitoring of the sensitivity of HPA antibody detection the panel of antisera should contain 'weak' reactive HPA antibodies (not obtained by dilution of strongly reactive HPA typing sera). A panel of sera shown to be inert for HPA and HLA antibodies should also be used.

- Kits for HPA typing should be validated for specificity on a batch basis using nine donors (three donors homozygous for each HPA allele together with three heterozygotes).

18.3 Donor testing

18.3.1 HPA typing

Donors whose products may be used for fetal/neonatal transfusions should be HPA typed twice using samples collected on different occasions. Further HPA typing at subsequent donations is not required after a confirmed type has been established. HPA typing of other donors need only be performed on one occasion and HPA-selected products may be issued on the basis of this 'unconfirmed' type.

18.3.2 Investigation of HPA antibodies

HPA antibody specificities should only be assigned when the sample investigated has been tested and a minimum of three positive and three negative reactions obtained. An antibody report can be issued at this stage. A donor with an HPA antibody should receive an HPA antibody card and an information leaflet. However, before an HPA antibody card and information leaflet is issued, the donor should be typed and found negative for that antigen.

18.4 Patient testing

18.4.1 HPA typing

Patients should be typed for HPA following the guidelines for donor HPA typing with the following exceptions:

- A provisional type can be issued on the basis of a genotype performed on one occasion. However, it is recommended that a second typing technique be used when quality exercises or routine practice have revealed technical problems when typing for particular polymorphisms. Typing of subsequent samples will allow a confirmed genotype to be reported.

- HPA typing of fetal amniocytes can be undertaken by molecular techniques using DNA isolated from non-cultured amniocytes and a provisional HPA genotype reported. The HPA genotype should be repeated on DNA extracted from cultured amniocytes and shown to be concordant with the first result.

18.4.2 Investigation of HPA antibodies

Patients should be investigated for HPA antibodies following the guidelines for donor investigation with the following exceptions:

- Laboratories serving populations with non-Caucasoid patients are advised to include cells in their panels which will aid the detection and identification of additional clinically significant antibodies (e.g. HPA-4, Naka/GPIV). If the acquisition of GPIV negative cells is not possible, an alternative approach is to establish assays capable of identifying GPIV antibodies that are controlled by appropriate positive control sera.

- Laboratories providing diagnostic testing for Neonatal Alloimmune Thrombocytopenia (NAITP) are advised to investigate cases with a clinical diagnosis suggestive of NAITP and a negative HPA antibody screen for antibodies against low-frequency or 'private' antigens. An effective approach is to use platelets from the child's father as an additional panel cell (paternal platelets should be HPA typed as a 'patient sample'). Alternatively, laboratories may refer such cases to a reference laboratory. In the event of a negative antibody screen in a case where NAITP is suspected and there is a potential HPA incompatibility between maternal and baby HPA types, laboratories are advised to repeat the antibody investigation 1 month after delivery.

- Laboratories providing diagnostic testing for platelet refractoriness should follow the algorithm for laboratory investigations of platelet refractoriness in Figure 16.1.

A patient with HPA antibodies should receive an HPA antibody card and, wherever possible, an information leaflet. However, before an HPA antibody card and information leaflet is issued, the patient should be typed and found negative for that antigen.

18.5 References

1. Metcalfe P, Watkins NA, Ouwehand WH, Kaplan C, Newman P, Kekomaki R, De Haas M, Aster R, Shibata Y, Smith J, Kiefel V, Santoso S. (2003). Nomenclature of Human Platelet Antigens. *Vox Sanguinis*, 85, 240–245.

Chapter 19
Tissue banking: general principles

19.1 Regulatory environment in the UK

The whole process of tissue banking is now covered by legislation. The EU Directive on Tissues and Cells (2004/23/EC)[1] and its associated Commission Directives (2006/17/EC and 2006/86/EC)[2,3] have been transposed into UK law as the Human Tissue (Quality and Safety for Human Application) Regulations 2007.[4] These regulations lay down standards of quality and safety for all aspects of banking of human tissues and cells intended for human applications. In addition, the Human Tissue Act 2004[5] applies throughout the UK with the exception of Scotland, where the Human Tissue (Scotland) Act 2006[6] applies.

All Tissue Establishments need to be licensed by the 'Competent Authority', which in the case of the UK is the Human Tissue Authority (HTA). Under the Human Tissue Act the HTA issues its expected standards in the form of 'Directions'[7] and 'Codes of Practice'[8] to Tissue Establishments. HTA expected standards are contained in the Guide to Quality and Safety Assurance for Human Tissues and Cells for Patient Treatment,[7] which is implemented via Directions and is periodically updated.

Every Tissue Establishment must designate a responsible person (termed the Designated Individual[4]) who shall be responsible for ensuring that all activities relating to human tissues and cells intended for human application are in accordance with the laws in force in the UK. It is therefore the responsibility of the Designated Individual to ensure that all the requirements of the HTA are met in a timely and comprehensive manner.

19.2 Reference documents for tissue banking

The advice contained in these guidelines is believed to represent acceptable practice at the time of writing. It is policy to revise these guidelines as new developments occur. However, it may not be possible to do so at the time of such change and the guidelines should therefore be used with due regard to current acceptable practice.

The guidelines in Chapters 19–21 apply to tissue banking activities within the Transfusion Services of the UK. They must be read in conjunction with the other sections of the guidelines including regulatory environment in the UK, quality in Blood and Tissue Establishments, microbiology tests for donors and donations and labelling of human tissue products.

Reference should be made to the current version of the JPAC *Donor Selection Guidelines*[9] available at www.transfusionguidelines.org.uk.

Other key documents relating to tissue banking are listed in the references at the end of this chapter.[10,11,12,13,14,15,16]

19.3 Data protection and confidentiality

Living donors and families of deceased donors must be told that information relating to the donation will be stored in accordance with the Data Protection Act (DPA)1998[17] and may be shared with relevant health professionals.

Tissue Establishments shall take the necessary measures to ensure that all data, collated within the scope of all their banking activities and to which third parties have access, have been rendered anonymous so that neither donor nor recipients remain identifiable.

19.4 References

1. Directive 2004/23/EC of the European Parliament and of the Council of 31 March 2004 on setting standards of quality and safety for the donation, procurement, testing, processing, preservation, storage and distribution of human tissues and cells. *OJ*, L 102, 07.04.2004, p48.

2. Commission Directive 2006/17/EC of 8 February 2006 implementing Directive 2004/23/EC of the European Parliament and of the Council as regards certain technical requirements for the donation, procurement and testing of human tissues and cells. *OJ*, L 038, 09.02.2006, p40.

3. Commission Directive 2006/86/EC of 24 October 2006 implementing Directive 2004/23/EC of the European Parliament and of the Council as regards traceability requirements, notification of serious adverse reactions and events and certain technical requirements for the coding, processing, preservation, storage and distribution of human tissues and cells. *OJ*, L 294, 25.10.2006, p32.

4. Statutory Instrument 2007 No. 1523 The Human Tissue (Quality and Safety for Human Application) Regulations 2007. Available at www.legislation.gov.uk/uksi/2007/1523/made.

5. Human Tissue Act 2004 (except Scotland). Available at www.legislation.gov.uk.

6. Human Tissue (Scotland) Act 2006. Available at www.show.scot.nhs.uk.

7. Human Tissue Authority: Directions given under the Human Tissue Act 2004 to establishments licensed under the Quality and Safety Regulations, available at www.hta.gov.uk/legislationpoliciesandcodesofpractice/htalegaldirections.cfm:

    - 003/2010 implementing the 'Guide to Quality and Safety Assurance for Human Tissues and Cells for Patient Treatment'

8. Human Tissue Authority: Codes of Practice, available at www.hta.gov.uk:

    - Code 1. Consent
    - Code 2. Donation of solid organs for transplantation
    - Code 5. Disposal of human tissue
    - Code 8. Import and export of human bodies, body parts and tissue
    - Code 9. Research

9. Joint UKBTS/NIBSC Professional Advisory Committee's (JPAC) *Donor Selection Guidelines*. Available at www.transfusionguidelines.org.uk:

    - Tissue donor selection guidelines: living donors (TDSG-LD)
    - Tissue donor selection guidelines: deceased donors (TDSG-DD).

10. SaBTO (2011). Guidance on the Microbiological Safety of Organs, Tissues and Cells used in Transplantation. Available at www.dh.gov.uk/en/Publicationsandstatistics/Publications/PublicationsPolicyAndGuidance/DH_121497.

11. Council of Europe (2010) *Guide to Safety and Quality Assurance for the Transplantation of Organs, Tissues and Cells*, fourth edition. Council of Europe Publishing.

12. Royal College of Ophthalmologists (2008). Standards for retrieval of human ocular tissue used in transplantation, research and training. Available at www.rcophth.ac.uk

13. Medicines and Healthcare products Regulatory Agency (2007). *Rules and Guidance for Pharmaceutical Manufacturers and Distributors 2007.* London: Pharmaceutical Press.

14. EC Guidelines to Good Manufacturing Practice Volume 4, Annex 1 (2008 revision): Manufacture of Sterile Medicinal Products. Available at http://ec.europa.eu/health/documents/eudralex/vol-4/index_en.htm.

15. Directive 98/79/EC of the European Parliament and of the Council of 27 October 1998 on *in vitro* diagnostic medical devices. *OJ*, L 331, 07.12.98, p1.

16. The Royal College of Pathologists and the Institute of Biomedical Science (2009). *The Retention and Storage of Pathological Records and Specimens*, fourth edition.

17. Data Protection Act 1998. Available at www.legislation.gov.uk.

Chapter 20
Tissue banking: selection of donors

20.1 General considerations

The overall responsibility for applying the policies for the selection and care of tissue donors lies with the tissue bank designated clinician, who must have relevant clinical experience and will be familiar with the various legal statutes and relevant documents which apply to tissue banking (see Chapter 19). The tissue bank designated clinician must consult with relevant specialist advisors as appropriate.

The designated clinician will rely on procedures and documentation that enable the appropriate medical and behavioural history to be acquired, to prevent microbial infection and transmission of disease (including malignant or neurodegenerative disease) to the recipient. Decisions on donor assessment should be consistent with JPAC *Donor Selection Guidelines*.[1]

Tissues must be procured, transported, processed, stored and distributed according to the requirements stated in these guidelines (the Red Book).

Procedures must be in place to document a complete audit trail from donor to recipient. Tissue banks must ensure that tissues can be traced from the donor to the point of issue. It is the responsibility of the hospital to document the fate of the tissue from its receipt to its use or discard. This will ensure that the audit trail can be followed in both directions. Clinicians caring for the recipients of tissues associated with risks identified following the issue of tissue must be informed where pertinent. Mechanisms should be in place to ensure that confidentiality is maximised.

UK Blood Transfusion Services tissue banks may collect tissues from donors referred to them by a third party such as a donor transplant coordinator or another tissue bank and may also refer donors to other tissue banking agencies such as a cornea or research bank. Whenever information regarding donor medical and behavioural history and/or consent for donation is obtained by, or on behalf of, a third party this must be subject to a written agreement between the parties involved. The agreement must specify what information is required regarding the medical and behavioural history of the donor and consent for donation, the standards for obtaining this information and the responsibilities of both parties in ensuring that the information is accurate and properly documented. The information should, as a minimum, be provided in accordance with the guidance in this document and the current JPAC *Donor Selection Guidelines*.[1] It is the responsibility of the designated clinician to determine the bank's policy for the referral of donors.

20.2 Consent

Consent must be obtained and documented by appropriately trained professionals competent in the issues and processes of tissue donation. No coercion or inducement to donate must be applied during the consent procedure. The statutory requirements for consent are detailed in the relevant national legislation, the Human Tissue Act (2004)[2] and the Human Tissue (Scotland) Act 2006.[3]

Further detailed guidance is laid out in the current version of the Human Tissue Authority Code of Practice on Consent[4] and in the Guide to Quality and Safety Assurance for Human Tissues and Cells for Patient Treatment.[5]

Living donors must be competent to give consent before donations can be accepted. Where donors are not competent, national legislation and the guidance of the Human Tissue Authority (HTA) must be followed. When a deceased person (while alive and competent) has explicitly consented to donation of organs and tissues then that consent is sufficient for the activity to be lawful. Where the wishes of the deceased are unknown, the Human Tissue Acts rank persons in a qualifying relationship for the purpose of obtaining consent to organ and tissue donation. The consent of the nominated representative or the highest ranking person at the time of death should be sought. In circumstances where this person does not wish to deal with the issue of consent, or is unable to do so, the next person in the ranking order is approached, but it is advisable to record this in the notes.

Consent must cover retrieval, testing, storage, discard and access to medical records. If the tissue may be used for research and development, or teaching, specific consent must be obtained for this as well. Explicit information must be given if tissues are to be retrieved for specific commercial use. Living donors and families of deceased donors must be informed that information relating to the donation will be stored in accordance with the Data Protection Act (1998)[6] and may be shared with relevant healthcare professionals.

For deceased donors, information to be supplied to the next of kin regarding various aspects of tissue donation which forms the basis of consent should include the following:

- that reconstruction will be performed following retrieval
- explicit information on which tissue is to be retrieved and the clinical purpose to which it is to be put
- if tissue is found to be unsuitable for clinical transplantation it will be discarded via local discard policies or, if permission is granted, it may be used for research or educational purposes
- that the donor will be tested for markers of microbial infection including HIV and after individual case assessment, those relevant contacts will be informed in the event of a relevant confirmed positive result
- that details of medical and behavioural history will be sought from additional professional sources and recorded.

Where the Coroner (the Procurator Fiscal in Scotland) is in legal possession of the body, permission must be requested to undertake the retrieval.

20.3 Medical and behavioural history

The information noted in the following two subsections for living and deceased donors should be reviewed by the designated clinician who is familiar with the relevant standards in the field of tissue banking (see Chapter 19).

20.3.1 For living donors

Medical and behavioural history must be sought by appropriately trained professionals and in compliance with the following guidance.

- Information may be obtained from the donor by either face-to-face interview or by recorded telephone interview by appropriately trained tissue bank staff. This must allow for the exclusion of lifestyle infectious risks. During interviews, a mechanism should be in place to ensure that confidentiality is maximised.

    - The interview must be conducted while the donor is free from the effect of anaesthetic, hypnotic or narcotic medication. The donor must be mentally competent to give an accurate history.

    - If the medical interview is not done at the time of admission for surgery, a system must be in place to capture any relevant medical and behavioural history changes that may occur in the interval between interview and donation.

    - A standard questionnaire to elicit the medical and behavioural history must be used.

    - Donors should be selected according to the JPAC *Donor Selection Guidelines*.[1]

    - The completed questionnaire must be retained as part of the tissue bank donor record.

    - The medical records, if available, must be consulted to review the medical and behavioural history and the medical examination.

Further medical history may be sought, where appropriate, from:

- the general practitioner

- any other relevant medical personnel.

20.3.2 For deceased donors

The cause of death and the medical and behavioural history should elicit whether the donor meets the selection criteria outlined in the JPAC *Donor Selection Guidelines*.[1] Modifications for the behavioural and medical history questions may be needed when accepting paediatric donors. Where the deceased donor is less than 18 months of age, or breast fed within the 12-month period prior to donation, the mother's risk for transmissible disease must also be evaluated. Information must be sought from the following sources by appropriately trained professionals and must be documented using a standard form:

- The donor's next of kin or other person identified as the most likely to be in possession of relevant information.

- The medical notes if the donor was admitted to hospital prior to death.

- The general practitioner.

- The post-mortem (where one is undertaken). If no post-mortem is undertaken, the cause of death of the donor, as ascertained from the medical notes, must be documented in the tissue bank donor record.

A record must be made of how the donor was identified (e.g. toe tag, wristband) and by whom.

The deceased donor's external appearance should be thoroughly examined at the time of retrieval. The appearance must be documented with respect to the donor's medical and behavioural history, including the presence of any obvious medical intervention, scars, tattoos, skin or mucosal lesions, jaundice, infection, trauma or needle tracks.

The date and time of death must be documented, and where applicable the time the body was refrigerated.

20.4 Tissue-specific donor considerations

Reference must be made to the JPAC *Donor Selection Guidelines*[1] document for ages and other specific donor requirements for different tissues.

20.5 Donor testing

The general principles of microbiological testing and the specific testing requirements for tissue donors are covered in Chapter 9. Testing must be completed in a licensed Tissue Establishment or under a third party agreement between the testing laboratory and the licensed Tissue Establishment. If a third party laboratory is used to perform any aspect of donor testing, the specific requirements and responsibilities of both parties in achieving them must be defined in a written agreement. Such testing should, as a minimum, be performed in accordance with the guidance in this document. There should be protocols for assuring the veracity and security of the sample, labelling, and supporting documentation. The time from sample acquisition to testing or freezing of the sample should be minimised and must be consistent with test kit manufacturers' recommendations or validated for the purpose. Due consideration should be given to dilution of the sample (see section 20.7).

Additional discretionary testing may be required (e.g. for malaria, Chaga's disease or West Nile Virus), dependent on the donor's travel history. RhD testing may be required on donors if the retrieved tissues will contain residual red cells or red cell membranes at the time of implantation.

The tissue bank should have a documented policy to follow in the case of donors with reactive screening tests. There should be protocols for alternative or confirmatory testing and acceptance or rejection of donations.

A positive result should be notified urgently to the source bank, Specialist Nurse Organ Donation or supplier of the tissue or cells so that clinicians in all centres that have received material from the same donor can be informed and take appropriate action. Where tissue or cells from a donor have been sent to other banks or centres, these banks or centres must be told about the positive result. Reports of positive tests should be included in the routine donor surveillance programmes and notified to the HTA (see section 21.8).

20.6 Living donor samples

All blood samples from living donors must be acquired using positive donor identification by an individual trained to ensure the security of the sample and supporting documentation. Living donors can be tested by either a single sample taken at the time of donation where testing includes a nucleic acid amplification technique (NAT) or by two samples including a post-quarantine sample where additional NAT testing is not required.

Where only a single sample is tested the 'donation sample' must be obtained at the time of donation or, if not possible, within 7 days post-donation.

Where two samples are tested the 'post-quarantine sample' is required after an interval of at least 180 days from the date of donation. In these circumstances of repeat testing, the donation sample can be taken up to 30 days prior to and 7 days after donation. When the donation blood sample is taken prior to the date of tissue donation a system must be in place to ensure that the pre-quarantine sample reflects the risk status at the time of donation.

For amnion donation only a maternal sample is required, i.e. a cord blood sample is not required.

20.7 Deceased donor samples

Appropriate mechanisms must be in place to ensure:

- The secure identification of samples obtained from hospital laboratories. Where there is doubt about the identity of a blood sample from a tissue donor (inadequate labelling), DNA profiling may be accepted as an accurate method for confirming the identity of the blood sample.

- Documentation of the date and time the sample was taken, the name of the individual and laboratory supplying the sample and sample storage conditions.

An ante-mortem blood sample, up to 7 days preceding death, is always preferable to a post-mortem sample for testing. Where no ante-mortem sample is available, then a post-mortem sample can be used. Samples for testing must not be taken more than 24 hours post-mortem and the time from sampling to testing or freezing of the sample should be minimised and must be consistent with the test kit manufacturer's recommendations or validated for the purpose.

The anatomical site from which the post-mortem sample was obtained must be documented. The sample appearance should be documented. If the sample appears dilute or grossly haemolysed, a repeat sample, preferably from an alternative site, should be obtained if possible. Tissue banks should have a protocol for post-mortem sampling, clearly defining preferred sites for sampling (e.g. cardiac puncture or femoral vessel puncture and avoiding sites close to intravenous lines).

Where a deceased donor with significant blood loss has received ante-mortem transfusions, a pre-transfusion sample should be used whenever possible for testing. If a pre-transfusion sample is not available, tissue banks must employ an algorithm incorporating the timing, nature and volume of the fluids infused and the donor's own blood volume to assess any resultant plasma dilution (see the JPAC *Donor Selection Guidelines*[1] for an example of a deceased donor intravenous fluid report form). Samples of blood estimated to be more than 50% dilute are not suitable for testing.

For post-mortem samples, concluded test results other than negative will debar tissues from release unless a superior sample can be obtained (e.g. obtained ante-mortem or closer to the time of death), and this sample is tested and negative results are obtained. The acquisition of the 'superior' sample must be subject to the same requirements given above.

In the case of deceased neonatal or infant tissue donors the following blood samples are required:

- A maternal sample is required when an infant is less than 18 months of age or when an older child has been breast fed within the 12-month period prior to donation.

- For still births and neonates less than 48 hours after birth, no sample is required.

- For neonates between 48 hours and 28 days after birth, a sample is only required if there are identifiable risks of possible viral transmission, e.g. receiving blood components/products or undergoing a surgical procedure.

- For infants more than 28 days after birth, a sample is always required.

20.8 Follow-up

There is a duty of care to the donor and/or donor's family. For donors who on confirmatory testing have positive or indeterminate results, there should be protocols in place for contacting, counselling and referring the donor, or relevant contacts of the deceased donor, for further investigation and treatment as appropriate.

For living donors this should be at a local level where the donor was recruited. Confidentiality must be ensured and the donor's permission sought prior to referral for further medical follow-up and assessment.

In the case of a deceased donor, the initial contact should be by the medical team who provided clinical care at the time of death, or if death occurred outside a healthcare facility by the Specialist Nurse Organ Donation or the Tissue Establishment. They should ensure that those close contacts of the deceased donor for whom results may have health implications are appropriately informed and counselled. Appropriate specialist referral should be offered.

20.9 Autologous tissue donation

The designated clinician should decide the policy in relation to the provision of an autologous service.

Autologous donors should be tested for the same microbiological markers as for an allogeneic living donor. Microbiological testing must include bacteriological culture where tissue does not undergo a validated terminal antimicrobial treatment. The medical history may be less relevant than for allogeneic donation of tissues. The rationale for any exceptions must be documented.

Separate storage must be used to avoid inappropriate issue. Autologous tissue must be securely segregated from allogeneic tissue at all stages from collection to issue. Autologous donations may not be transferred to the allogeneic bank.

A system must be in place to enable the hospital to recognise that the tissue is autologous. The autologous tissue must be labelled with the donor/recipient name, hospital number and date of birth.

20.10 Archiving of donor samples

An archive blood sample should be kept for look-back investigations in the event of an adverse reaction. This must be for a minimum of 11 years after the expiry date of the tissue with the longest storage life.

Tissues can be held for a number of years prior to issue. During this period in storage there may be changes to the mandatory microbiology test requirements and improvements in screening assays for mandatory or other markers. Consideration should be given for an additional blood sample archive for tissues with a long expiry for possible future testing that is not currently available.

A policy regarding the need for re-testing of the tissue inventory needs to be established. Any policy adopted must be operationally feasible and will depend on both the maximum storage period of the tissue and the probability of the tissue being issued. When new, or significantly improved, mandatory tests are introduced consideration should be given to the re-testing of archive samples from the donors of tissue still in issuable stock. Where there is no archive sample available to test, a risk assessment must be performed. It should include factors such as the seriousness of the infection, any viral inactivation procedures performed on the tissue, the effect on inventory of discarding such tissues and the severity of impact of possible tissue shortages on recipients.

20.11 Release criteria

For allogeneic donors the concluded result of all microbiological assays, with the exception of syphilis and anti-HBc, must be negative for a tissue to be released from quarantine for issue.[7] For donors who are found to be 'repeat reactive' in any screening assay but for whom subsequent testing confirms lack of infection, the initial reactivity in the screening assay is due to non-specific reactivity and any tissue products from this donation may be safely released for clinical use.

In the case of a deceased infant donor where a maternal sample is found to be positive for any mandatory marker of infection, the donation must not be used irrespective of the test result for the infant.

Donors with a positive anti-HBc may be considered as eligible provided an anti-HBs has been documented at more than 100 IU/L at some time.

Donors with reactive confirmatory tests for the presence of treponemal infection should be fully assessed, taking into account the results of confirmatory (reference) testing and medical history. The presence of current (active) infection will exclude the use of tissues from such donors. Where the assessment leads to the conclusion that the risk of active infection is remote, then non-cardiovascular tissues may be used. The presence of serological marker patterns of treponemal infections (e.g. IgM positivity) should not be used as a sole criterion to determine the presence of active infection (and therefore their eligibility). Any reactive results obtained on confirmatory testing should be discussed with staff experienced in interpreting treponemal test results, before a decision is made to use tissues.

For autologous donors positive test results will not necessarily prevent the tissues or cells or any product derived from them being stored, processed and reimplanted, if appropriate isolated storage facilities are available to ensure no risk of cross-contamination with other grafts and/or no risk of mix-ups at issue.

20.12 References

1. Joint UKBTS/HPA Professional Advisory Committee's (JPAC) *Donor Selection Guidelines*. Available at www.transfusionguidelines.org.uk.

2. Human Tissue Act 2004 (except Scotland). Available at www.legislation.gov.uk.

3. Human Tissue (Scotland) Act 2006. Available at www.show.scot.nhs.uk.

4. Human Tissue Authority Code of Practice 1. Consent. Available at www.hta.gov.uk.

5. Human Tissue Authority Guide to Quality and Safety Assurance for Human Tissues and Cells for Patient Treatment. Available at www.hta.gov.uk.

6. Data Protection Act 1998. Available at www.legislation.gov.uk

7. SaBTO (2011). *Guidance on the Microbiological Safety of Organs, Tissues and Cells used in Transplantation*. Available at www.dh.gov.uk/en/Publicationsandstatistics/Publications/PublicationsPolicyAndGuidance/DH_121497

Chapter 21
Tissue banking: tissue retrieval and processing

21.1 General considerations

Tissue banks should have dedicated processing and storage facilities designed and operated to prevent contamination, cross-contamination, mislabelling and deterioration of tissues.

All processes which affect the safety or quality of tissues must be validated.

21.1.1 Equipment – retrieval/processing

All equipment which affects the safety or quality of tissues must be validated.

Where possible single-use instruments must be used.

If it is impractical or not possible to use single-use instruments and reusable equipment has to be used then the use must be risk assessed to ensure that all required mitigating actions are considered. Tissue bank reusable instruments and other items which come into direct contact with donor tissue during retrieval and processing must be thoroughly washed and sterilised between uses. These must be fully traceable to the individual tissue donor/batch and allow tracking through decontamination, sterilisation and use. These instruments should be washed and sterilised according to NHS Estates Health Technical Memoranda (HTM) 2010,[1] 2030[2] and 2031.[3] Instruments must not be allowed to dry out before washing prior to sterilisation. Prompt removal of residual blood and tissues is an important aspect of decontamination, particularly with regard to Creutzfeldt-Jakob Disease (CJD).

21.1.2 Incoming materials and solutions

All purchased materials and solutions which affect the tissue quality and safety must be inspected on receipt to ensure compliance with specification.

21.1.3 Use of third parties

UK Blood Transfusion Services tissue banks may use third parties to perform tissue retrieval, processing steps such as irradiation, tissue evaluation such as bacterial tests, quality control tasks such as environmental monitoring or tissue storage, transport and distribution. Wherever such tasks are performed by or on behalf of a third party, this must be subject to a written agreement between the parties involved. This must specify the processes to be performed, the applicable standards and specifications, and the responsibilities of both parties in achieving the desired outcome. The processes should be performed, as a minimum, in accordance with the guidance given in HTA Direction 003/2010.[4]

21.1.4 Tissue contamination

In the event of a healthcare worker sustaining an injury such that his/her blood comes into contact with the tissue, the tissue must be discarded.

21.2 Retrieval

21.2.1 Retrieval times and preliminary storage

For eye donation retrieval must be completed within 24 hours after death and the body should preferably be refrigerated. For all other tissues retrieval should be as soon after death as possible. If the body has not been refrigerated, procurement of tissues must be completed within 12 hours after death. If the body has been refrigerated within 6 hours of death, procurement should preferably start within 24 hours and must be completed within 48 hours of death.

Tissues must be placed at a temperature of 0–10°C within 4 hours of retrieval.

21.2.2 General considerations for tissue retrieval

Every effort must be made to minimise contamination of tissue during procurement.

The procurement facility must be suitable for procurement of tissues and must be risk assessed prior to commencement of tissue retrieval.

A local sterile field must be created using sterile drapes. An appropriate antibacterial skin preparation agent must be used before commencing the retrieval.

All instruments used during the retrieval must be sterile and should be stored on a back table which is covered with a sterile drape. Where possible, single-use equipment should be used.

Staff conducting the retrieval must be appropriately gowned in sterile clothing, and wear sterile gloves and protective masks.

Every effort should be made to minimise the number of people present during deceased tissue retrieval and to ensure that a post-mortem is not proceeding during the retrieval.

Where possible the retrieval should precede any post-mortem examination of the donor. In cases referred to the Coroner (or the Procurator Fiscal in Scotland), the Coroner's consent must be obtained to enable the retrieval of tissues.

21.2.3 Deceased donor reconstruction

It is integral to the maintenance of the dignity of the donor that the body is cleaned and reconstruction is carefully undertaken. Whenever long bones are removed they must be replaced with appropriate prostheses. All incisions should be neatly sutured.

For similar reasons, skin must not be procured from the neck, arms, face or other areas that may affect funeral viewing.

Every effort should be made to ensure that appropriate advice on the handling of deceased donors after retrieval should be made available for mortuary and funeral home staff.

21.2.4 Labelling of donations

At the time of donation, the container for each category of tissue (e.g. skin, bone or heart valves) must be labelled with the nature of the contained tissue and a barcoded tissue or donor identification (ID) label as appropriate.

The accompanying donation record must be labelled with the same tissue or donor identification number(s), key donor identifiers (name, date of birth etc.), and the date of collection prior to removal from the retrieval site. Bacteriology and blood samples, together with accompanying documentation where relevant, must be labelled according to agreed local procedures such that the results can be linked to the correct donor/tissue while still preserving anonymity where required.

A double container system is required for all tissues retrieved. The containers must not be opened until ready for use or further aseptic processing at a facility approved by the tissue bank.

21.3 Transportation conditions from retrieval site to Tissue Establishment

Transportation systems must be validated to show maintenance of the required storage temperature.

The requirement for transport solution needs to be validated with respect to the preservation and characteristics required of the tissue to be transported.

For viable tissue the grafts should be placed into a transport solution with due regard to its effects on the ability of cells to propagate or metabolise. There must be adequate control of buffering capacity, osmolarity and tissue oxygenation. External contamination and desiccation must be avoided.

The type, lot, manufacturer and the expiry date of the transport solution must be documented.

21.4 Bacteriostasis and disinfection

21.4.1 Tissue without terminal antimicrobial processing

Tissue must be subjected to one of the following treatments, as soon as possible and within 24 hours of retrieval:

- antibiotic disinfection
- an alternative disinfection method
- frozen storage at –20°C or lower.

In the case of tissue taken from heart-beating donors in the operating theatre at the time of organ retrieval, this period may be extended to 48 hours.

21.4.2 Tissue with terminal antimicrobial processing

Bone from living donors which is refrigerated within 4 hours of retrieval but not frozen until 24–48 hours after retrieval must be subjected to terminal antimicrobial processing.

Tissue with terminal antimicrobial processing must be subjected to one of the treatments detailed in the above section within 24 hours of retrieval with a maximum of 72 hours following death. A summary of the guidance regarding temperature/time relationships contained in these guidelines is given in Table 21.1.

Table 21.1 Temperature/time relationships for banked tissues

Retrieval	If the body has not been refrigerated, procurement of tissues must be completed within 12 hours after death.
	If the body has been refrigerated within 6 hours of death procurement should preferably start within 24 hours and must be completed within 48 hours of death.
Retrieved tissue	Must be placed at an ambient temperature of 0–10°C within 4 hours of retrieval.
Bacteriostasis	Freezing tissue to at least −20°C within 24 hours of retrieval (or up to a maximum of 72 hours of death) can be used as a bacteriostatic treatment.
	Bone from living donors which is not frozen until 24–48 hours after retrieval must be subjected to terminal antimicrobial processing.
Long-term storage	**Frozen* non-viable tissue** may be stored:
	1. At −20°C or lower for up to 6 months.
	2. At −40°C or lower for up to 5 years. Temporary storage of frozen musculoskeletal tissue between −20°C and −40°C is limited to 6 months in total. Grafts stored at this temperature must then be transferred to −40°C or colder to give an expiry of up to a maximum of 5 years from donation.
	Cryopreserved** viable tissue should be stored:
	1. At −135°C or lower to claim a 10-year expiry for all grafts to maintain a reasonable inventory of size-matched grafts (e.g. heart valves and menisci). Other cryopreserved tissues should have a 5-year expiry.
	Glycerol-preserved tissue:
	1. Skin preserved in high-concentration (>90%) glycerol may be stored at 0–10°C for up to 2 years.
	2. Amnion preserved in low-concentration (50%) glycerol may be stored below −40°C for up to 2 years.
	Freeze-dried tissue may be stored at ambient temperature for up to 5 years.
Transportation and local storage	**Frozen* tissues** must be transported and stored locally prior to clinical use, at −20°C or lower in order to have the designated expiry (specified above).
	Cryopreserved** tissues may be transported in the vapour phase of liquid nitrogen (<−135°C) or on dry ice (−79°C). If tissues are transported on dry ice they should continue to be stored locally at around −80°C for a maximum of 6 months.
For the purposes of this guidance, the following definitions apply:	
* Frozen tissue – tissue frozen and stored under conditions unlikely to be compatible with preservation of cells.	
** Cryopreserved tissue – tissue treated with a cryoprotectant and/or cooled at a controlled rate in order to preserve cells.	

21.4.3 Positive bacteriology or mycology

It is the responsibility of the designated medical officer or designated microbiologist to develop written policies regarding the selection and conduct of tests for bacterial and fungal contamination and the acceptance criteria for specific tissues.

Where tissues are shown to carry viable bacteria or fungi they may be suitable for clinical use (e.g. skin grafts) depending on microbial types and densities of growth on culture. For other tissues the material may be approved for use provided that a validated antimicrobial processing technique is used.

21.5 General guidelines for tissue processing

Processing must not change the physical properties of the tissue so as to make it unacceptable for clinical use. Processing steps must be validated to demonstrate that the final product does not have any clinically significant residual toxicity.

21.5.1 Aseptic processing facilities

Facilities for aseptic processing must comply with the *Rules and Guidance for Pharmaceutical Manufacturers and Distributors 2007*[5] and EC Guidelines to Good Manufacturing Practice.[6] They must provide separate work areas with defined physical and microbiological parameters. Facilities must have:

- floors, walls and ceilings of non-porous smooth surfaces that are easily sanitised
- temperature control
- air filtered through high-efficiency particulate air (HEPA) filters with appropriate pressure differential between zones, which must be documented
- a documented system for monitoring temperature, air supply conditions, particle numbers and bacterial colony-forming units (environmental monitoring)
- a documented system for cleaning and disinfecting rooms and equipment
- a documented system for gowning and laundry
- adequate space for staff and storage of sterile garments
- access limited to authorised personnel
- documented system for general staff hygiene practices.

21.5.2 Tissue not destined for terminal microbial processing

Critical work areas are those where tissue is manipulated openly either following a disinfection or sterilisation step or in those cases where tissue has been procured aseptically and will not be further disinfected or sterilised. Critical work areas on which sterile containers, aseptically procured tissue or disinfected tissue are exposed to the environment, must have an air quality of Grade A and should have a Grade B background. (For further information see *Rules and Guidance for Pharmaceutical Manufacturers and Distributors 2007*[5] and the EC Guidelines to Good Manufacturing Practice.[6]) Any lowering to this standard in the background environment (as long as it is compliant with EU requirements) must be documented and it must be demonstrated that the chosen environment achieves the quality and safety required, at least taking into account the intended purpose, mode of application and immune status of the recipient.

Wherever possible, representative samples of tissue should be removed and tested for bacterial and fungal contamination using protocols authorised by the designated medical officer or designated microbiologist. Swabs or other validated non-destructive sampling methods should be used where it is impossible to remove tissue without damaging the graft. Microbiological inclusion/exclusion criteria should be developed by the designated medical officer or designated microbiologist in accordance with national policy.

Where tissues are processed in batches, procedures must ensure that no cross-contamination between batches can occur. Key process parameters and acceptance limits must be identified and validated. A full record of each process applied to each tissue or batch must be retained.

21.5.3 Tissue destined for terminal microbial processing

Work areas in which tissue materials and containers are prepared should have an environment with air quality of at least Grade C in the vicinity of exposed tissue.

Terminal antimicrobial processing must follow the filling of the final container. The procurement, processing and filling environment must be of sufficient quality to minimise the microbial contamination of the tissue to ensure that the subsequent antimicrobial processing is effective.

The tissue in its final container must be subjected to a validated procedure utilising an agent such as gamma irradiation. The processing method and dose of the sterilant should be validated as sufficient to bring about at least a six logarithms reduction in a recognised marker resistant organism (e.g. *Clostridium* sp. for irradiation).

21.5.3.1 Terminal sterilisation

Sterilisation is a statistical phenomenon, expressed as the probability of microorganisms surviving the procedure. The sterility assurance level (SAL) is the probability of a microorganism on one item within a batch or within a defined population. The accepted level for considering medical devices to be 'sterile' is a SAL of 10^{-6} (i.e. less than one item per million items will have a surviving microorganism on it). For medical devices, the microorganisms under consideration are contaminants (i.e. bacteria and fungi and their spores). Unless specifically stated, viruses are not routinely considered.

Because of the large numbers involved, demonstrating SAL of 10^{-6} must use procedures that extrapolate from smaller batches. For sterilisation procedures that show a $\log_{10}$/linear decrease in microbial viability, extrapolation can be achieved using the D-value (decimal reduction value) concept.

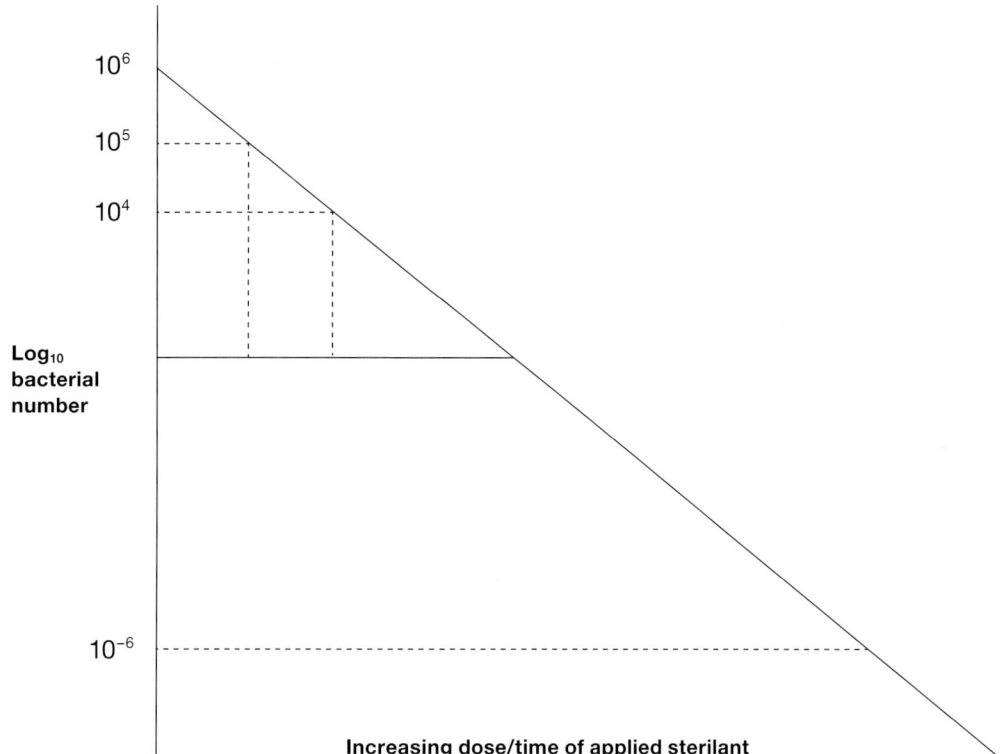

Figure 21.1 An example of increasing inactivation of bacteria related to increasing the dose of the sterilant

In the example shown in Figure 21.1, each log reduction requires an additional unit of the sterilant to be applied, hence D-value = 1.0. Therefore moving from an initial bioburden of 10^6 bacteria to a SAL of 10^{-6} would require 12 × D-value of the sterilant.

In practice, the processing that is applied to tissue grafts prior to application of the terminal sterilisation step often reduces the bioburden to close to zero. Therefore application of a sterilisation procedure sufficient to provide a 6-log reduction of bacteria is often satisfactory to achieve a SAL of 10^{-6}.

Very often, validation studies will be carried out using the microorganism that is known to be most resistant to the sterilisation procedure (often bacterial spores). This is therefore a 'worst-case' validation. Achieving a SAL of 10^{-6} for this microorganism will guarantee a significant overkill for more sensitive microbes.

21.5.3.2 Validation of terminal sterilisation

Whenever a novel terminal sterilisation step is introduced the following validations need to be addressed:

- That the sterilisation technique achieves a SAL of 10^{-6} for the most resistant microorganisms.

- That the sterilisation technique can be applied to the tissue graft in its final packaging without subsequent exposure, and that the integrity of the packaging is not adversely affected by the process.

- That the sterilisation technique does not adversely affect the essential properties of the graft and does not leave toxic residuals.

- That the sterilisation technique inactivates all categories of microorganisms commonly found on tissue grafts including vegetative Gram positive and Gram negative bacteria, vegetative fungi, and bacterial and fungal spores. This must be demonstrated either by literature review or validation.

21.5.4 Gamma irradiation

Gamma irradiation must be performed in a controlled manner to ensure that all tissue receives at least the minimum specified dose of radiation. This requires the use of standard packaging materials and irradiator load configuration and is usually validated using calibrated dosimeters placed throughout the load. The dose should never be less than 15 kGy, unless pre-irradiation processing has been validated to consistently yield a low microbial bioburden such that there is the required assurance, in accordance with medical device standards, that the dose will result in the tissue being sterile.

Tissue must be irradiated in its final packaging, which must bear a suitable indicator to demonstrate that it has been irradiated. This must be checked before release of the tissue.

If a dose in excess of 25 kGy is required, then consideration must be given to the possible detrimental effect on the biological and physical properties of the tissue.

Many viruses are resistant to irradiation and therefore any claim of viral inactivation must be supported by validation data obtained using appropriate marker viruses.

21.5.5 Pooling

Pooling of tissues from different donors is not permitted.

21.5.6 Preservation methods

Where specific attributes of a tissue are claimed, the process should be validated to show these attributes are preserved.

21.5.6.1 Freezing

For the purposes of this guidance this term applies to tissues that are frozen and stored under conditions that are unlikely to be compatible with preservation of cells. Frozen tissue must be stored below –20°C and the length of storage permitted depends on the temperature the tissues are stored at (see Table 21.1).

21.5.6.2 Cryopreservation

For the purposes of this guidance this term applies to tissues that are treated with a cryoprotectant and/or cooled at a controlled rate in order to preserve cells. Cryopreserved tissue must be stored below –135°C. For storage at higher temperatures, validation must be performed to demonstrate that the required properties of the graft are maintained for the stated expiry.

21.5.6.3 Freeze-drying

Where tissues are freeze-dried, a sample of each type of tissue from each freeze-drying run must be analysed for residual water which must be less than 5% (weight/weight) of the dry weight of the graft or equivalent residual water activity of between 0.2 and 0.5 Aw.

21.5.6.4 Glycerolisation

Where tissues are preserved by high concentrations of glycerol the procedure should be validated to demonstrate achievement of the specified glycerol concentration within the tissue or an acceptable range within the tissue.

21.5.7 Solutions

Rinse solutions, antibiotic mixtures, nutrient media and cryopreservation solutions must be stored at a specified temperature and with a storage period consistent with functional requirements. They must be discarded if not used within 24 hours of opening. Any solutions coming into direct contact with tissues during retrieval or processing must be sterile.

21.6 Tissue storage

Refrigeration devices containing tissue shall be suitable for the use intended and procedures for monitoring such devices shall be validated so that tissues are maintained at the required storage temperature. Continuous monitoring and recording of temperature, together with suitable alarm systems, shall be employed on all storage refrigerators, freezers and liquid nitrogen tanks.

Every effort should be made to avoid cross-contamination of material stored in liquid nitrogen vessels. Wherever possible, there should be specifically designated pieces of equipment (e.g. nitrogen level rulers, portable thermometers) for each vessel. Where this is not possible (e.g. liquid nitrogen delivery hoses) and the item has to be used for more than one vessel, it should not come into contact with the liquid phase or the sides of the vessel.

Frozen and cryopreserved tissue should be double wrapped during storage. The seals and the material employed must be validated for their use at the designated storage temperature and the conditions of use, to demonstrate integrity of the packaging and labelling. This is crucially important for storage in liquid nitrogen vessels because of the high levels of accumulated microbial contaminants found within these vessels.

Quarantined and released tissue must be stored in physically segregated, clearly designated locations distinct from each other.

21.6.1 Tissue release

Prior to any tissue being cleared for issue, all relevant records including donor records, processing and storage records, and post-processing quality control test results must have been reviewed, approved and documented as acceptable by the individual(s) responsible according to the relevant local standard operating procedures. Responsibilities for setting policies for exceptional release of tissues reside with the designated medical officer.

21.6.2 Tissue discard

There must be a documented policy for the discard of tissue unsuitable for clinical use. Records should include details of date and method of discard and reason for discard. Tissues for discard should be appropriately handled and disposed of in a manner compliant with local control of infection guidelines.

21.6.3 Labelling and packaging of tissues for issue

Packaging must ensure integrity and maintain sterility of the contents of the final container, and must also comply with current legislation.

The container must be labelled with the graft-specific identification (batch and shipment number if applicable), expiry date and supplying tissue bank, storage instructions and barcoded product description and instruction to see pack insert, as a minimum. In addition, more detailed information should be provided either on the label or package insert or both as follows:

- sizing information

- antimicrobial processing procedure used (if applicable)

- preservative used and its concentration (if applicable)

- special instructions (e.g. 'Do not freeze'), thawing, dilution instructions

- presence of known sensitising substances

- type and calculated quantity of antibiotics added during processing (if applicable)

- any other potential residual processing agent

- RhD type (where appropriate)

- a statement that the tissue was prepared from a donor who was non-reactive for current mandatory markers of infection, with the added rider that all biological tissue carries some risk of disease transmission

- results and findings from clinically relevant bacteriological cultures performed on the tissue before final packaging

- storage instructions

- instructions for reconstitution (if appropriate)

- a warning on loss of package integrity

- instructions on dealing with queries, reporting adverse events/reactions and return or disposal of unsuitable or unused tissue

- a statement that tissue use must be authorised by a medical/dental practitioner

- a statement should accompany each tissue product stating that it may not be sterilised after leaving the tissue bank

- a statement should accompany each package stipulating that each package is for single-patient use only

- if the package insert carries graft-specific information it must be labelled with the unique graft-specific identification code

- instructions to the user regarding the need for a documented system for the tracking and follow-up of the fate of the tissue

- when cells are known to be positive for a relevant infectious disease marker, it must be marked as a BIOLOGICAL HAZARD.

21.6.4 External labelling of the shipping container

For transport, the primary container must be placed in a shipping container that must be labelled with at least the following information:

- identification of the originating Tissue Establishment, including an address and telephone number

- identification of the organisation responsible for human application of destination, including address and telephone number

- a statement that the package contains human tissue/cells and HANDLE WITH CARE

- where living cells are required for the function of the graft, such as stem cells, gametes and embryos, the following must be added: 'DO NOT IRRADIATE'

- recommended transport conditions (e.g. keep cold, in upright position etc.)

- safety instructions/method of cooling (when applicable).

21.6.5 Distribution

All reasonable efforts must be made to ensure that tissues are sent to qualified individuals/organisations who have accepted responsibility for their proper handling and use. A written agreement must be in place between the Tissue Establishment and the organisation ordering the tissue.

Where tissue is transported in a refrigerated or frozen condition, adequate safeguards should be taken to ensure that the tissue remains at the designated temperature. Monitoring of temperature should be undertaken wherever practicable but if not, the method should at least have been validated to show that appropriate temperatures are maintained.

21.7 Tracking of tissues

Each Tissue Establishment shall ensure that it has the ability to locate and identify all tissues/cells during any step from procurement through to distribution to recipient or disposal and vice versa. This traceability shall also apply to all relevant data relating to products and materials coming into contact with these tissues and cells.

Tissue Establishments shall have effective and accurate systems to uniquely identify and label tissues/cells received and distributed.

Tissue Establishments shall keep the data necessary to ensure traceability at all stages. Data required for full traceability shall be kept for a minimum of 30 years after clinical use. Data storage may also be in electronic form. Data that must be kept are shown in Table 21.2 (based on Annex VI, Directive 2006/86/EC).[7]

Table 21.2 Minimum donor/recipient data set to be kept

A. BY TISSUE ESTABLISHMENTS
Donor identification
Donation identification that will include at least: • Identification of the procurement organisation or Tissue Establishment • Unique donation identification number • Date of procurement • Place of procurement • Type of donation (e.g. single or multi-tissue; autologous or allogeneic; living or deceased).
Product identification that will include at least: • Identification of the Tissue Establishment • Type of tissue and cell/product (basic nomenclature) • Pool number (if applicable) • Split number (if applicable) • Expiry date • Tissue/cell status (i.e. quarantined, suitable for use etc.) • Description and origin of the products, processing steps applied, materials and additives coming into contact with tissues and cells and having an effect on their quality and/or safety • Identification of the facility issuing the final label.
Human application identification that will include at least: • Date of distribution/disposal • Identification of the clinician or end user/facility.
B. BY ORGANISATIONS RESPONSIBLE FOR HUMAN APPLICATION
• Identification of the supplier Tissue Establishment • Identification of the clinician or end user/facility • Type of tissues and cells • Product identification • Identification of the recipient • Date of application.

21.8 Notification of serious adverse events and reactions

Tissue Establishments in the UK are required to report adverse events to the Human Tissue Authority (HTA) through the Serious Adverse Events and Reactions system. For the purposes of reporting, a serious adverse reaction (SAR) is defined as an unintended response, including a communicable disease, in the donor or in the recipient associated with the procurement or human application of tissues and cells that is fatal, life-threatening, disabling or incapacitating or which results in, or prolongs, hospitalisation or morbidity. A serious adverse event (SAE) is defined as any untoward occurrence associated with the procurement, testing, processing, storage and distribution of tissues and cells that might lead to the transmission of a communicable disease, to death or life-threatening, disabling or incapacitating conditions for patients or which might result in, or prolong, hospitalisation or morbidity.

Tissue Establishments shall ensure that there is a system in place to report, investigate, register and transmit information about serious adverse events and reactions. A root cause analysis should be performed. Moreover, each Tissue Establishment shall ensure that an accurate, rapid and verifiable procedure is in place which will enable it to recall from distribution any product which may be related to an adverse event or reaction.

21.9 Additional guidelines for skeletal tissue retrieval and processing

21.9.1 Procurement of surgically removed bone

A system of documentation must be in place to ensure that theatre staff are clearly informed that a particular patient has or has not consented to bone donation. This may be by enclosing a copy of the consent form in the patient's notes, or some equivalent method.

Where bones are retrieved during surgery by theatre staff on behalf of the tissue bank, these staff must follow a protocol provided by the tissue bank in accordance with third party agreements.

The removed bone should be placed, as quickly as possible, in a sterile container and labelled in a manner to distinguish it from cleared issued bone.

Documentation must be completed in theatre, detailing the time of bone retrieval and providing the identity of the staff members carrying out the retrieval and labelling.

If the donated bone is not destined for terminal antimicrobial processing, it must be cultured for microbial contamination at the time of collection, using a collection and transport system provided by, or approved by, the tissue bank. Bone sampling must be carried out immediately prior to closing the bone container.

Tissue samples for culture should comprise of chips of bone from the cut end of the bone, which should be placed in appropriate transport or culture media. The bone should be finally packaged in a double sterile container.

A secure system utilising barcodes for the identification and linkage of the donation to the donor and samples must be in place.

The bone container, tissue samples and blood samples, if collected at this time, must each be clearly labelled with the barcoded donation numbers and stored at appropriate temperatures until collection.

Alternatively, protocols can be put in place to arrange for the hospital blood bank or other appropriate laboratory, to separate serum from the blood samples and to store it and the donation at –20°C or lower, for collection at a later date. Testing should be performed within 1 month of sampling. Note: If tissues are stored by a hospital for more than 48 hours then the hospital requires to be licensed by the HTA, as storage cannot be covered by a 'third party agreement'.

Bone which is not subject to antimicrobial processing can only be released for use if cultures for aerobic and anaerobic bacteria, and fungi are negative.

Where environmental contaminants are detected on surgically retrieved bone, this bone may be further processed and subjected to terminal sterilisation, e.g. gamma irradiation (>1.5 megarads = >15 kGy) (see section 21.5.4).

21.9.2 Procurement of skeletal tissues from deceased donors

If iliac crest is to be retrieved, it should be taken last in case the bowel is perforated and should be stored in a separate container. Where osteochondral allografts are to be retrieved, care should be taken to avoid drying of articular surfaces. It is best to retrieve the joint entirely and to dissect it later in the laboratory.

21.9.3 Processing of skeletal tissues

Cycles of thawing and freezing must be minimised. Skeletal tissues should not be heated above 60°C and tendons and costal cartilage should not be warmed above 30°C.

Osteochondral allografts, such as proximal or distal femur or femoral hemicondyles, are cryopreserved with a cryoprotectant (such as DMSO) on the articular surfaces and cooled following appropriate cryopreservation protocols. Cryopreservation of allografts must begin within 48 hours of procurement. These allografts must not be exposed to gamma irradiation and must therefore be procured and processed aseptically.

21.10 Cardiovascular tissue retrieval and processing

21.10.1 General

This section predominantly relates to the banking of heart valves.

21.10.2 Sizing and evaluation of cardiovascular tissue

Aortic and pulmonary valves should be sized at the annulus and the internal diameter recorded in millimetres.

The length of the aortic conduit, main pulmonary artery and right and left pulmonary artery remnants should be recorded.

Detailed description of the condition of the valve must be recorded in the donor processing records, which should include a grading system or schematic representation.

Valve descriptions and evaluation must accompany the allograft distribution and be made available to the surgeon on request.

Heart valves and vessels should be processed using a disinfection process which has been shown to produce decontaminated tissues.

Disinfection time must not exceed that specified in a validated disinfection regime.

21.10.3 Bacteriological testing of tissue

Where tissues are exposed to a decontamination step an assessment of the bacteriological status prior to decontamination must be performed.

Processed tissue must be subjected to bacterial (including *Mycobacterium tuberculosis*) and fungal testing using validated techniques. Each bank should develop a list of exclusion criteria based on type and number of contaminating organisms prior to and following decontamination.

21.10.4 Cryopreservation

Currently accepted optimal procedures involve controlled rate cooling of cardiovascular tissues in the presence of cryoprotectant.

21.10.5 Storage and warming of cardiovascular tissues

For material stored at –135°C or below, if during warming the tissue is warmed too rapidly between the storage temperature and –100°C, fractures can occur. A validated method of warming (e.g. on dry ice) must be used to minimise the risk. This must ensure that the valve has reached a temperature above –100°C before thawing in a 37°C water bath.

Material stored at –135°C, which is subsequently transported with solid carbon dioxide (–79°C), should be maintained in a mechanical freezer (at –80°C) if not used immediately. Thereafter, a maximum storage time of 6 months will pertain.

21.10.6 Distribution

Cryopreserved valves and vessels must be transported either in solid carbon dioxide at –79°C or in a container maintaining a temperature of –135°C or lower. Cardiovascular tissue must not be submerged in liquid nitrogen during transport.

21.11 Skin retrieval and processing

21.11.1 Skin retrieval

Skin sites should be shaved if necessary and treated with an antimicrobial agent such as chlorhexidine.

Samples of skin must be cultured for aerobic and anaerobic bacteria and fungi prior to and following decontamination.

21.11.2 Skin processing

Skin can be processed to provide an acceptable graft in a number of ways. These include cryopreservation, high-concentration glycerolisation and other methods. The specification for any skin product should clarify the required properties.

21.12 Ocular tissue retrieval and storage

21.12.1 Eye retrieval

An 'NHSBT Tissue Retrieval Site Risk Assessment' form must be completed by the eye retriever to ensure the suitability of the retrieval site. This must be done for every eye retrieval as circumstances may change even within the same premises.

Eye retrieval must be carried out by a person who is trained and competent in enucleation. Either this individual must be employed by an HTA-licensed eye bank or there must be a third party agreement in place between the eye bank and the individual's employing authority.

Enucleation should be carried out as soon as possible, but no longer than 24 hours after death. The eye retriever must be satisfied that lawful consent/authorisation has been obtained and that at the time of retrieval there is no known medical reason to suggest that the eyes should not be retrieved. Sterile, single-use instruments must be used and disposed of safely after the retrieval. The NHS Blood and Transplant (NHSBT) Human Tissue Transport Box contains all the required documentation, including an enucleation protocol, and a set of sterile, single-use instruments. All required documentation must be fully completed by the eye retriever, including the NHSBT Ocular Tissue Donor Information form and body map.

The NHSBT enucleation protocol must be followed.[8] After enucleation a stump of optic nerve at least 5 mm long must remain attached to the eye, which is then secured in a plastic eye stand. The eye stand and eye (cornea uppermost) are placed on top of a moist cotton wool ball or gauze swab and placed in a sterile pot (moist chamber). The eye must not be immersed in any liquid in the moist chamber. The moist chambers are then packed in an NHSBT Human Tissue Transport box together with a plastic bag containing melting ice. At least 1 kg of ice is needed to keep the contents of the transport box below 5°C for up to 24 hours during transportation to the eye bank. The donor's eye sockets should be packed with cotton wool and lids closed over plastic eye caps to restore the original profile of the lids. The final cosmetic appearance is of critical importance as family or friends may wish to view the body. Any bleeding or bruising resulting from the enucleation must be noted on the body map.

21.12.2 Ocular tissue storage

Corneas may be stored for up to 2 weeks at 4°C in an appropriate hypothermic storage solution. Alternatively, the great majority of corneas in the UK are stored for up to 4 weeks in organ culture at 34°C. The corneal endothelium is examined by light microscopy a few days before use to ensure its suitability for transplantation in patients with corneal endothelial disease/deficiency. Organ-cultured corneas are delivered to hospitals in medium containing 5% dextran to reverse the stromal oedema that occurs during storage. Corneas with an inadequate endothelium may still be suitable for anterior lamellar grafts. These corneas may also be transferred to 70% ethanol and stored at room temperature for up to 12 months for use in glaucoma surgery. Sclera, which is also stored in 70% ethanol for up to 12 months, is used for glaucoma or other reconstructive surgery. Ocular surface stem cells may be isolated from the limbus and expanded in *ex vivo* culture for treating limbal stem cell deficiency.

21.13 References

1. Health Technical Memorandum (HTM) 2010 Sterilization. Available at www.tsoshop.co.uk/bookstore.asp.

2. Health Technical Memorandum (HTM) 2030 Washer-Disinfectors. Available at www.tsoshop.co.uk/bookstore.asp.

3. Health Technical Memorandum (HTM) 2031 Clean Steam for Sterilization. Available at www.tsoshop.co.uk/bookstore.asp.

4. Human Tissue Authority Direction 003/2010 implementing the *Guide to Quality and Safety Assurance for Human Tissues and Cells for Patient Treatment* available at www.hta.gov.uk/legislationpoliciesandcodesofpractice/htalegaldirections.cfm

5. Medicines and Healthcare products Regulatory Agency (2007). *Rules and Guidance for Pharmaceutical Manufacturers and Distributors 2007.* London: Pharmaceutical Press.

6. EC Guidelines to Good Manufacturing Practice Volume 4, Annex 1 (2008 revision): Manufacture of Sterile Medicinal Products. Available at http://ec.europa.eu/health/documents/eudralex/vol-4/index_en.htm.

7. Commission Directive 2006/86/EC of 24 October 2006 implementing Directive 2004/23/EC of the European Parliament and of the Council as regards traceability requirements, notification of serious adverse reactions and events and certain technical requirements for the coding, processing, preservation, storage and distribution of human tissues and cells. *OJ*, L 294, 25.10.2006, p32.

8. NHS Blood and Transplant Organ Donation & Transplantation Directorate Ocular Tissue Advisory Group OTAG(09)29 'Optimisation of Eye Retrieval'.

Chapter 22
Haemopoietic progenitor cells

22.1 Introduction

Cellular therapy is now covered by a variety of legislation. The EU Directive on Tissues and Cells (2004/23/EC) and its associated Commission Directives (2006/17/EC and 2006/86/EC) have been transposed into UK law as the Human Tissue (Quality and Safety for Human Application) Regulations 2007. For advanced therapy medicinal products there is EU Directive 2001/83/EC with its subsequent amendments and Regulation (EC) No. 1394/2007 on advanced therapy medicinal products. The Human Tissue Act 2004, Human Tissue (Scotland) Act 2006 and Directions or Codes of Practice issued by the Human Tissue Authority also apply. In addition, there are a number of key international standards for haemopoietic stem cells, notably the FACT-JACIE and the NetCord-FACT Standards. The lists of publications in sections 22.1.1 to 22.1.5 have been grouped according to their origins.

The guidelines in this chapter apply to the donation, collection, testing, processing, cryopreservation, storage and distribution of haemopoietic progenitor cells (HPC) and therapeutic cells (TC) within the UK Blood Transfusion Services (UKBTS). HPCs include bone marrow, peripheral blood and cord blood progenitor cells. The guidelines must be read in conjunction with the other sections of the book including those that apply to quality systems, quality assurance and testing of donors. These guidelines are applicable to stem cell donor registries and to bone marrow, peripheral blood and cord blood collection and processing facilities.

22.1.1 European Union Directives/guidelines

1. Directive 2004/23/EC of the European Parliament and of the Council of 31 March 2004 on setting standards of quality and safety for the donation, procurement, testing, processing, preservation, storage and distribution of human tissues and cells. *OJ*, L 102, 07.04.2004, p48. Available at www.transfusionguidelines.org.uk.

2. Commission Directive 2006/17/EC of 8 February 2006 implementing Directive 2004/23/EC of the European Parliament and of the Council as regards certain technical requirements for the donation, procurement and testing of human tissues and cells. *OJ*, L 038, 09.02.2006, p40. Available at www.transfusionguidelines.org.uk.

3. Commission Directive 2006/86/EC of 24 October 2006 implementing Directive 2004/23/EC of the European Parliament and of the Council as regards traceability requirements, notification of serious adverse reactions and events and certain technical requirements for the coding, processing, preservation, storage and distribution of human tissues and cells. *OJ*, L 294, 25.10.2006, p32. Available at www.transfusionguidelines.org.uk.

(Note: The EU Directive on Tissues and Cells and its associated Commission Directives are referred to collectively as the EU Directives on Tissues and Cells in this chapter.)

4. Regulation (EC) No. 1394/2007 of the European Parliament and Council on advanced therapy medicinal products and amending Directive 2001/83/EC and Regulation (EC) No. 726/2004. Available at http://eur-lex.europa.eu/LexUriServ/LexUriServ.do?uri=OJ:L:2007:324:0121:0137:EN:PDF.

5. Directive 2001/83/EC of the European Parliament and Council on the Community code relating to medicinal products for human use. Available at http://eur-lex.europa.eu/LexUriServ/LexUriServ.do?uri=OJ:L:2001:311:0067:0128:EN:PDF.

6. Commission Directive 2003/63/EC amending Directive 2001/83 on the Community code relating to medicinal products for human use. Available at http://eur-lex.europa.eu/LexUriServ/LexUriServ.do?uri=OJ:L:2003:159:0046:0094:EN:PDF.

7. Regulation (EC) No. 726/2004 of the European Parliament and of the Council laying down Community procedures for the authorisation and supervision of medicinal products for human and veterinary use and establishing a European Medicines Agency. Available at http://eur-lex.europa.eu/LexUriServ/LexUriServ.do?uri=OJ:L:2004:136:0001:0033:EN:PDF.

8. EC Guidelines to Good Manufacturing Practice Volume 4, Annex 1 (2008 revision): Manufacture of Sterile Medicinal Products. Available at http://ec.europa.eu/health/documents/eudralex/vol-4/index_en.htm.

9. Directive 2001/20/EC of the European Parliament and of the Council on the approximation of the laws, regulations and administrative provisions of the member states relating to the implementation of good clinical practice in the conduct of clinical trials on medicinal products for human use. Available at http://eur-lex.europa.eu/LexUriServ/LexUriServ.do?uri=OJ:L:2001:121:0034:0044:en:PDF.

10. Commission Directive 2005/28/EC laying down principles and detailed guidelines for good clinical practice as regards investigational medicinal products for human use, as well as the requirements for authorisation of the manufacturing or importation of such products. Available at http://eur-lex.europa.eu/LexUriServ/LexUriServ.do?uri=OJ:L:2005:091:0013:0019:EN:PDF.

11. The European Medicines Agency Committee for Medicinal Products for Human Use (CHMP) prepares scientific guidelines, in consultation with the Competent Authorities of the EU member states, to help applicants prepare marketing-authorisation applications for medicinal products for human use. Guidelines are intended to provide a basis for practical harmonisation of the manner in which the EU member states and the Agency interpret and apply the detailed requirements for the demonstration of quality, safety and efficacy contained in the EU Directives. Available at www.ema.europa.eu/ema/index.jsp.

22.1.2 International Standards

12. International Standards for Cellular Therapy Product Collection, Processing, and Administration. Fifth edition (2012) from the Foundation for the Accreditation of Cellular Therapy (FACT) and the Joint Accreditation Committee of ISCT-Europe and EBMT (JACIE). Available at www.jacie.org.

13. International Standards for Cellular Therapy Product Collection, Processing, and Administration Accreditation Manual. Fifth edition (2012). Available at www.jacie.org.

14. NetCord-FACT International Standards for Cord Blood Collection, Processing and Release for Administration. Fourth edition (2010). Available at www.factwebsite.org.

15. NetCord-FACT Cord Blood Accreditation Manual. Fourth edition (2012). Available at www.factwebsite.org.

16. World Marrow Donor Association (WMDA) promotes a range of standards, guidelines and recommendations to facilitate the exchange of haemopoietic stem cells across international borders. Available at www.worldmarrow.org.

22.1.3 Human Tissue Authority

17. Human Tissue Act 2004 (except Scotland). Available at www.legislation.gov.uk. The Human Tissue Act 2006 (Scotland). Available at www.show.scot.nhs.uk.

18. Statutory Instrument 2007 No. 1523 The Human Tissue (Quality and Safety for Human Application) Regulations 2007, implementing the EU Directives on Tissues and Cells. Available at www.legislation.gov.uk/uksi/2007/1523/made.

19. Human Tissue Authority Guide to Quality and Safety Assurance for Human Tissues and Cells for Patient Treatment (implemented by HTA Directions: 003/2010), explains the requirements under the EU Tissues and Cells Directives. Available at www.hta.gov.uk.

20. Human Tissue Authority (HTA). Codes of Practice for: Consent (Code 1); for Disposal of Human Tissue (Code 5); for Donation of Allogeneic Bone Marrow and Peripheral Blood Stem Cells for Transplantation (Code 6). Available at www.hta.gov.uk.

22.1.4 Histocompatibility, donor selection and microbiology documents

21. Hurley CK (1999). Histocompatibility testing guidelines for haematopoietic stem cell transplantation using volunteer donors: report from the World Marrow Donor Association. Quality Assurance and Donor Registries Working Groups of the World Marrow Donor Association. *Bone Marrow Transplant*, 24(2), 119–121.

22. European Federation for Immunogenetics (EFI) 'Standards for histocompatibility testing' version 5.6.1 (2010). Available at www.efiweb.org.

23. National Marrow Donor Program (USA) Standards, 20th edition, March 2009. Available at www.marrow.org

24. Joint UKBTS/NIBSC Professional Advisory Committee's (JPAC) *Donor Selection Guidelines* for either cord blood donors or bone marrow/peripheral blood stem cell donors are available at www.transfusionguidelines.org.uk.

25. SaBTO (2011). Guidance on the microbiological safety of human organs, tissues and cells used in transplantation. Advisory Committee on the Safety of Blood Tissues and Organs. Available at www.dh.gov.uk//en/Publicationsandstatistics/Publications/PublicationsPolicyAndGuidance/DH_121497

22.1.5 UK legislation

26. Caldicott Report (1997). Available at www.dh.gov.uk/prod_consum_dh/groups/dh_digitalassets/@dh/@en/documents/digitalasset/dh_4068404.pdf.

27. Data Protection Act 1998. Available at www.legislation.gov.uk/ukpga/1998/29/contents.

22.2 Terminology

For the purposes of these guidelines, the terms shall, will, or must mean that the guideline is to be complied with at all times. The terms may and should indicate an activity that is recommended or advised, but for which there may be effective alternatives.

The cellular therapy products described in these guidelines are referred to as haemopoietic progenitor cells HPC-A, HPC-M and HPC-C to denote their collection by apheresis or from marrow and cord blood respectively or as therapeutic cells (TC), the most commonly used of which is TC-T cells (T), often referred to as donor lymphocyte infusions (DLI).

22.3 Policy and procedure requirements

Policies and procedures must include all aspects of the operation including donor selection, assessment, consent, microbiological testing, collection, labelling, system of numbering, processing, quality management and improvement, proficiency testing, storage, including alternative storage strategies if the primary storage device fails, transportation, outcome analysis, audits, expiry dates, emergency and safety procedures, equipment and supplies, maintenance and monitoring, cleaning procedures, personnel training, disposal of medical and biohazard waste, release procedures, including criteria for exceptional release, references, tolerance limits, corrective actions, recall, returns and discard policy. A risk management approach must be demonstrated.

The medical director/advisor and laboratory director/manager must review and approve all policies, procedures and research protocols annually to determine that they are clinically appropriate and consistent with the requirements of users of the service. They should seek to maximise safety for both donors and recipients.

Procedures carried out by third parties (e.g. donor assessment and harvesting centres, clinical transplant units and testing laboratories) must be described by written agreements. These must define and document relationships between the facility and the third party. The details of the agreement including responsibilities must be clearly specified, documented and agreed between parties. The agreement must include an option for audit of procedures carried out by the third party. Documented procedures to review these agreements should be in place.

All clinical and laboratory facilities should conform to the relevant EU Directives and both FACT-JACIE and NetCord-FACT Standards as appropriate. Laboratories must participate in appropriate recognised external quality assurance schemes. All clinical and laboratory facilities must be compliant with the requirements of the EU Clinical Trials Directive. Documentation of all research protocols performed by the facility must be maintained. This must include copies of research and ethics committee approvals for all relevant procedures.

22.4 Safety requirements

Each HPC-processing facility must be operated in a manner to minimise risks to the health and safety of employees, donors and recipients. Suitable facilities and equipment must be available to maintain safe operations.

There must be procedures for microbiological, chemical and radiation safety, as appropriate, and a system for monitoring training and compliance.

HPC and TC collections must be handled and discarded with precautions that recognise the potential for exposure to infectious agents.

22.5 Adverse events and reactions

Facilities must ensure that there is a system in place to detect, report, investigate, document and follow up all errors, adverse events and reactions affecting donors and those which could affect the quality of HPC components and which may be attributable to their collection and processing.

These systems must also apply to any serious adverse events and reactions observed after administration of HPC components.

Documentation of these events shall be reviewed by the facilities' directors as appropriate.

The Designated Individual must ensure that these events are notified to the HTA within 24 hours of discovery.

Facilities must ensure that appropriate corrective actions are taken and that recall procedures are in place to enable it to recall any component(s) related to serious adverse events and reactions.

22.6 Donor selection, consent and testing

22.6.1 Allogeneic HPC-M donors

22.6.1.1 General principles

- Registries must have detailed policies and procedures for the testing and assessment of donors of HPC and TC. These must be in accordance with the requirements of the EU Directives on Tissues and Cells, FACT-JACIE Standards and the WMDA.

- Counselling: Relevant information must be given to potential donors at appropriate times. This shall include an explanation of the risks of the procedure; benefits for the intended recipient; tests to be performed to protect the health of the donor and recipient; the policy of informing donors of significant abnormal results; the possible need for second donations of HPC or TC; the right to withdraw from the donation; the risk of death for the recipient if the donor withdraws after the recipient's conditioning therapy has started; anonymity policy; insurance arrangements; reimbursement of expenses.

- Consent: The donor must be competent to give and have given valid consent before conditioning therapy is initiated in the recipient. Consent must be obtained in accordance with the requirements of the Human Tissue Act and the HTA's Codes of Practice on consent, and donation of allogeneic bone marrow and peripheral blood stem cells for transplantation.

22.6.1.2 Medical history, physical examination and testing

- The donor medical assessment must be performed according to the requirements of the EU Directives on Tissues and Cells, FACT-JACIE Standards and the WMDA.

- Anonymity must be maintained between donors and recipients in accordance with the requirements of EU Directive 2004/23/EC. The British Bone Marrow Registry (BBMR) and the Welsh Bone Marrow Donor Registry (WBMDR) must have robust policies for donor anonymity and follow-up in accordance with the requirements of the WMDA, FACT-JACIE and NetCord-FACT Standards and the relevant EU Directives.

22.6.2 Allogeneic HPC-A donors

HPC-A may be collected after mobilisation with a licensed G-CSF preparation.

The requirements of section 22.6.1 also apply. A donor of HPC-A must be found fit for both apheresis and G-CSF administration and may also be assessed for fitness to undergo bone marrow harvest in the event of failure to mobilise stem cells.

22.6.3 Autologous HPC-M and HPC-A donors

The assessment and counselling of patients is not within the scope of these guidelines. However, consent must be obtained in accordance with the requirements of the HTA. The requirements for processing, preservation, storage and testing of autologous donations are described in sections 22.9, 22.10 and 22.11.

22.6.4 Repeat donations of allogeneic HPC-A, HPC-M or first or repeat donations of TC

These are requests either for further donations of HPC, for the same or a different patient, from donors who have in the past given an HPC donation, or for a TC donation for the same patient where an HPC donation has already been given. Individual assessment of each request is required. This must include further medical assessment with appropriate testing, counselling and consent.

22.6.5 Allogeneic HPC-C donors

- HPC facilities/cord blood banks must have detailed policies and procedures for the assessment and testing of donor mothers and infant donors of HPC-C. These must be in accordance with the requirements of the EU Directives on Tissues and Cells, NetCord-FACT Standards and the WMDA.

- Maternal assessment must be performed by appropriately trained staff, according to the requirements of the EU Directives on Tissues and Cells, NetCord-FACT Standards and the WMDA.

- Infant assessment must be performed by appropriately trained staff, according to the requirements of the EU Directives on Tissues and Cells, NetCord-FACT Standards, SaBTO and the WMDA.

- Testing requirements, see section 22.11 Maternal samples taken at time of collection of the HPC-C (Day 0 to +7) shall be tested in accordance with the requirements of the EU Directives on Tissues and Cells, NetCord-FACT Standards and the WMDA.

- Consent. Detailed information must be provided to potential donor mothers prior to requesting consent, in terms and translations relevant to the mother. Consent for collection must be obtained prior to harvest of the cord blood. Consent must be obtained in accordance with the requirements of the Human Tissue Act, the HTA's Codes of Practice for consent and donation of organs, tissue and cells for transplantation, the EU Directives on Tissues and Cells and NetCord-FACT Standards.

22.7 Collection facilities for HPC-A, HPC-M, HPC-C and TC

22.7.1 General

HPC-A, HPC-M, HPC-C and TC should only be collected in a hospital facility or Blood Service apheresis unit with appropriate experience (see section 5.8) and which meets the standards required by the EU Directives on Tissues and Cells, FACT-JACIE Standards and NetCord-FACT Standards as appropriate. The facility will be headed by a medical director/advisor and a collection facility director with appropriate experience as described in the above standards. The collection facility shall have an organisational structure and operational procedures appropriate for the activities carried out. There must be an organisational chart which clearly defines accountability and reporting relationships. The medical director/advisor shall have responsibility and authority for all clinical aspects of the programme including compliance with national and local guidelines as well as ensuring compliance with regulatory requirements.

The collection facility director is responsible for the operational management and technical aspects of the service. The medical director/advisor may also act as the collection facility director. There shall be adequate numbers of staff whose training and competency to perform the assigned procedures must comply with the requirements of the EU Directives on Tissues and Cells, FACT-JACIE Standards and NetCord-FACT Standards.

There must be a documented quality management system applied to all activities, and a designated quality manager.

There must be a Designated Individual as defined by the EU Directives on Tissues and Cells/Human Tissue Act.

22.7.1.1 HPC-M donors

HPC-M donors should be assessed and managed in accordance with the aforementioned guidance. Specific points of importance are:

- A consultant anaesthetist should take responsibility for the care of the donor during the harvest procedure.
- There should be intensive care (or equivalent) and resuscitation facilities on-site.

22.7.1.2 HPC-A donors

HPC-A donors should be assessed and managed in accordance with the aforementioned guidance. Specific points of importance are:

- Physicians prescribing human growth factors must be experienced in their use.
- Donors and recipients undergoing progenitor cell mobilisation must have access to advice and medical supervision 24 hours a day.

Venous access

- Peripheral veins should ordinarily be used for venous access for donors.
- Where access via peripheral veins is not feasible and appropriate consent is obtained, central venous catheterisation (e.g. via the femoral or other route) may be considered.
- The placing of central catheters should only be undertaken in hospital facilities with access to intensive care and radiology facilities by highly trained staff who regularly perform this procedure.
- Collection centres must ensure that the adequacy of central venous catheterisation has been confirmed.

22.7.1.3 HPC-C collections

HPC-C collections should be managed in accordance with the aforementioned guidance. Specific points of importance are:

- For unrelated collections there must be a written agreement defining the responsibilities and expectations between the cord blood bank and the obstetric department of the collection hospital.
- For directed allogeneic or autologous collections, harvested in a non-fixed collection facility, there must be a written agreement related to HPC-C collection, transport, processing, testing, storage and release, between the referring consultant and the HPC facility.
- Delivery practices must not be modified in an attempt to facilitate HPC-C collections.
- There must exist a documented system for identification of the HPC-C product and for confirming the link with the mother.

22.8 Component definitions

22.8.1 Definitions

Unmanipulated: HPC as obtained at collection and not subject to any manipulation.

Manipulated: Subjected to an *ex vivo* process that selectively removes/enriches, expands or functionally alters HPCs.

- Minimally manipulated: Processing that does not alter the relevant biological characteristics of cells or tissues.

- More than minimally manipulated: Processing that does alter the relevant biological characteristics of cells or tissues.

Investigational medicinal product (IMP): A pharmaceutical form of an active substance or placebo being tested or used as a reference in a clinical trial, including a product with a marketing authorisation when used or assembled in a way different from the authorised form, or when used for an unauthorised indication, or when used to gain further information about the authorised form. These products require a separate IMP manufacturer's licence from the Medicines and Healthcare products Regulatory Agency (MHRA).

Advanced therapy medicinal product (ATMP): An ATMP is a medicinal product which is:

- a gene therapy medicinal product as defined in Part IV of Annex 1 to Directive 2001/83/EC; or

- a somatic cell therapy medicinal product as defined in Part IV of Annex 1 to Directive 2001/83/EC; or

- a tissue engineered product as defined in Article 2 1 (b) of the ATMP Regulation.

The MHRA is the Competent Authority for the assessment of applications for clinical trial authorisations and the associated manufacturer's licence for investigational ATMPs. It is also the Competent Authority for ATMPs which are prepared and used under the hospital exemption scheme (laid down in Article 3 (7) of the ATMP Regulation) and made and supplied under the 'specials' scheme.

22.8.2 Products

HPC, apheresis (HPC-A): HPC collected from the peripheral blood using an apheresis technique usually after receiving a haemopoietic growth factor.

HPC marrow (HPC-M): HPC aspirated from the iliac crests, sternum or other bones.

HPC cord blood (HPC-C): HPC from umbilical cord ± placenta at time of delivery.

Therapeutic cells (TC): Cell products harvested or manufactured for the purpose of providing therapeutic benefit.

- TC, T cells (TC)

- TC, dendritic cells (DC)

- TC, marrow

- TC, whole blood

- TC, apheresis

- TC, T regulatory cells (T-Reg)
- TC, tumour-derived
- TC, mesenchymal stem cell (MSC)
- TC, natural killer (NK)
- TC, cytotoxic lymphocytes (CTL)
- Other therapeutic cells

22.8.3 Product modifications

B cell depleted: Cells processed by negative selection for B lymphocytes.

Buffy coat enriched: Cells remaining after depletion of mature erythrocytes and plasma by sedimentation or centrifugation using devices, supplies and techniques validated for this purpose.

CD34 selected: Enriched cells processed by positive selection for CD34 antigen bearing cells.

Cryopreserved: Cells frozen using devices, supplies and techniques validated to maintain viability.

Density enriched: Primarily mononuclear cells remaining after depletion of mature erythrocytes, polymorphonuclear cells and plasma by separation of the cell on the basis of density. This is achieved using devices or reagents validated for the separation of cells based on density.

***Ex vivo* expanded:** Cells that have been cultured *in vitro* for the purpose of producing and/or enriching for a specific functional subset. Note: *Ex vivo* expanded cells may require an IMP or ATMP manufacturer's licence from the MHRA.

Gene manipulated: Cells that have been processed to alter their own genes or introduce new genetic material.

Plasma and RBC reduced: Cells remaining after depletion of mature erythrocytes and a portion of plasma by sedimentation and/or centrifugation using devices, supplies and techniques validated for this purpose

Plasma reduced: Cells remaining after a portion of plasma has been depleted by sedimentation or centrifugation using devices, supplies and techniques validated for this purpose.

RBC reduced: Cells remaining after depletion of mature erythrocytes by sedimentation and/or centrifugation using devices, supplies and techniques validated for this purpose.

T cell depleted: Cells processed by negative selection for T lymphocytes.

Tumour cell depleted: Cells processed by negative selection for tumour cells.

22.9 Haemopoietic progenitor cell processing standards

22.9.1 Personnel and facilities

Processing facilities must comply with the requirements of the EU Directives on Tissues and Cells, FACT-JACIE Standards and NetCord-FACT Standards. There shall be a medical director/advisor who will have responsibility and authority for all clinical aspects of the programme including compliance with national and local guidelines as well as ensuring compliance with regulatory requirements.

There will be a laboratory director/manager who is responsible for the operational management and technical aspects of the service. There should be adequate numbers of staff whose training and competency to perform the assigned procedures must comply with the requirements of appropriate regulations and standards.

There must be a Designated Individual as defined by the EU Directives on Tissues and Cells/Human Tissue Act.

The HPC-processing facility shall have an organisational structure and operational procedures appropriate for the activities carried out. There must be an organisational chart which clearly defines accountability and reporting relationships. There must be a documented quality management system applied to all activities, and a designated quality manager.

22.9.2 Procedures

- Before processing there should be a written request from the transplant physician. This is not required for unrelated cord blood collections.

- Processing should be performed according to written procedures and policies. All procedures must be validated prior to implementation. Aseptic techniques must be employed. Any deviation from such written procedures shall be documented and reviewed.

- Documented process simulation must be routinely undertaken to demonstrate that all processes are adequate and staff and facilities are fit for purpose.

- Before material is accepted from a third party, including receipt from abroad, the laboratory accepting the donation should, wherever possible, ensure that standards equivalent to those in UK guidelines have been met. Material should be inspected upon receipt and the condition of the product recorded.

- Where appropriate the HPC donation should be passed through a sterile non-reactive aggregate filter to remove fat, clots or bone spicules that may be present. A closed system must be used wherever practical.

- Processing and transplant facilities must agree and validate the adequacy of dose (total nucleated cells, mononuclear cells, CD34 positive cells and/or CFU-GM (colony-forming unit – granulocyte/macrophage) as appropriate for each source of HPC) required to achieve reliable and sustainable engraftment. Tests for cell dose and viability should be performed as in section 22.11.

22.10 Storage of cellular therapy products

Policies must be in place for the storage of all material whether or not destined for cryopreservation, e.g. HPC-M undergoing red cell depletion and for other HPCs prior to cryopreservation. Details should be specified for all types of storage conditions. These should cover:

- labelling
- primary and secondary containers
- storage temperature and duration
- cell concentration

It is recommended that donations with a nucleated cell concentration above 200×10^9/L are diluted to less than 200×10^9/L, preferably with autologous plasma. HPC-A donations must be placed at $4 \pm 2°C$ if they are for liquid storage and/or are not being processed immediately. It is recommended that the final concentration after addition of the cryoprotectant is less than 100×10^9/L.

- transport if appropriate.

Where donations of known virology or bacteriology positive material are stored, appropriate risk assessments ensuring adequate controls are in place must be completed.

22.10.1 Duration

Facilities storing HPC components shall establish policies for the duration and conditions of storage and indications for discard. Patients, donors and associated transplant centres should be informed about these policies and consent obtained where appropriate.

22.10.2 Alarm systems

- Storage devices shall have alarm systems that are continuously active.

- Alarm systems shall have audible signals.

- If laboratory personnel are not always present in the immediate area of the storage device, a remote alarm device shall be required at a location staffed 24 hours a day. Alternatively an auto-dial facility connecting to an on-call member of staff may be satisfactory.

- Alarms shall be set to activate at temperatures, or an unsafe level of liquid nitrogen, to allow time to salvage components.

- There shall be a written procedure to be followed if the storage device fails.

- A procedure for notifying laboratory personnel should be in place.

- Alarm systems shall be checked periodically for function.

- Additional storage devices of appropriate temperature shall be available for component storage if the primary storage device fails.

22.10.3 Inventory control

There shall be an inventory control system to enable component and quality control vials to be located. It should include the donor name or unique identifier, date of collection, type of storage device and location within it, and state the number of containers and vials and number issued, dates of issue and numbers of containers and vials remaining.

22.10.4 Cryopreservation

- **Archive samples** Aliquots of the HPC component, processed and stored under the same conditions as the HPC component, must be available for additional testing as necessary.

- Methods should be validated, taking into account critical pre-freeze variables such as temperature, duration of storage, cell density and type of cryoprotectant.

- A secondary container, 'double bagging', must always be used to prevent cross-contamination between donations and to effectively quarantine the unit.

- The containers must be clearly and unambiguously labelled using labels that have been validated for use under the required storage conditions. The data on the labels must be in accordance with FACT-JACIE and NetCord-FACT Standards.

- Cryopreservation of the HPC product must be with an established cryoprotectant (e.g. 10% DMSO), used in a validated procedure with defined times and temperatures of exposure to specified concentrations.

- Established conditions of time and temperature of exposure of the HPC component to the cryoprotectant must be observed. These must be specific to the cryoprotectant system used. Validated storage conditions for the cryoprotectant must be observed.

Frozen HPCs should be stored at a sufficiently low temperature to ensure recovery of living cells after the intended preservation period. HPC donations are generally stored for named patients in low volumes using containers with a high surface area. To minimise the risk of transient warming events that may reduce viability and to maximise the time available to salvage donations should a storage device fail a temperature below −150°C should be used.

It is recommended that the vapour phase of liquid nitrogen is used to reduce the risk of cross-contamination. It is recognised, however, that this is associated with a greater temperature fluctuation and measures should be taken to ensure that the paragraph above applies. Some facilities may employ total or partial immersion in liquid phase to store HPC donations. Whatever method of storage is used it must always be assumed that liquid nitrogen is microbially contaminated and secondary enclosure must be employed.

For vapour phase the storage vessels should be fitted with a minimum of two temperature probes that are linked to a remote central monitoring system manned continuously. For liquid phase storage the vessel should be fitted with a minimum of a single probe. Records must be kept of these temperatures.

If liquid nitrogen refrigeration is used an automatic filling mechanism or a standardised manual procedure must be provided to ensure and document that adequate levels of liquid nitrogen are maintained.

22.11 Testing of haemopoietic progenitor cell donors and components including therapeutic cells

22.11.1 Infectious disease marker testing

This must be done in accordance with the requirements of the EU Directives on Tissues and Cells, SaBTO, FACT-JACIE and NetCord-FACT.

The minimum current requirements include testing for HIV, HTLV I/II, HBV, HCV and syphilis. Additional testing may be required in some cases, e.g. for malaria and toxoplasmosis. Table 22.1 indicates the requirements for the timing of testing for each type of HPC, while Chapter 9 contains further information on microbiology testing procedures.

Table 22.1 Requirements for the timing of testing

Test	Allo HPC-A/ HPC-M/TC	Auto HPC-A/ HPC-M	HPC-C donor mother	HPC-C
ABO + RhD	Test at each donation	Test at first donation		Day 0 to Day +7
anti-HIV 1/2 antibody	Day −30 to Day 0	Day −30 to Day 0	Day −7 to Day +7	Prior to release
anti-HCV antibody	Day −30 to Day 0	Day −30 to Day 0	Day −7 to Day +7	Prior to release
anti-HTLV I/II/ (pooled) antibody	Day −30 to Day 0	Day −30 to Day 0	Day −7 to Day +7	Prior to release
HCV RNA (pooled)	Day −30 to Day 0	Day −30 to Day 0	Day −7 to Day +7	Prior to release
HBsAg	Day −30 to Day 0	Day −30 to Day 0	Day −7 to Day +7	Prior to release
anti-HBc antibody	Day −30 to Day 0	Day −30 to Day 0	Day −7 to Day +7	Prior to release
CMV	Day −30 to Day 0	Day −30 to Day 0	Day −7 to Day +7	Prior to release
Pregnancy test	−7 days preconditioning			
Malaria	Where clinical indication	Where clinical indication	Where clinical indication. All mothers where there is risk	
Haemoglobinopathy, i.e. sickle cell	Where clinical indication	Where clinical indication		Prior to release
Syphilis screen*	Day −30 to Day 0	Day −30 to Day 0	Day −7 to Day +7	
Bacteriology testing	If manipulation	If manipulation		On final product
FBC	Before each apheresis procedure	Before each apheresis procedure		Pre and post process

* Confirmatory tests should be performed if screen positive

Additional tests must be undertaken for quarantined HPC-C products where a Day 180 repeat test has not been performed on the mother. The following tests should be performed on the mother's initial sample to permit release:

- HIV PCR   pooled/single
- HCV PCR   pooled/single
- HBV PCR   single

Mechanisms should be in place to ensure that archived material/samples can be re-tested at the time of issue of donation for all current markers of infection including the latest generation of assays.

22.11.2 HLA typing

- At initial registration: HLA-A, -B, -DR type by a Clinical Pathology Accreditation (CPA) and European Federation for Immunogenetics (EFI) accredited laboratory. As a minimum these antigens should be defined at low/medium resolution level using DNA techniques.

- Confirmatory typing: Must be performed on a sample drawn independently of that used for initial registration. HLA-A, -B, -C, -DRB3, -DRB4, -DRB5 and -DQB1 types should be defined, at a minimum, to medium resolution using DNA techniques. HLA-DRB1 should be defined to the allele level by DNA techniques. High/allele resolution typing for HLA-A, -B, -C, -DRB3, -DRB4, -DRB5, -DQB1 and -DPB1 can also be performed as required by the transplant protocol.

For cord blood donations it is recommended that a maternal sample is HLA typed to confirm identity. High-resolution typing of cord blood units shall take place when requested by a transplant centre. In cord blood banking, prior to the release of a cord blood unit for transplantation a sample obtained from a contiguous segment of the cryopreserved cord blood unit must be tested to verify HLA type or short tandem repeat (STR) can be performed according to NetCord-FACT Standards.

22.11.3 ABO and RhD typing

For allogeneic donors of HPC-A and HPC-M, ABO and RhD typing must be performed on samples taken from the donor or cell therapy component at the time of each collection. For autologous donors of HPC-A and HPC-M, ABO and RhD typing must be performed on samples taken from the donor or cell therapy component at the time of first collection. For HPC-C the ABO and RhD type of each donation shall be determined.

22.11.4 Clonogenic assays

Clonogenic assays (e.g. CFU-GM) may be undertaken as part of a quality programme or when specifically indicated or requested by the transplant physician. Consideration should be given to performing surrogate tests for viability prior to conditioning on a representative archive sample of any cryopreserved HPC components. For cord blood units CD34+ cells should be enumerated according to NetCord-FACT Standards and progenitor cell assays should be assessed on a thawed sample before release of the unit for transplant.

22.11.5 Sterility

Bacteriological and fungal screening employing aerobic and anaerobic conditions must be performed on the final HPC component after processing and before cryopreservation, unless validation studies demonstrate that bacteriological screening of waste processing material, such as plasma or erythrocytes, are equivalent to screening of the final product. All positive cultures should be subsequently identified and antibiotic sensitivities performed if the material is to be put to clinical use.

22.11.6 Test samples

Archival samples must be stored for reference and any future testing that may be required as described in the EU Directives on Tissues and Cells, FACT-JACIE Standards and NetCord-FACT Standards. Documentation must be kept to ensure security and accurate retrieval of the stored samples when required. Storage conditions must:

- maintain cell viability (below −150°C)
- be suitable to obtain material for the preparation of 50 mg DNA.

22.12 Labelling, packaging, transportation and temperature controls

The requirements for these are described in the HTA's Guide to Quality and Safety Assurance for Human Tissue and Cells for Patient Treatment, FACT-JACIE Standards and NetCord-FACT Standards and the requirements for labelling are summarised in Tables 22.2 and 22.3.

Table 22.2 Label content adapted from FACT-JACIE

Element	Partial label	Label at completion of collection	Label during processing	Label at completion of processing	Label at distribution	Inner and outer shipping container
Unique identifier of product	AF	AF	AF	AF	AF	
Proper name of product	AF	AF	AF	AF	AF	
Recipient name and identifier	AF (if applicable)	AF (if applicable)	AF (if applicable)	AF (if applicable)	AF (if applicable)	
Date, time collection ends and (if applicable) time zone		AF		AC	AC	
Approximate volume		AF		AC	AC	
Name and volume or concentration of anticoagulant and other additives		AC		AC	AC	
Donor identifier and (if applicable) name		AF		AT	AT	
Identity and address of collection facility or donor registry		AC		AC	AC	
Recommended storage temperature		AT		AT	AT	
Biohazard label		AC (if applicable)		AC (if applicable)	AC (if applicable)	AC (if applicable)
Identity and address of processing facility				AF	AF	
ABO and Rh of donor				AC	AC	
Red blood cell compatibility testing results				AC	AC (if applicable)	
Statement 'Properly identify intended recipient and product'				AC	AC	
Statement 'Warning; this product may transmit infectious agents'				AF	AF	
Expiration date				AF (if applicable)	AF (if applicable)	
Expiration time				AF (if applicable)	AF (if applicable)	

Element	Partial label	Label at completion of collection	Label during processing	Label at completion of processing	Label at distribution	Inner and outer shipping container
Statement 'For autologous use only' **or** Statement 'For use by intended recipient only'				AF (if applicable) AF (if for allogeneic recipient)	AF (if applicable) AF (if for allogeneic recipient)	
Statement 'Do not irradiate'				AT	AT	
Statement 'Not for infusion' including reason				AT (if applicable)	AT (if applicable)	
Name and address of receiving institution						AT
Name and telephone number of contact person at receiving institution						AT
Statement 'Medical specimen'						AT
Statement 'Do not X-ray'						AT
Name, address and telephone number of shipping facility						AT

AF = affixed, AT = attached or affixed, AC = accompanying or attached or affixed

22.13 Release

Prior to HPCs being cleared for issue, all relevant records, including donor records, processing and storage records, and post-processing quality control tests must have been reviewed, approved and documented as acceptable by the individual(s) responsible according to the relevant local standard operating procedures. Responsibility for setting policies for exceptional release and for issuing products on concession resides with the medical director/advisor.

Records must demonstrate that before cells are released the product specification is met and verified according to a written procedure by a person authorised by the Designated Individual.

For clinical use of a product that has not met its specification, exceptional release-specific authorisation must be given by the facility medical director or designee.

For cord blood donations release occurs at two stages:

- Following completion of testing and donor selection when donations are formally banked and made available for search.
- At issue for transplantation.

Table 22.3 Label content for HPC-C adapted from NetCord-FACT

Label element	Partial label	Label at completion of collection	Shipping container labelling for transport from collection	Label at completion of processing	Label at cord blood unit release	Dry shipper labelling at issue
Unique numeric or alphanumeric identifier	AF	AF		AF	AF	
Proper name HPC, Cord Blood	AF	AF	AF	AF	AF	
Product modifiers				AC	AC	
Statement 'Directed donor' (directed allogeneic and autologous HPC-C units)	AF	AF		AF	AF	
Collection centre identifier		AF	AT			
Date of collection		AF		AC	AC	
Time of collection		AC				
Name and volume or concentration of anticoagulant and other additives		AF		AC	AC	
Recommended storage temperature		AT		AF	AF	
Donor name (directed allogeneic and autologous HPC-C units)		AF		AF	AF	
Recipient's name, unique identifier or family (directed allogeneic and autologous HPC-C units) – if applicable		AF			AF	
Volume or weight of the HPC-C unit at the end of collection				AC	AC	
Volume or weight of the HPC-C unit at the end of processing				AC	AC	
Date of cryopreservation				AC	AC	
ABO group and Rh type				AC	AC	
HLA phenotype				AC	AC	
Number of nucleated cells post-processing				AC	AC	
Gender of HPC-C infant donor				AC	AC	
Identity of the cord blood bank				AF	AF	
Statement 'Properly identify intended recipient and product'					AT	
Statement 'For use by intended recipient only' (allogeneic HPC-C units)					AT	
A statement indicating that leucoreduction filters should not be used					AT	

Label element	Partial label	Label at completion of collection	Shipping container labelling for transport from collection	Label at completion of processing	Label at cord blood unit release	Dry shipper labelling at issue
Statement 'Do not irradiate'					AT	
Statement 'For non-clinical use only' (if applicable)					AT	
Biohazard labels – if applicable		AF	AF	AT	AT	
Date of distribution					AC	AF
Shipping facility name, address, telephone number			AF			AF
Receiving facility contact details			AF			AF
Identity of person or position responsible for receipt of shipment			AF			AF
Statement 'Do not X-ray'						AF
Statement 'Medical specimen', 'Handle with care'						AF
Statement indicating HPC-C for transplantation						AF
Shipper handling instructions						AF

AF = affixed, AT = attached or affixed, AC = ccompanying or attached or affixed

22.14 Transportation

The methods used to transport frozen components to the hospital must have been shown to maintain integrity of the component and to provide the temperature specified for storage. Liquid nitrogen dry shippers are suitable. Only components that were stored either partially or completely submerged in liquid nitrogen may be submerged in liquid nitrogen for transport.

22.15 Thawing and infusion

- The units should be thawed in a manner that has been established as appropriate for the overall preservation technique.

- Infusion documentation shall facilitate tracking of the product from the donor to recipient. A component infusion form shall be issued with the product and completed for each component infused. A copy should be returned to the processing laboratory.

- There must be an effective recall procedure in place defining responsibilities and actions to be taken including notification to the Competent Authority (HTA).

- Procedures must be in place for the documentation of returned products, defining acceptance criteria into the inventory.

22.16 Disposal of haemopoietic progenitor cells

- Appropriate prospective consent for discard should have been obtained. Prior to collection there shall be a written agreement between the processing facility and the donor defining the length of storage and circumstances for disposal or transfer of cellular therapy products to an alternative facility.

- The medical director/advisor of the processing facility, in consultation with the patient's transplant physician, must approve of component discard and method of disposal.

- There must be written documentation of the recipient's death or no further need for any component before it is discarded. Written instructions from the transplant physician should be obtained. The records for discarded components must indicate the component discarded, date of discard and method of disposal.

- The method of disposal and decontamination must meet the UK laws, current codes, rules and regulations for disposal of biohazardous materials.

22.17 Records

22.17.1 General requirements

- All patient records and results should be maintained to the requirements of the Caldicott Report (1997) and the Data Protection Act (1998).

- Records shall be accurate, legible and indelible.

- Records must be made concurrently with each step of the harvesting, processing, testing, cryopreservation, storage, issue and transplant or disposal of each component in such a way that all the steps may be accurately traced from donor to recipient.

- All records and communications between the collection, processing and transplant centres must be regarded as privileged and confidential. Safeguards to assure this confidentiality must be established and followed.

- Records required for full traceability must be kept for a minimum of 30 years after clinical use, in an appropriate and readable storage medium.

- Records including raw data, such as original temperature monitoring records, which are critical to the safety and quality of the tissues and cells, must be kept for at least 10 years after any expiry date, clinical use or disposal of the tissues and cells.

22.17.2 Records to be maintained

The requirements for these are described in the EU Directives on Tissues and Cells, FACT-JACIE Standards and NetCord-FACT Standards. Records of the following must be kept:

- donor and patient details
- collection and processing
- storage, issue and administration
- compatibility testing
- quality control

- personnel, training, continued education, competency testing
- incidents, errors and corrective action taken.

22.17.3 Records in cases of divided responsibility

If two or more facilities participate in the collection, processing or distribution of the product, the records of the processing facility shall show clearly the extent of its responsibility.

Chapter 23
Specification for the uniform labelling of blood, blood components and blood donor samples

23.1 Introduction

23.1.1 General information

The information contained in this chapter is intended to inform all persons involved in labelling blood and blood components of the specifications for uniform labelling. It is intended for users, software developers and suppliers of pre-printed labels.

The specification covers labels required by the United Kingdom Blood Transfusion Services (UKBTS) for the labelling of blood donation (collection) packs, satellite packs, associated samples and documentation. It utilises barcodes to encode information in addition to eye-readable symbols.

Blood pack labelling is in a period of transition as the established Codabar system is replaced with the International Society of Blood Transfusion (ISBT) international standard ISBT 128. Currently the UKBTS use ISBT 128 data structures for the donation identification number (DIN) and the blood group code.

Where this document refers to ISBT 128 cross-reference should be made to the ICCBBA Inc. (www.iccbba.org) ISBT 128 Standard Technical Specification which gives detailed information on data structures and labelling. This chapter interprets relevant sections of the Technical Specification in the light of UK requirements, and in some cases it limits the available options or deviates from the Technical Specification. In all such cases, this chapter takes precedence.

Further migration to ISBT 128 involves converting and/or adding more data structures and adopting the ISBT 128 definitions. The timetable for further changes is currently under consideration and development.

Note: Barcodes included in all figures are not readable and are for visual purposes only.

23.1.2 The purpose of a standardised, structured coding system

The objective is to reduce the dangers of incompatible blood transfusions caused by human error and a central part of the label design is machine-readable coding of essential information.

Each blood donation pack, plus connected satellite packs and associated samples and documentation, must be identified by a **unique** identification number applied at the time of donation. Additionally each pack requires identification by labelling showing the ABO group, RhD type and the component type. Such a system will ensure unique identification of every blood component, and help secure association between donations and samples.

Further adoption of an international coding system such as ISBT 128 will facilitate the movement of blood components across national and international boundaries.

23.1.3 Applicability

All blood pack/sample labels for use by the UK Blood Establishments must comply with the specifications in this document.

23.1.4 Referenced document

ISBT 128 Standard Technical Specification. See current version on the ICCBBA website (www.iccbba.org).

23.2 The labelling system

The labelling system for blood and blood components comprises the following elements:

- **The base label:** The label applied to the blood pack by the manufacturer of the blood pack or harness (see Chapter 26) and other critical consumables (see Chapter 27).

- **The donation identification number label:** A label bearing the ISBT 128 (donation identification number – ICCBBA Data Structure 001) with a barcode and eye-readable equivalent. Produced in sets these labels ensure the accurate and unique identification of a donation event (can include donation, sample(s) and documentation). Allocated at the point of donation, this number is fundamental to the secure audit trail for blood components.

- **The batch identification number label:** Also a label bearing the unique ISBT 128 (ICCBBA Data Structure 001) with a barcode and eye-readable equivalent. Applied to identify pooled blood components (prepared from a number of donations), for instance pooled platelets.

- **The blood group label:** A label bearing the ISBT 128 (nationally assigned data structure – see ICCBBA specification table RT003) defined short form unit identifier barcode, the ISBT 128 (Blood Groups [ABO and RhD] – ICCBBA Data Structure 002) blood group barcode and the Codabar expiry date barcode. This label also contains eye-readable information and label text on blood group, expiry and other blood characteristics. This label is applied by the Blood Establishments prior to a component's release into stock.

- **The component label:** A label currently utilising the Codabar component barcode, together with component-specific information. Applied at the time of component manufacture by the Blood Establishments.

The labels indicated in the second to fifth points above are all affixed onto the base label (see Chapter 26).

The final or complete arrangement of labels is shown in Figure 23.1. This diagram is for orientation purposes only. See under the appropriate sections for details of each label content and layout.

All labels must conform to the recommendations set out in the appropriate section of the ISBT 128 Standard Technical Specification unless specifically stated otherwise in this document.

Linear barcodes specified as ISBT 128 must comply with the Code 128 Bar Code Symbology and Application Specification. Barcodes specified as Codabar must be built to Codabar ABC standard with a recommended density of 10 (ten) characters per 25 mm. Any use of ISBT Data Matrix 2D barcodes will need to comply with the ICCBBA specifications and be authorised by the Joint UKBTS/HPA Professional Advisory Committee (JPAC) on advice from its Standing Advisory Committee on Information Technology (SACIT).

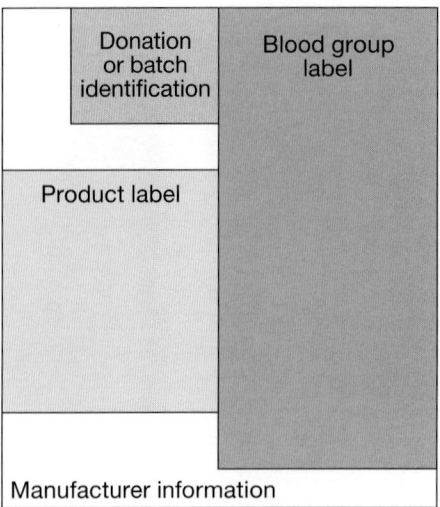

Figure 23.1 Layout of labels on the manufacturer's base label

All labels must be:

- self-adhesive using a non-invasive biocompatible adhesive (see ISO 10993 series – expanded in Chapter 26)

- tamper-evident (i.e. removal must deface the label)

- smear-resistant

- resistant to water, alcohol and humidity

- capable of being affixed readily to paper documents, base label material and sample containers (e.g. plastic or glass). Once applied, winging ('winging' is defined as the lifting of a label from the surface to which it is applied) must not exceed 2.5 mm as the maximum linear distance of the label not adhering to the surface at any label edge, measured after 24 hours of refrigeration at 4°C

- capable of withstanding a temperature range of –80°C to +56°C after application to the blood pack. This range may be extended by the ordering authority at the time of order

- capable of being applied without slippage during use where subject to temperature variation, e.g. tubes/packs stored in a vehicle and then used at normal ambient temperature, such equipment being by definition 'damp'

- non-flaking ('flaking' is defined as disintegration of the label or print material potentially affecting readability) regardless of instrumentation used for reading

- where sets of pre-printed labels are purchased from a vendor or created 'in-house' by appropriate systems, they must be printed at a quality standard that overall has a decodability of 'C' or above to be acceptable for use (ISO/IEC 15416 Barcode Quality Specification, 2000).

23.3 Barcode reading and interpretation

Barcoding is carried out to ensure the accuracy of transmitted information. To gain the maximum benefit from such coding, systems reading and interpreting the codes need to ensure that valid codes have been scanned. The following minimum checks should be carried out by the receiving application software:

- Ensure that the barcode identifiers (ICCBBA data identifiers) are correct for the code being read. For example, ISBT 128 Component code (ICCBBA Data Structure 003) would be expected to have a data identifier of '=<'.

- Ensure that the format (length and character types) of the received data string matches the defined format for the expected code. For example ISBT 128 Component code (ICCBBA Data Structure 003) should be ten characters long (two data identifiers plus eight data characters).

- Ensure that where checksums are used to validate correct data transmission, they are checked and valid.

- Any barcode scanning devices used to read linear ISBT 128 barcodes must conform to the industry standard ISO/IEC 15417: 2007 (E): Information technology – Automatic identification and data capture techniques – Code 128 barcode symbology specification.

23.3.1 ISBT 128 barcoding

Code 128 and Data Matrix (2D code) are high-density alphanumeric barcode symbologies which have been adopted by ICCBBA for the provision of a worldwide unique numbering and coding system for blood and blood components. ICCBBA defines the data structures of this system, the supporting reference databases and application-specific information. The specification for concatenation support provided by standard Code 128 has been modified at the request of ICCBBA to incorporate the need for spatial and/or temporal limitation on concatenated reading (refer to ICCBBA Technical Specification). Barcode readers used for reading these codes must comply with this specification.

23.3.1.1 The importance of data identifiers in ISBT 128 data structures

ISBT 128 barcodes comprise two main elements:

- The data identifier characters that identify which ISBT 128 data structure is being transmitted

- The data characters which provide the data values to be interpreted in accordance with the definition of the appropriate structure.

In order to accurately interpret information from an ISBT 128 barcode, it is essential that application software carries out the following steps before interpreting the data values:

- Analyse the data identifiers to ensure that the barcode entered is of the correct type

- Verify that the data length and format match that defined for the barcode type and included ISBT structure(s).

Failure to carry out these checks could lead to incorrect assignment of critical information.

23.3.1.2 Concatenation

Concatenation for the purpose of this requirement is defined as:

The reading of two horizontally adjacent barcodes together as a single input using a barcode-scanning device.

Concatenation requirements for ISBT 128 are laid out in the ICCBBA ISBT 128 Standard Technical Specification. Where concatenated codes are to be read, it is essential that the barcode readers used support concatenation.

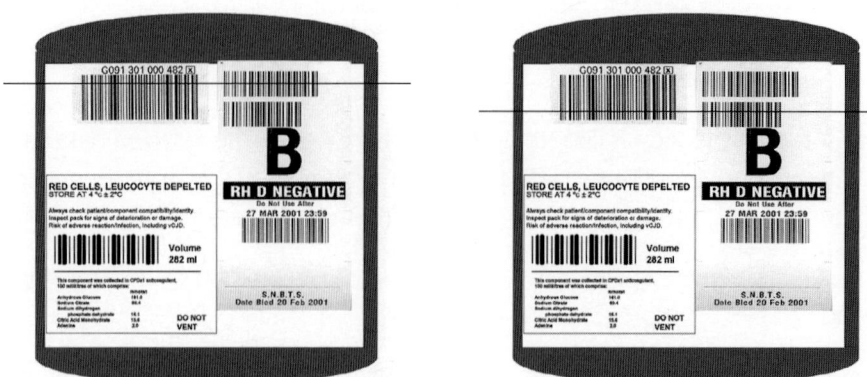

Figure 23.2 Two concatenation processes. On the left the donation identification number (DIN) with nationally defined structure, and on the right the DIN with the ABO/Rh blood group barcode

In the UK correct blood group labelling can be confirmed by up to two concatenation processes (see Figure 23.2).

- Concatenation of the donation identification number (ICCBBA Data Structure 001) with the short form unit identifier printed on the blood group label (this nationally defined code is a non-ICCBBA defined structure but is ICCBBA registered – see section 23.3.1.3 on National ISBT 128 definitions). This concatenation is mandatory for all UK Blood Establishments.

- Concatenation of the donation identification number (ICCBBA Data Structure 001) with the blood group (ICCBBA Data Structure 002) printed on the blood group label. (This concatenation is at the discretion of the Blood Establishment providing it can demonstrate other safety measures are in place.)

23.3.1.3 National ISBT 128 definitions

National bodies are permitted by ICCBBA to allocate nationally defined codes identified by data identifiers of '&' followed by a lower-case alpha character. Within the UK this responsibility lies with SACIT (Standing Advisory Committee on Information Technology).

The following national codes have been assigned by SACIT.

Short form donation identification number (Version 1)

&a

Defined for the shortened form of a donation number used on demand-printed group labels for concatenated read with the donation number as part of label verification. This code must not be used as the primary identifier of a component. The code structure is:

&annnnnn

Where:

&a   are the ISBT 128 data identifiers

nnnnnn is the six-digit unit serial number from the donation number definition (ICCBBA Data Identifier 001).

Short form donation identification number (Version 2)

&b

Defined for the shortened form of a donation number used on demand-printed group labels for concatenated read with the donation number as part of label verification. This code must not be used as the primary identifier of a component. The code structure is:

&bnnnnnnk

Where:

&b	are the data identifiers
nnnnnn	is the six-digit unit serial number from the donation number definition (ICCBBA Data Identifier 001)
k	is a single-digit iteration number, used to assist in controlling labelling where more than one labelling process takes place (e.g. an additional group label has to be placed over the initial label to display additional testing information such as CMV (cytomegalovirus) status).

Note: Where the counter is not utilised, its default value is 0.

Patient sample identification number for patient samples

&d

Defines a sample identification number for patient samples. The data structure is:

&daaaaayynnnnnnff

Where:

&d	are the data identifiers
aaaaa	is the facility identifier. The first character will always be zero. Values in the range 09900 to 09999 are assigned for use by NHSBT.
yy	is the nominal year of collection (slippage of 1 month either side of the end of year is permitted)
nnnnnn	is a six-digit sequence number
ff	are barcode check characters. These are derived from a two-digit checksum calculated from the data sequence aaaaayynnnnnn as described in the ICCBBA 128 Technical Specification for ISBT 128.

In the eye-readable form of this number, the checksum is represented as a single boxed character.

23.3.1.4 Codabar ABC barcoding

The Codabar ABC barcoding encodes the following characters:

- ten numerics {0, 1, 2, 3, 4, 5, 6, 7, 8, 9}
- six control characters {-, $, ., +, :, /}
- four start/stop (or pause) characters {a, b, c, d}.

Control codes

Within Codabar there are alpha characters assigned as start/stop characters. In some instances these are accompanied by a numeric (0–9), thus forming left-hand/right-hand control codes. These are used to identify the type of data encoded between the controls.

The assigned alpha characters are a, b, c, d.

Where an alpha character is accompanied by a numeric character, the combination will normally constitute the complete left/right-hand control and needs to be treated as such in decoding. Within the UK, however, there are instances where the numeric constituent of the left-hand control has been utilised as part of the data message (see section 23.6).

Codabar is only used in blood component labelling for component coding and expiry date representation.

23.3.1.5 Barcode specifications

Barcode dimensions

The minimum acceptable height for barcodes on labels in the UK is 6 mm. The standard density of the encoded characters is 0.4 character per mm. Inter-character gaps must be a minimum of 0.2 mm to provide adequate resolution between characters. Gap dimensions are not critical as each character is read independently and gaps do not carry information. The barcode is a series of straight parallel lines perpendicular to a base reference line.

Individual characters must not be misaligned by more than five degrees from adjacent characters.

A minimum border ('quiet zone') of 2.5 mm must be allowed at each end of the encoded message (but see section 23.4.1). The border above and below the code is not critical, but will normally include eye-readable information, the printing of which must not touch the code. Maximum depression or embossment of the printed barcode must not exceed 0.05 mm.

Optical parameters

The symbol is insensitive to the light-scattering properties of the substrate, except to the extent to which background reflectance is affected. Background diffuse reflectance is not specified as a separate parameter as it is integral in the definition of contrast (see below). However, a background diffuse reflectance of at least 70% (optical density 0.1) in the 500–950 nm range is necessary.

Contrast

Defined as the nominal difference in the diffuse reflectance between the background and the ink film, this should be at least 50% as measured over the 500–950 nm range. Measurements should be averaged over an area equivalent to a 0.2 mm diameter circle. A print contrast ratio of at least 90% is recommended.

Voids and ink specks

The missing ink coverage or 'white' spots within the bars or the extraneous dark specks between bars must not exceed 0.05 mm diameter, or subtend more than 25% of the area within a 0.10 mm diameter circle.

Edge roughness

The maximum area of edge irregularities subtending a 0.1 mm diameter circle must not exceed 25% of the area of that circle. The area of irregularity is to be measured with respect to the nominal bar edge.

Ink fill uniformity

Variation in ink film reflectance across the character should not exceed 5% within the same character.

Ink fill-in

Must not expand individual bars within characters to dimensions exceeding the tolerance specified for dimensional parameters ('see Barcode dimensions' above).

23.4 Donation identification numbers (DIN)

23.4.1 General structure

The donation identification number ('donation number') – ICCBBA Data Structure 001, plays a critical role in the safety of the blood supply. It provides a unique identification number which cross-references blood components and samples taken at the time of donation.

An example set of identification numbers is shown in Figure 23.3. Barcode density information is provided in the ICCBBA ISBT 128 Standard Technical Specification. The structure of the donation identification number is described further below. The example shows labels of various sizes and densities due to their use. If required, a tag can be incorporated in the labels designed for the blood tubes to facilitate the placing on the tube straight by users. This alignment is critical for blood samples being tested in analysers where the barcodes are read 'in situ' by internal barcode readers.

The donation identification number contains the facility code from where the donation has originated. These codes can be viewed on the ICCBBA website.

Blood Establishments can optionally add text below each number in the set to show from which Blood Establishment the donation originated.

Figure 23.3 ISBT 128 donation number sets (with and without Blood Establishment text)

23.4.1.1 General

All labels should have tamper evidence designed into the numbers sets to reduce the chance of a label being removed and re-stuck, i.e. any tampering with a label should deface the label making it unusable.

Labels should be self-adhesive using a non-invasive biocompatible adhesive (see ISO 10993 series – expanded in Chapter 26).

23.4.1.2 Requirements for pre-printed labels

Donation identification number (DIN) labels must be generated in primary sets under strictly controlled conditions which ensure that all the labels in a set bear the same number, and that each set is unique. It is the responsibility of the manufacturer of the label sets to undertake appropriate quality control measures to ensure these conditions are met.

The required number of individual labels comprising a set, the configuration of the labels and the commencing number for the print run, must be defined by the ordering authority at the time of order.

Quality control of sequential print must be organised to obviate the possibility of duplication within a print run, and also to avoid the misplacement of the various cutting devices which would cause any set to contain two different numbers.

Any unusable numbers or missing numbers **must not be replaced**.

Any roll/pad containing an incomplete sequence for any reason must have the discrepancy marked at the beginning of the roll/pad, or the manufacturer must supply a separate list of missing numbers. The total permissible missing numbers must not exceed 1% of the quantity ordered. Each roll/pad should not contain more than six missing numbers per 200 sets.

Pre-printed barcodes on number sets should be of decodability level no less than B to reduce label mis-reads.

The layout of the eye-readable numbers should follow the 4,3,3,3,1 format (see Figure 23.4).

Labels printed should have the correct facility identification code.

No barcodes within the number sets should have a height of less than 6 mm.

A quiet zone of at least 2 mm either side of each barcode is included in the label design.

Any incorporated check digits must be correct. This includes both barcode-incorporated and eye-readable check digits included in the design.

All adhesives used in production of these labels must be non-invasive biocompatible (see ISO 10993 series – expanded in Chapter 26).

Label colour: The labels must be printed black on a white background. Where required by the ordering establishment, part of an order may incorporate a coloured stripe (usually to assist in the identification of new (first-time) donors or sample-only donations). A colour must be selected which will not interfere with the efficiency of any barcode reader in decoding essential information.

23.4.1.3 Requirements for demand-printed labels

Additional donation identification labels may be demand-printed at the point of use.

Where demand-printing is used to generate additional labels for an existing set, the label must only be generated in direct response to the electronic input of a number from the original set.

Where demand-printing is used to generate new label sets, there must be controls to prevent number duplication.

Where ICCBBA flag characters are adopted within ICCBBA Data Structure 001, they must be used in accordance with the standard, and if they are incorporated within final component donation numbers, they must have been authorised by JPAC on advice from SACIT.

Locally printed barcodes should be of decodability grade level not less than C to reduce label mis-reads (see ISO 15416:2001).

The layout of the DIN eye-readable numbers printed should follow the 4,3,3,3,1 format (see Figure 23.4 and section 23.4.2).

Where applicable, labels printed should have the correct facility identification code.

No barcodes should be created with a height of less than 6 mm.

A quiet zone of at least 2 mm either side of each barcode is included in the label design.

Any incorporated check digits must be correct. This includes both barcode-incorporated and eye-readable check digits included in the design.

23.4.2 ISBT 128 donation identification number (DIN) barcode and text

Labels will follow the ISBT 128 Specification for Data Structure 001 with the exception of the eye-readable presentation.

The eye-readable presentation of the donation identification number must be presented in 4,3,3,3,1 format with the check character boxed (see Figure 23.4).

It is strongly recommended that all characters are of equal size and weight. The font used should be selected to clearly distinguish between similar alpha/numerics (e.g. 0 and O, 1 and I), and should be as large as possible within the constraints of label size.

Where keyboard entry of donation number is used, the full number and check character should be entered, and application software should verify the string format and check character value. Use of pre-programmed 'hot keys' is not an acceptable alternative.

Calculation of checksums and the corresponding check characters for the ISBT 128 numbers is described in the ICCBBA Technical Specification.

Note: Currently the UK standard only incorporates the modulus 37,2 check digits. If future developments include the flag characters in the donation number, they must be placed on the label at 90 degrees to the eye-readable text between the six-digit unit serial number and the eye-readable check digit. When the checksum is replaced with flag characters the eye-readable check digit **must** always be included in the label format. Any use of flag characters must be authorised through JPAC on advice from SACIT (see Figure 23.4, right).

Figure 23.4 Labels showing the use of flag characters. On the left, the label shows the eye-readable format 4,3,3,3,1 layout with the check digit in a box, and on the right, the same label shows the use of the flag character

23.5 Blood group labels

These labels are required for the purpose of blood group identification on the blood collection and satellite packs. The blood group can fall into one of eight classifications as shown in Table 23.1. Alternative labels, for use in special circumstances, are also described.

The blood group label is part of a complete overstick label and must be attached to the blood collection pack and/or satellite pack in the appropriate place immediately adjacent to the donation number. This is to allow a continuous straight-line read of the combined labels.

Label dimensions are defined below:

44 mm ±1 mm wide × 99 mm ±1 mm deep

(range 43–45 mm wide × 98–100 mm deep)

23.5.1 Label colour

All labels must be produced in black and white. All characters must be solid black on white except for RhD negatives where the ABO character must be in outline, and the 'RhD NEGATIVE' must be in solid white on a black background.

23.5.2 Printing

Group labels must be demand-printed at the point of labelling. The label must be generated in response to the electronic entry of a donation number and, once affixed to the blood pack, must be verified by the concatenated electronic entry of the codes from the donation number label and the group label. Valid blood group labels must only be generated for units which have been fully tested and are suitable for transfusion.

23.5.3 Information content

The label design is illustrated in Figure 23.5. The content is described in the subsections below from the top down.

23.5.3.1 Group label verification number

This must be printed at the top left-hand side of the label in barcode format only. It must be an ISBT 128 number, complying with one of the national definitions (&a or &b; see section 23.3.1.3). The distance of the barcode from the left-hand edge of the label must not be less than 2.5 mm or more than 4 mm.

The barcode must be between 7 mm and 10 mm high.

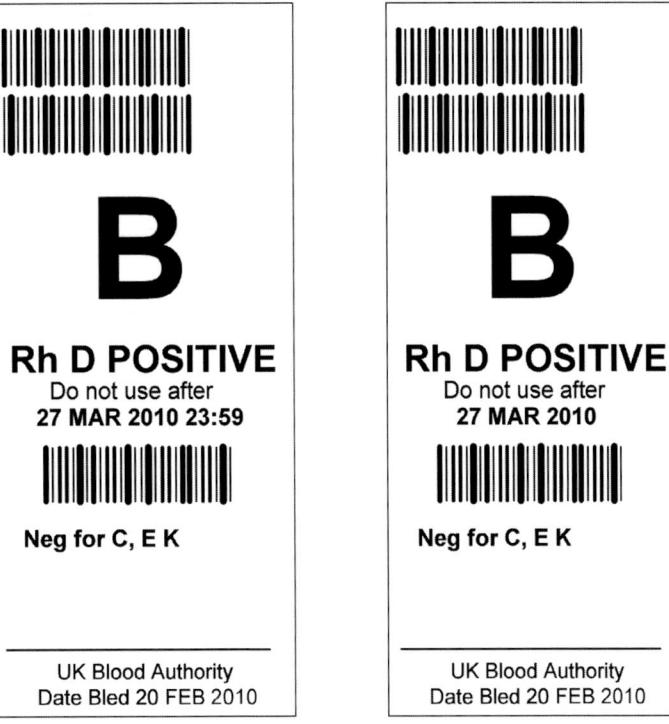

Figure 23.5 ABO/Rh blood group label layouts showing 'Do not use after' with and without time

23.5.3.2 Expiry day/month

The day and month of expiry may be included in the top right-hand corner (optional) of the label in eye-readable form and, if present, this must be in a DD/MM format. The text must be at least 2.5 mm away from the printed barcodes.

23.5.3.3 Blood group

The blood group barcode must be positioned below the group label verification number barcode separated by a gap of between 1 mm and 5 mm. The left-hand edges of the codes must be aligned. The blood group barcode must be between 7 mm and 10 mm high.

The format of the ISBT 128 group code will follow IDSBT 128 Data Structure 002 (see ICCBBA Standard Technical Specification).

In Data Structure 002, the value that holds the ABO/RhD and usage information is held in 2 characters labelled as 'gg'. The UK values of 'gg' for standard donations (without donation use limitations) are indicated in Table 23.1.

For donations using these group codes, the eye-readable blood group must be presented in two parts. The ABO group must be printed immediately below the group barcode. The characters must be solid black for RhD positives, and outline for RhD negatives.

The RhD status must be indicated immediately below the group barcode and eye-readable ABO. The text must be 'RhD POSITIVE' in solid black characters, or 'RhD NEGATIVE' in solid white characters enclosed in a black rectangular background.

The UK values of 'gg' used where donation use limitations apply are indicated in Table 23.2.

The eye-readable text associated with these codes is illustrated in Table 23.3 using O RhD POSITIVE as an example.

Table 23.1 Standard blood group classifications

Text	gg value	Text	gg value
O RhD POSITIVE	51	O RhD NEGATIVE	95
A RhD POSITIVE	62	A RhD NEGATIVE	06
B RhD POSITIVE	73	B RhD NEGATIVE	17
AB RhD POSITIVE	84	AB RhD NEGATIVE	28

Table 23.2 Usage limitation

ABO RhD blood groups	Usage – Directed donation only (gg value)	Usage – Emergency use only (gg value)	Usage – Directed donation, crossover permitted (gg value)	Usage – Autologous donation, crossover permitted (gg value)	Usage – Autologous use only (gg value)
O Rhesus D POSITIVE	47	48	50	52	53
O Rhesus D NEGATIVE	91	92	94	96	97
A Rhesus D POSITIVE	58	59	61	63	64
A Rhesus D NEGATIVE	02	03	05	07	08
B Rhesus D POSITIVE	69	70	72	74	75
B Rhesus D NEGATIVE	13	14	16	18	19
AB Rhesus D POSITIVE	80	81	83	85	86
AB Rhesus D NEGATIVE	24	25	27	29	30

Table 23.3 Blood group and donation use label text

gg	Label text
47	DIRECTED USE ONLY O RhD POSITIVE
48	EMERGENCY USE ONLY O RhD POSITIVE
50	DIRECTED (Eligible for Crossover) O RhD POSITIVE
52	AUTOLOGOUS (Eligible for Crossover) O RhD POSITIVE
53	AUTOLOGOUS USE ONLY O RhD POSITIVE

23.5.3.4 Expiry date or 'Do not use after'

The expiry date must be presented in eye-readable and barcode formats. The eye-readable text must be printed with characters of no less than 3 mm height. The content as a minimum must comprise the day number, the month represented by its first three characters, and the four-digit year (e.g. 1 FEB 2010). Where a system can include time to be printed as part of the eye-readable text it must be recorded after the year in the 24-hour format (e.g. 1 FEB 2010 23:59).

Currently the expiry date is coded using a Codabar barcode. The barcode must have a start code of 'a2' and a stop code of '4a'. The data content must be the last three digits of the year, and a three-digit Julian day number; thus 1 Feb 2010 would be represented by '010032', i.e. the 32nd day of the year.

While the current practice may allow the use of either 'Expiry date' or 'Do not use after' to identify when the component expires, consideration should be given to adopt 'Do not use after'.

23.5.3.5 Additional information (standard donations)

Additional information may appear immediately below the expiry date in an area no less than 10 mm and no more than 25 mm high. The data content of this section is at the discretion of the labelling authority, but is available for providing additional information on phenotypes, CMV status etc. Some UK Blood Establishments use a Codabar barcode of a8738a to indicate anti-CMV negative in addition to the eye-readable description.

23.5.3.6 Collection facility identification

The identification of the collecting facility may be indicated in eye-readable format below the additional information section of the group label. Alternatively, this information may be printed as part of the donation identification number (see section 23.4). The text content will be identified by the relevant national service and may comprise one or two lines of text.

23.5.3.7 Date bled

This must be printed in eye-readable form only at the bottom of the label. The characters must be no less than 3 mm high. The format must be day number as two digits, first three characters of the month name, and the four-digit year, e.g. 01 JAN 2010. Where a system can include time to be printed as part of the eye-readable format, it must be recorded after the year in the 24-hour format (e.g. 1 JAN 2010 23:59).

23.5.3.8 Label design for units with use limitations

An example of a blood group label design for units labelled with use limitations is shown in Figure 23.6. The lower section, used for additional information on standard labels, is used to indicate recipient information. It is important to recognise that this information is for identification of the recipient for which the donation is intended, but does not replace the need for crossmatch labelling or documentation.

Note: The NHS No. is in use in England; other countries will have an equivalent patient identification system that will be used in its place. Where this is the case, the numbering system used must be clearly identified so as not to introduce any ambiguity.

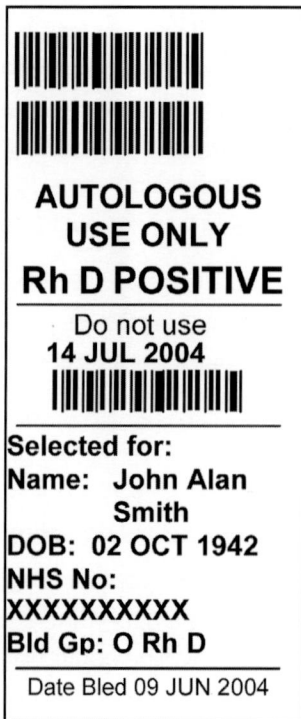

Figure 23.6 Label for unit with use limitations

23.5.3.9 Alternative labels

There are five status labels defined for use in the 'blood group label' location. The specification for these labels is divided into two sections, one for essential information which must be present on the label as specified, and one for optional information which may be added if desired.

All labels are to be demand-printed black on white.

The labels covered by this section of the specification are:

- HOLD label for use on donations where testing information is outstanding.

- NOT FOR TRANSFUSION label for use on units which are microbiology negative but not suitable for transfusion.

- RED CELLS NOT FOR CLINICAL USE label for use on donations which are microbiology negative but where the red cell component is unsuitable for transfusion.

- BIOHAZARD label for use on donations found to be microbiology positive.

- EMERGENCY USE ONLY label for use on donations which are to be issued for transfusion prior to completion of all mandatory testing.

23.5.3.10 'HOLD' label specification

Essential information

ISBT 128 barcode: ISBT 128 group code (ICCBBA Data Structure 002) where gg = 'Mq'. Positioned to allow concatenated read with an adjacent donation number.

Text: The word 'HOLD' in upper-case letters of minimum height 6 mm

Text: The words 'FURTHER INVESTIGATION REQUIRED' in upper-case letters of minimum height 3 mm.

Optional information

Text: The word 'Reason:' followed by a free-format message giving the reason for hold

Text: Identification text of the testing centre

Text: The words 'Date Bled:' followed by the date bled.

23.5.3.11 'NOT FOR TRANSFUSION' label specification

Essential information

ISBT 128 barcode: ISBT 128 group code (ICCBBA Data Structure 002) where gg = 'Md'. Positioned to allow concatenated read with an adjacent donation number.

Text: The words 'NOT FOR TRANSFUSION' in upper-case letters of minimum height 4 mm.

Optional information

Text: The word 'Reason:' followed by a free-format message

Text: The words 'Blood Group' followed by the ABO/RhD type if known

Text: Identification text of the testing centre

Text: The words 'Date Bled:' followed by the date bled.

23.5.3.12 'RED CELLS NOT FOR CLINICAL USE' label specification

Essential information

ISBT 128 barcode: ISBT 128 group code (ICCBBA Data Structure 002) where gg = 'Mf'. Positioned to allow concatenated read with an adjacent donation number.

Text: The words 'PLASMA USE ONLY' in upper-case letters of minimum height 2 mm

Text: The words 'RED CELLS NOT FOR CLINICAL USE' in upper-case letters of minimum height 4 mm.

Optional information

Text: The word 'Reason:' followed by a free-format message

Text: The words 'Blood Group' followed by the ABO/RhD type

Text: Identification text of the testing centre

Text: The words 'Date Bled:' followed by the date bled.

23.5.3.13 'BIOHAZARD' label specification

Essential information

ISBT 128 barcode: ISBT 128 group code (ICCBBA Data Structure 002) where gg = 'Mb'. Positioned to allow concatenated read with an adjacent donation number.

Text: The word 'BIOHAZARD' in upper-case letters of minimum height 4 mm

Text: The words 'HIGH RISK' in upper-case letters of minimum height 6 mm

Symbol: Biohazard warning symbol of minimum height 20 mm

Text: The words 'INACTIVATE BEFORE DISPOSAL' in upper-case letters of minimum height 2 mm.

Optional information

Text: Identification text of the testing centre

Text: The words 'Date Bled:' followed by the date bled.

23.5.3.14 'USE IN EMERGENCY ONLY' label specification

Essential information

ISBT 128 barcode: Under ISBT 128 it is necessary to include the historical ABO/RhD type within the barcode. This is achieved by using the modified ISBT 128 group code, where gg is as defined in Table 23.2. Positioned to allow concatenated read with an adjacent donation number.

Text: The words 'BLOOD GROUP NOT CONFIRMED, USE IN EMERGENCY ONLY' in upper-case letters of minimum height 4 mm

Text: The words 'UNCONFIRMED BLOOD GROUP:' followed by the unconfirmed ABO/RhD type if known

Text: The words 'DATE BLED:' followed by the date of collection

Text: The words 'EXPIRY DATE:' followed by the expiry date. Minimum text height 2 mm

Optional information

Text: Identification text of the testing centre

Text: Free-format additional status information such as 'Mandatory Microbiology Tests Negative'.

23.6 Component labels

23.6.1 General description

These labels are for use on blood collection packs and/or satellite packs. Each label will display a component description printed in bold text, a Codabar barcode and additional information. All information is printed in black on a white background. These labels may be pre-printed or produced using a demand-printed system where the information is transferred electronically from a host system.

23.6.2 Label dimensions

Label dimensions are defined below:

   55 mm ±1 mm wide × 55 mm +1/−3 mm deep

   (range 54–56 mm wide × 52–56 mm deep)

23.6.3 Label specification

The label must meet the following specifications:

- The barcode height must be no less than 10 mm with a 2 mm quiet zone each side of it.

- The barcode must have the eye-readable code textually displayed to accompany the barcode.

- The textual component description must be in bold characters and be exactly as is registered in the UK portfolio.

- Use of abbreviations must be authorised by the Standing Advisory Committee on Blood Components (SACBC) or JPAC groups.

- A UK JPAC agreed instruction statement must be included.

- The volume of the component must be textually displayed on the label as either the exact or as a nominal volume in millilitres (mL).

- Any storage or special instructions for storage must be included.

- The recipe for any included anticoagulant or additive must be indicated on the label in textual form.

- Where the component is part of a split component, the split should be identified as Pack 1, Pack 2 etc. textually on the label.

- If the component has a reference number (i.e. CT number), it should be included on the label in textual form with or without version number as a suffix.

Figure 23.7 shows an example of a component label layout.

23.6.4 Component barcodes

All components have an individual barcode. The barcode comprises three main elements:

- a start code 'a0'

- a five-character code to uniquely denote the component

- a stop code '3b'.

23.6.5 Component code reference table

The current component code reference table is held and managed by SACIT. The table includes:

- the text defining the component. Where possible this text is the same as that defined in Chapter 7 of these guidelines

- the start code for the component

- the code for the component, e.g. 04260

- the stop code for the component.

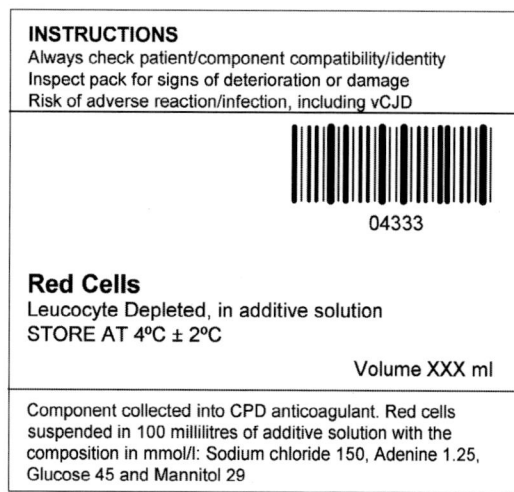

Figure 23.7 Example of a component label layout

23.6.6 Allocation of new component codes

In the event of a UK Blood Establishment requiring a code for a component that will be issued on a regular basis, the following steps must be carried out:

- A request form for a new component code, including a component being trialled, must be completed and sent to SACBC. This committee will determine if the component is a 'new' component or if it is covered by an existing component registration. If it is a new component it will be reviewed by SACBC members and if agreed, the product will be accepted.

- SACBC will authorise the component to be part of the UK component portfolio and it will then be numbered with a new unused Codabar component code.

Chapter 24
Specification for the uniform labelling of human tissue products using ISBT 128

24.1 Introduction

The ISBT 128 Standard is an internationally defined coding system for the barcoding of information on blood components, progenitor cells and tissues. Designed by the International Society of Blood Transfusion (ISBT) Working Party on Automation and Data Processing, the responsibility for the worldwide management and distribution of the ISBT 128 Technical Specification and associated databases now resides with the International Council for Commonality in Blood Banking Automation Inc. (ICCBBA).

A specification for the use of the coding system for the description of tissue products has been agreed by ICCBBA (ICCBBA Product Code Database, available from the website www.iccbba.org).

Some UK tissue bank facilities use Codabar product codes at present. The use of Codabar product codes for UK tissues will be phased out over time and the ISBT 128 product coding will be fully adopted in its place.

This chapter details the manner in which internationally agreed ISBT 128 tissue donation identification numbers, blood group codes and product description codes will be incorporated into tissue labelling systems in the UK where ISBT 128 is in use. The document cross-references the UK database of tissue product description label text which is maintained by the Joint UKBTS/HPA Professional Advisory Committee (JPAC) Standing Advisory Committee on Tissues and Cellular Therapy Products. The labelling of stem cell donations and products is outside the scope of this document.

The ICCBBA ISBT 128 Technical Specification is provided to companies and Blood Transfusion Services that have registered with ICCBBA, or may be downloaded directly from the ICCBBA website (www.iccbba.org).

24.1.1 The ISBT 128 Technical Specification: summary

The ISBT 128 Technical Specification:

- describes the standard layout for a blood group label

- defines the data identifiers for barcodes used in the tissue bank environment

- defines the data structures that carry information, i.e. how a particular barcode will be recognised by a reader, how many characters there are, and whether the characters are letters, numbers or both

- includes tables that define how complex barcodes should be translated, such as ABO/Rh blood groups.

24.2 The labelling system

The labelling system for retrieved tissues and tissue products comprises the following elements:

- **Base label:** The label applied to the retrieved tissue container following tissue retrieval and/or to the final container following tissue processing. It includes guide marks (preferably corner marks to prevent interference with barcode reading) to assist in the positioning of overstick labels. Retrieved tissue may be from living donors (retrieved during surgery) or from cadaveric donors (retrieved after death). It is noted that in the majority of cases, tissue is transferred during processing to a secondary/final container. In these circumstances a new base label is applied to the final container.

- **Donation identification number label:** A label bearing the ISBT 128 donation number barcode (ICCBBA Data Structure 001). Produced in sets, these labels ensure the accurate and unique labelling of all tissue donations and samples. Allocated at the point of donation, this number is fundamental to the secure audit trail for tissues. Where a retrieved tissue is processed without pooling or is issued unprocessed, the original donation number barcode is used to identify it to the point of implantation. This label will bear the title of the Service supplying the tissue, unless this is included on another label.

- **Batch/pool identification number label:** A label bearing an ICCBBA Data Structure 001 donation identification barcode. These labels are demand-printed when different tissues from one donor are pooled for processing. They ensure the accurate and unique identification of tissues once they have been pooled through to the individual resulting tissue grafts/units each of which bears the same identification number. Ideally, the number sequence used for batch/pool identification numbers should be different from donation number sequences and should be easily identifiable as batches/pools. This label will bear the title of the Service supplying the tissue, unless this is included on another label.

- **Product label:** A label bearing the ISBT 128 tissue product barcode (ICCBBA Data Structure 003) together with tissue product information, applied at the time of tissue retrieval and final tissue product manufacture. Where individual tissue units have been produced from a pool of tissues (from one or more donors) the product barcode can be used to individually identify up to 999 splits from the pool. This label can include unit-specific information.

- **Tissue status label:** A label indicating the status of a particular product in barcoded and eye-readable form. This is equivalent to the blood group label in blood banking. The following status labels can be applied and all use ISBT 128 coding (ICCBBA Data Structure 002):

  - FIT FOR CLINICAL USE (RhD NOT SPECIFIED)
  - QUARANTINE – NOT YET RELEASED FOR CLINICAL USE
  - RhD POS – FIT FOR CLINICAL USE
  - RhD NEG – FIT FOR CLINICAL USE
  - MUST BE STERILISED
  - FOR *IN VITRO* R & D ONLY
  - BIOHAZARDOUS
  - DISCARD
  - SEE OUTER CONTAINER FOR PRODUCT STATUS (for cryopreserved products)

- AUTOLOGOUS USE – FIT FOR CLINICAL USE
- AUTOLOGOUS USE – QUARANTINE.

The tissue status label will also bear the nationally defined unit identifier in barcode form (this is a non-ICCBBA defined data structure allocated by JPAC's Standing Advisory Committee on Information Technology (SACIT) to meet ICCBBA guidelines) and other donation-specific information (e.g. date of donation or retrieval site). This label will be applied by the tissue provider prior to release into stock, allocation for R&D or discard. (The only exception is the 'See outer container' label, which will be applied to the base label before the product is cryopreserved.) These labels are positioned to allow concatenation between the unit identifier barcode on the base label and the short form identifier and the rhesus/status barcodes on the status label.

- **Expiry date label:** A label indicating the date by which the tissue must be processed (if in quarantine), issued (if in issue stock) or used (if dispatched for clinical use). Different expiry date labels may be overstuck on products at different times. For example, some banks shorten the shelf life of products once they are issued from a bank due to concerns relating to appropriate long-term storage and control in hospitals.

The labels indicated above are all affixed onto a base label, except in the case of cryopreserved products where two status labels may be used: one on the product container itself (applied before cryopreservation), 'See outer container for product status', and one on the outer container giving the product status. In this case, a new base label, product label and expiry label should all be attached to the outer container. The arrangement of labels depends on the product and container type. Two options are shown in Figures 24.1 and 24.2; each would require a different base label. These diagrams are for orientation purposes only: see under the appropriate sections for details of each label content and layout.

The four basic quadrant labels may be printed as combination labels; for example, the donation number label and the product description label may be printed as a single vertical strip label and affixed to cover the left-hand half of a square base label. Similarly, expiry date information may be printed on a status label so that the two right-hand quadrants are printed as a single strip.

24.3 General requirements

24.3.1 Label quality

Labels used for tissue and sample labelling must be:

- self-adhesive using a non-invasive adhesive
- tamper-evident (i.e. removal must deface the label)
- smear-resistant and non-fading
- resistant to water and humidity
- capable of being affixed readily to paper or other base label material, plastic surfaces, glass (particularly glass tubes of 12 mm diameter) without winging ('winging' is defined as the lifting of a label from the surface to which it is applied). Winging should not exceed 2.5 mm as the maximum linear distance of the label not adhering to the tube at any label edge, measured after 24 hours of refrigeration at 4°C

- capable of withstanding a temperature range of –80°C to +56°C after application to the tissue container. This range may be extended by the ordering authority at the time of order. This condition must extend to the printed text which must not deteriorate due to thermal conditions. Where products are stored at lower temperatures, labels will be sealed into plastic pockets on the container

- capable of being applied without slippage to tubes etc. subject to temperature variation prior to use, for example tubes/packs stored in a vehicle and then used at normal ambient temperature, such equipment being by definition 'damp'

- non-flaking when read using a hand-held light-pen touching the label.

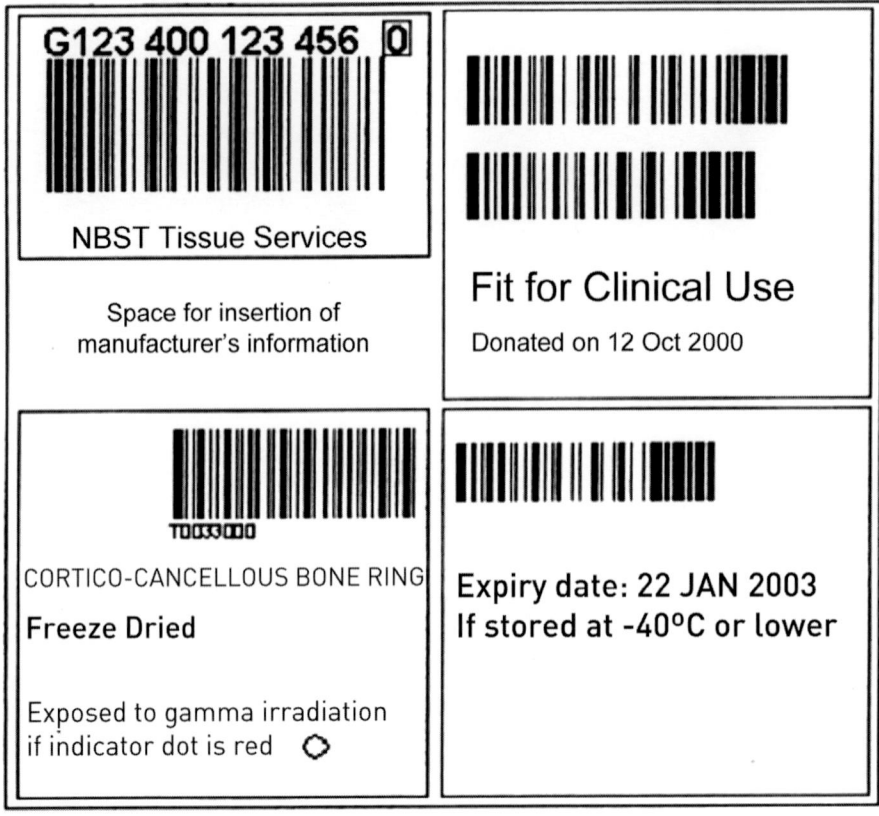

Figure 24.1 Label positioning: option 1 (example; see cautionary note in text)

Figure 24.2 Label positioning: option 2 (example; not to scale)

24.3.2 Printing requirements: eye-readable information

The ICCBBA ISBT 128 Technical Specification (latest version can be downloaded from the ICCBBA website www.iccbba.org) stipulates that 'Every bar code, with the exception of the donation identification number (ICCBBA Data Structure 001), should be accompanied by an exact eye-readable representation of the data characters in the bar code'. In the UK this requirement is not being implemented for the short form unit identifier, and is currently optional for the blood group/status code and expiry date code.

Requirements for each type of label are defined in the appropriate sections.

24.3.3 Printing requirements for barcodes

All barcodes will be printed as specified in the ICCBBA ISBT 128 Technical Specification.

24.3.4 Concatenation

Concatenation for the purpose of this requirement is defined as:

The reading of two horizontally adjacent barcodes together as a single input using a barcode-scanning device.

Concatenation requirements for ISBT 128 are laid out in the ICCBBA ISBT 128 Technical Specification and further expanded in ICCBBA Technical Bulletin No. 5. Where concatenated codes are to be read it is essential that the barcode readers used support concatenation of Code 128 barcodes with the defined temporal/spatial limitations of ISBT 128.

In the UK release status labelling will be confirmed by concatenation of the donation identification number (ICCBBA Data Structure 001) with the non-ICCBBA defined unit identifier (nationally defined – see section 24.3.5) and donation ID. The relevant data identifiers are specified within the appropriate sections of this document. For further details refer to the ICCBBA ISBT 128 Technical Specification (www.iccbba.org).

24.3.5 National ISBT 128 definitions

National bodies are permitted by ICCBBA to allocate nationally defined codes identified by data identifiers of '&' followed by a lower-case alpha character. Within the UK this responsibility lies with SACIT (Standing Advisory Committee on Information Technology).

The following national codes have been assigned by SACIT which will be applied in tissue labelling.

Short form donation identification number (Version 1)

&a

Defined for the shortened form of a donation number used on demand-printed status labels for concatenated read with the donation number as part of label verification. This code must not be used for any other purpose. The code structure is:

&annnnnn

Where:

&a are the ISBT 128 data identifiers

nnnnnn   is the six-digit unit serial number from the ISBT 128 donation number definition (ICCBBA Data Structure 001).

Short form donation identification number (Version 2)

&b

Defined for the shortened form of a donation number used on demand-printed status labels for concatenated read with the donation number as part of label verification. This code must not be used for any other purpose. The code structure is:

&bnnnnnnk

Where:

&b   are the data identifiers

nnnnnn   is the six-digit unit serial number from the ISBT 128 donation number definition

k   is a single-digit iteration number, used to assist in controlling labelling where more than one labelling process takes place (e.g. an additional group label has to be placed over the initial label to display additional testing information such as CMV (cytomegalovirus) status).

24.4 Tissue product labels

24.4.1 The base label

The base label dimensions are to be at least 110 mm wide by 104 mm high on all tissue containers/labels where the square format is used. Where the horizontal format is used they will be at least 220 mm wide by 52 mm high.

It is noted that where tissues are stored in very small containers, the base label may be attached to a secondary container. In these circumstances, the inner container will be labelled with the donation number barcode to provide a link to the label on the outer packaging.

The guide marks on Figures 24.3 and 24.4 are required to assist positioning of later labels.

24.4.1.1 Square format

The top left-hand quadrant will be used for the application of a donation identification number label. The space below this on the left-hand side of the label between 25 mm and 40 mm from the top edge must be left blank. This space may be pre-printed, for certain donations, by the company supplying the container with the lot/batch number of the container. This text must be visible at all times.

The bottom left-hand quadrant will be overstuck with a product description label.

The top right-hand quadrant will have pre-printed text indicating that the donation is in quarantine, as follows:

   QUARANTINE

   NOT YET RELEASED FOR CLINICAL USE

The top right-hand quadrant will be overstuck with a status label once its status has been determined (for cryopreserved products, this quadrant can be overstuck with a 'See outer container for product status' label). The status label can then be applied to a secondary container.

The bottom right-hand quadrant will be overstuck with an expiry date label which relates to expiry date prior to issue or to expiry date following issue.

24.4.1.2 Horizontal format

The same four quadrants will be used but the order in this case will be as shown in Figure 24.4.

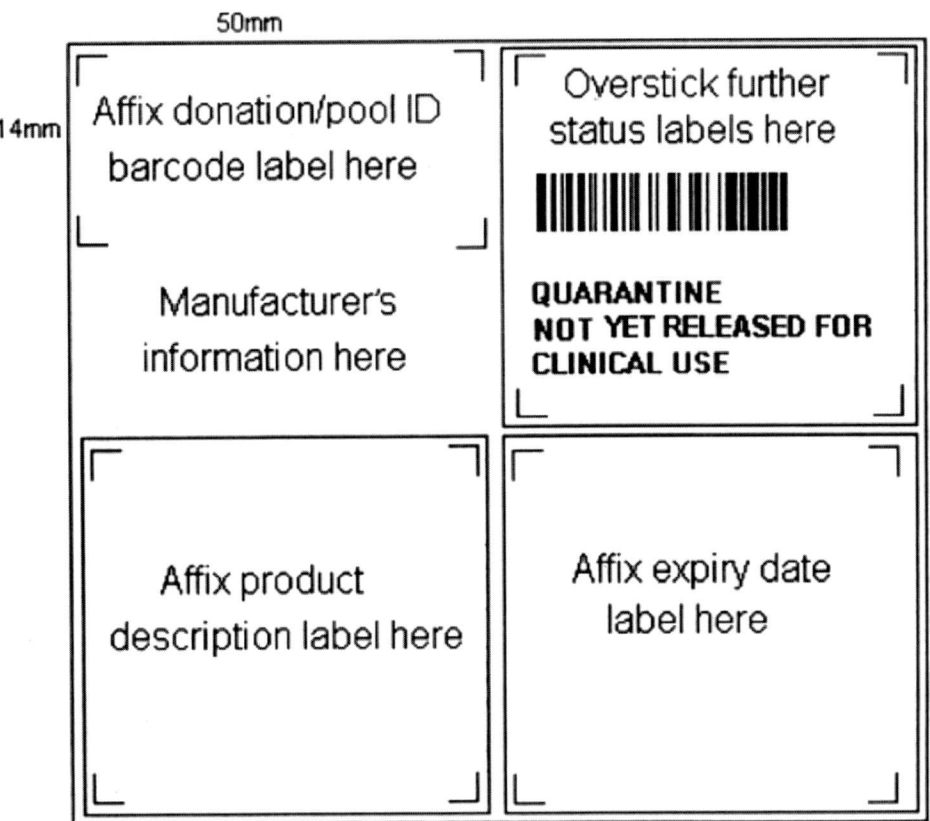

Figure 24.3 Base label design: square format

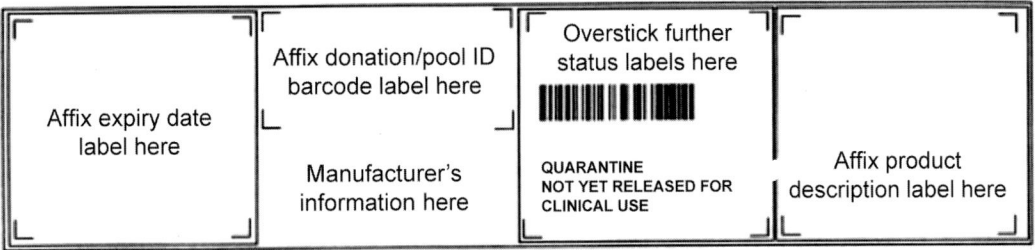

Figure 24.4 Base label design: horizontal format (not to scale)

24.4.2 Donation and pool identification number labels

The donation identification number plays a critical role in the safety of the tissue supply. It provides a unique identification number which cross-references tissue donations and products and samples taken at the time of donation. Where tissue products are not further processed, they are issued with the same donation identification number label.

Donation identification number labels must be generated in sets under strictly controlled conditions which ensure that all the labels in a set bear the same number, and that each set is unique. It is the responsibility of the manufacturer of the label sets to undertake appropriate quality control measures to ensure these conditions are met.

Figure 24.5 Donation identification number label set

Pool identification number labels are generated on demand when donations are processed together, whether from one or more donors.

As tissues are usually transferred from their original containers to secondary and tertiary containers during processing, it is a requirement that donation and pool identification numbers can be printed on demand.

An example set of identification numbers is shown in Figure 24.5. Barcode density information is provided in the ISBT 128 Technical Specification. The structure of the donation identification number is described further below.

For identification number labels to be applied to tissue products, the dimensions of the label are as indicated in Figure 24.6. As with all barcodes, there should be a minimum 'quiet zone' of 2.5 mm between the edge of the label and the start of the barcode. This label is affixed to the top left-hand section of the base label.

The donation identification number complies with ICCBBA Data Structure 001. The country/collection facility identification codes included within this data structure are allocated by ICCBBA and a list of these can be downloaded from ICCBBA's website. Any tissue service site within the UK requiring a new facility code must make a request first to SACIT before applying to ICCBBA for registration.

The collection year characters (6 and 7) should correspond to the last two digits of the year in which collection took place. In practice, this cannot be readily achieved using pre-printed labels without considerable wastage. Within the UK it is therefore permissible to allow a maximum variation of 1 month either way, i.e. it is permissible to use the previous year's collection year characters up to 31 January in the current year, and to use donation numbers with the following year's collection year characters from 1 December in the current year.

The use of ICCBBA Data Structure 001 allows either an inclusion of the modulus 37,2 check digits or the ability to use the last two characters as process control flags. At present all UK donation identification numbers incorporate the modulus 37,2 check digits. If the check digits are not used and process control flags are used in their place, they must be registered and authorised by SACIT prior to their use.

The algorithm for calculating 37,2 check characters can be found in the ICCBBA ISBT 128 Technical Specification. Users will need to take into account that units imported from countries outside the UK may well use these flag characters for process control as permitted in the specification.

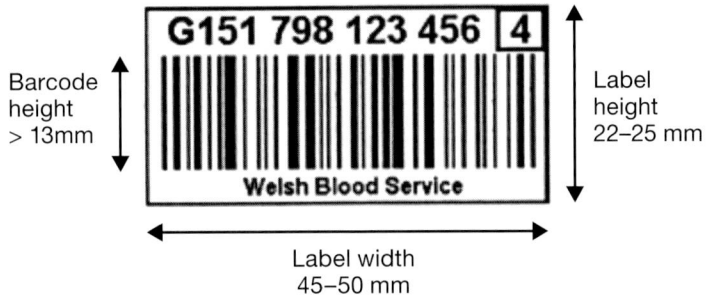

Figure 24.6 Donation number label dimensions

Figure 24.7 Donation number showing process control/flags characters

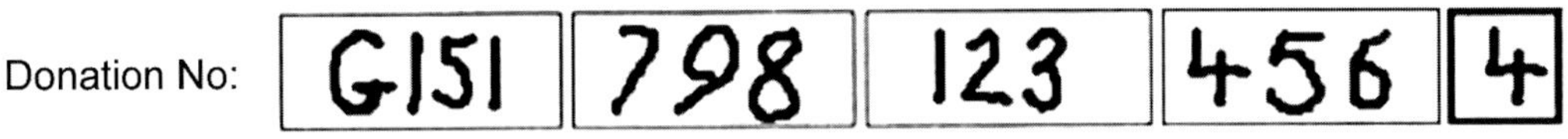

Donation No: | G151 | 798 | 123 | 456 | 4 |

Figure 24.8 Form boxes designed to enable accurate recording

The eye-readable format of the donation identification number in the UK comprises the data characters excluding the flag characters, followed by the manual entry check character. The layout differs from that in the ICCBBA ISBT 128 Technical Specification in that all characters of the number must be of equal size and weight. Printing of the six-digit unit serial number in larger or bold characters is not permitted. Software manufacturers should ensure that only the eye-readable format is presented in screen displays.

If process control flags are used within the donation identification number, they must be displayed as per the standard between the last digit and the boxed eye-readable check digit (i.e. 90 degrees to the rest of the number) as shown in Figure 24.7.

The number should be displayed with the characters grouped in a 4,3,3,3,1 arrangement. It is recommended that the check character be enclosed in a box where this is possible. The check character set uses the characters I and 1, 0 and O, and the font selected should be one which allows easy differentiation between these characters.

Where the donation identification number has to be recorded manually, form designs that assist accurate recording, such as the use of boxes to encourage correct character grouping, are recommended. An example is given in Figure 24.8.

The full eye-readable donation identification number, including check character, must be recorded and entered in all cases. The use of pre-programmed shortcut keys ('hot' keys) or pre-printing of part of a number is not acceptable.

24.4.3 The product label

The product label (50–55 mm wide by 50–52 mm high) is affixed to the left lower quadrant of the square base label or the right-hand side of the horizontal base label, if printed as a single quadrant (it may be printed as a combined label with another quadrant). A start product label is attached to all base labels at the time of tissue retrieval. If the tissue remains in the same container until the time of issue for implantation, it is issued with this product label. If it is subjected to further processing while remaining in its original container (e.g. gamma irradiation) the start product label is overstuck with the appropriate final product label before application of a status label. If it is transferred to another container following processing, a new base label is attached and the appropriate final product label is attached to the lower half of the base label following processing. The template for the product label is shown in Figure 24.9.

Codes for tissues and tissue products should only be used if they are registered with ICCBBA, approved by the Standing Advisory Committee on Tissues and Cellular Therapy Products (SACTCTP) and the Standing Advisory Committee on Information Technology (SACIT).

New tissue donations and tissue products will have codes assigned as required by SACIT in liaison with SACTCTP and ICCBBA. Requests for new codes should be made in writing or by e-mail to the Chair of SACIT with notification to the Chair of SACTCTP.

Updates of the Human Tissue Code Database can be obtained from the ICCBBA website (www.iccbba.org).

The first two lines of text contain the tissue component class and modifier, for example:

> CORTICO-CANCELLOUS BONE RING
>
> Freeze-dried

Lines 3 to 7 describe various attributes, where relevant, though one of these can be used to provide further product description information (see section 24.4.5). It is not necessary to include the unit of issue attribute details. Space will be available next to the method of sterilisation attribute where exposure 'dots' can be applied. The significance of the dot colour need not be detailed on the label but can be explained in the package insert. The volume/dimension field will contain either the actual or nominal tissue volume or other relevant dimensions (e.g. length, depth etc.). Immediately under the product barcode will be the unique reference number of the label which will correspond to the eye-readable barcode without the data identifier characters.

An example of a product label is given in Figure 24.10.

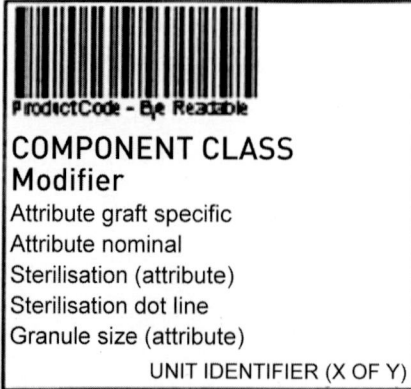

Figure 24.9 Tissue product label template

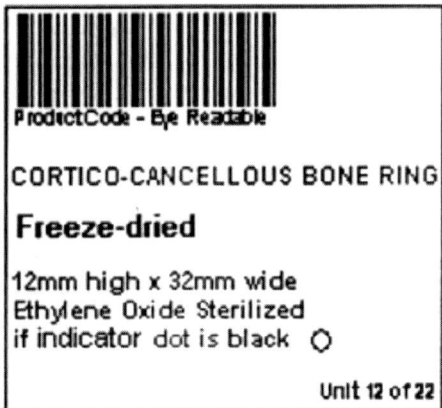

Figure 24.10 Product label (example)

Figure 24.11 Tissue release status label

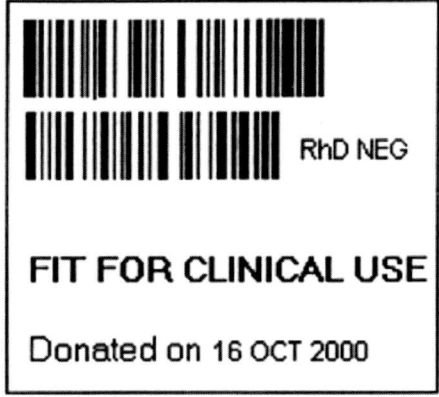

Figure 24.12 Status label (example)

24.4.4 The tissue status label

The tissue status label is a demand-printed label (50–55 mm wide by 50–52 mm high). The overall layout of the label is shown in Figure 24.11. This label can include graft-specific information such as date and site of donation.

An example of a status label is given in Figure 24.12.

The elements of the label content from top to bottom are described in the following sections.

24.4.4.1 Non-ICCBBA defined data structure – unit identifier (short form ID)

The tissue status label is unique to a specific donation. To ensure that it is affixed to the correct container a barcode, the nationally defined identification code, is printed on the label. This is used by the Service in a concatenated read with the donation identification number at the time of labelling. (Note: Although this is a non-ICCBBA defined data structure, it is ICCBBA authorised and controlled in the UK through the SACIT committee.)

The structure of the short form unit identifier is defined in section 24.3.5. Either the '&a' or '&b' versions of the code can be used.

Barcode indicating product status and the statement of product status

The statement of product status (which appears below the barcode) will be one of those listed in Table 24.1.

The barcode giving the product status is taken from the ICCBBA ISBT 128 Technical Specification.

24.4.4.2 Donation-specific information

Specific information which applies to the donation may be included on this label. This includes the RhD blood group and the date of donation.

The RhD blood group is only relevant where red cells remain in the final tissue product and where the product is supplied for female recipients of childbearing age.

Below the short form unit identifier is printed the RhD blood group barcode for certain products. The text relating to RhD type will be printed to the right of the status barcode. Where the RhD type is indicated, products will always be fit for clinical use.

Within the UK the blood group data structure will reflect that given in the ICCBAA Data Structure 002:

    =%ggre

Where:

'gg' is the ABO/Rh/status code. The default ABO/Rh codes or the special message codes described in the ICCBBA ISBT 128 Technical Specification will be used as indicated. The characters r and e from this data structure are not used in the UK at this time and are both set to 0 (i.e. 00).

For example, an RhD positive unit will code as:

    =%T100

The barcode and text content of these labels is described in section 24.4.5.

Date of donation can also be included on this label following the conventions described for expiry dates. This information does not need to be barcoded; it is represented in text only and must comprise the day number, the month represented by its first three characters, and the four-digit year (e.g. 1 FEB 2002).

24.4.5 Status label definitions

For each of the special message codes indicated in the status label section an associated status label is defined. The specification for these labels is divided into two sections: one for essential information which must be present on the label as specified, and one for optional information which may be added if desired. All labels are to be demand-printed black on white.

Table 24.1 Statements of product status

Statement	Status code
FIT FOR CLINICAL USE (RhD NOT DEFINED)	T3
QUARANTINE NOT YET RELEASED FOR CLINICAL USE	Mq
RhD POS FIT FOR CLINICAL USE	T1
RhD NEG FIT FOR CLINICAL USE	T2
MUST BE STERILIZED	T6
BIOHAZARDOUS	Mb
DISCARD	Md
FOR IN VITRO R & D ONLY	Mr
SEE OUTER CONTAINER FOR PRODUCT STATUS	T5
AUTOLOGOUS USE FIT FOR CLINICAL USE	Ma
AUTOLOGOUS USE QUARANTINE	T4

24.4.5.1   T3   'FIT FOR CLINICAL USE' (RhD not specified)

Essential information

Barcode: ISBT 128 group code, where gg = 'T3'. Positioned to allow concatenated read with an adjacent donation number

Text: The words 'FIT FOR CLINICAL USE' in upper-case letters of minimum height 4 mm.

24.4.5.2   Mq   'QUARANTINE – NOT YET AVAILABLE FOR CLINICAL USE'

Essential information

Barcode: ISBT 128 group code where gg = 'Mq'. Positioned to allow concatenated read with an adjacent donation number

Text: The words 'QUARANTINE' in upper-case letters of minimum height 6 mm

Text: The words 'NOT YET RELEASED FOR CLINICAL USE' in upper-case letters of minimum height 3 mm.

Optional information

Text: The word 'Reason:' followed by a free-format message giving the reason for hold.

24.4.5.3   T1   'RH D POS – FIT FOR CLINICAL USE'

Essential information

Barcode: ISBT 128 group code where gg = 'T1'. Positioned to allow concatenated read with an adjacent donation number

Text: The words 'RhD POS' in upper-case letters (except the 'h') of minimum height 6 mm to appear to the right of the status barcode

Text: The words 'FIT FOR CLINICAL USE' in upper-case letters of minimum height 3 mm.

24.4.5.4 T2 'RhD NEG – FIT FOR CLINICAL USE'

Essential information

Barcode: ISBT 128 group code where gg = 'T2'. Positioned to allow concatenated read with an adjacent donation number

Text: The words 'RhD NEG' in upper-case letters (except the 'h') of minimum height 6 mm to appear to the right of the status barcode

Text: The words 'FIT FOR CLINICAL USE' in upper-case letters of minimum height 3 mm.

24.4.5.5 T6 'MUST BE STERILIZED'

Essential information

Barcode: ISBT 128 group code where gg = 'T6'. Positioned to allow concatenated read with an adjacent donation number

Text: The words 'MUST BE STERILIZED' in upper-case letters of minimum height 3 mm.

Optional information

Text: The word 'Reason:' followed by a free-format message.

24.4.5.6 Mb 'BIOHAZARDOUS'

Essential information

Barcode: ISBT 128 group code where gg = 'Mb'. Positioned to allow concatenated read with an adjacent donation number

Text: The word 'BIOHAZARDOUS' in upper-case letters of minimum height 4 mm

Text: The words 'HIGH RISK' in upper-case letters of minimum height 6 mm

Symbol: Biohazard warning symbol of minimum height 20 mm.

24.4.5.7 Md 'DISCARD'

Essential information

Barcode: ISBT 128 group code where gg = 'Md'. Positioned to allow concatenated read with an adjacent donation number

Text: The words 'DISCARD' in upper-case letters of minimum height 4 mm.

Optional information

Text: The word 'Reason:' followed by a free-format message.

24.4.5.8 Mr 'FOR IN VITRO R & D ONLY'

Essential information

Barcode: ISBT 128 group code where gg = 'Mr'. Positioned to allow concatenated read with adjacent donation number

Text: The words 'FOR IN VITRO R & D ONLY' in upper-case letters of minimum height 3 mm.

24.4.5.9 T5 'SEE OUTER CONTAINER FOR PRODUCT STATUS'

Essential information

Barcode: ISBT 128 group code where gg = 'T5'. Positioned to allow concatenated read with adjacent donation number

Text: The words 'SEE OUTER CONTAINER FOR PRODUCT STATUS' in upper-case letters of minimum height 3 mm.

24.4.5.10 Ma 'AUTOLOGOUS USE (FIT FOR CLINICAL USE)'

Essential information

Barcode: ISBT 128 group code where gg = 'Ma'. Positioned to allow concatenated read with adjacent donation number

Text: The words 'AUTOLOGOUS USE' to appear in upper-case letters of minimum height 4 mm

Text: The words 'FIT FOR CLINICAL USE' to appear in upper-case letters of minimum height of 4 mm.

24.4.5.11 T4 'AUTOLOGOUS USE (QUARANTINE)'

Essential information

Barcode: ISBT 128 group code where gg = 'T4'. Positioned to allow concatenated read with adjacent donation number

Text: The words 'AUTOLOGOUS USE' to appear in upper-case letters of minimum height 4 mm

Text: The words 'QUARANTINE' to appear in upper-case letters of minimum height 4 mm.

24.4.6 The expiry date label

An expiry date label will be applied to base labels at the time of tissue retrieval and whenever another base label is used. A final expiry date label may be applied at the time of issue if the bank follows a policy of shortening the shelf life at the time of issue.

The use of a barcoded version of expiry date is optional. If used, it should follow either ICCBBA Data Structure 004 or 005 (it should be noted that Data Structure 004 will be stood down in the near future and only Data Structure 005 will be valid).

24.4.6.1 For ICCBBA Data Structure 004

=>cyyjjj

Where => are the data identifiers, 'c' designates the century (e.g. 9 for 1999; 0 for 2000); 'yy' designates the year and 'jjj' is the Julian date (i.e. the number of the day in the year, e.g. 022 is 22 JAN).

24.4.6.2 For ICCBBA Data Structure 005

&>cyyjjjhhmm

Where &> are the identifiers, cyyjjj are as Data Structure 004 and hhmm signifies the hour and minutes the product expires. It should be noted the default expiry for a product with a lifespan counted in full days will be 23:59, i.e. the product will expire on the last day at 23:59.

24.4.6.3 Other information

The expiry date must be presented in eye-readable format. Additional text will follow each expiry date and will be specific for each product. For instance:

> 22 JAN 2003 if stored at −40°C or lower

The eye-readable text must be printed with characters of no less than 3 mm height. The content must comprise the day number, the month represented by its first three characters, and the four-digit year (e.g. 1 FEB 2002).

The use of the date format DD MMM YYYY avoids problems which may arise due to national differences in the order of the elements of numerically expressed dates. The accepted month abbreviations are JAN, FEB, MAR, APR, MAY, JUN, JUL, AUG, SEP, OCT, NOV, DEC.

The expiry date label should also include the following text:

> See package insert for further information

Unit-specific product information such as product weight may also be included on the expiry date label. For example:

> 84 g

Where the expiry date label is printed as a quadrant label on its own it should also have the short form donation number barcode identifier (see section 24.3.5). This is not necessary where the label is printed as part of a status label (already including this identifier). An example of an expiry date label is shown in Figure 24.13.

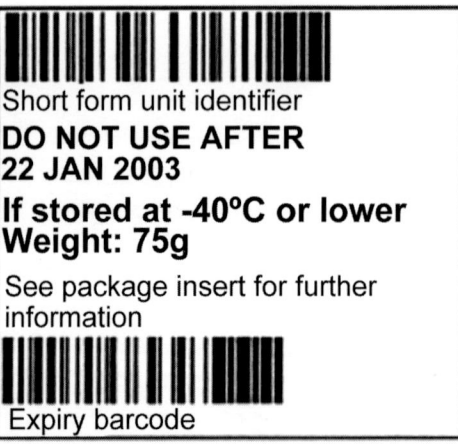

Figure 24.13 Expiry date label (example)

Chapter 25
Standards for electronic data interchange within the UK Blood Transfusion Services

25.1 Introduction

UK Blood Establishments and hospital blood bank computer systems have developed to provide sophisticated control of information on donors, blood components and patients, with secure methods of information transfer utilising barcodes and electronic data capture. However, secure information transfer between Blood Establishments and their customer hospitals has been limited to the barcoded information incorporated on the blood packs, and is of restricted scope.

In the future it is hoped that international electronic data interchange standards such as HL7 (not for profit organisation setting standards for healthcare IT communication in UK – www.hl7.org.uk) will be developed and adopted by Blood Establishments. The Joint UKBTS/HPA Professional Advisory Committee (JPAC) Standing Advisory Committee on Information Technology (SACIT) will continue to monitor developments by special interest groups in this area. Currently the International Society of Blood Transfusion (ISBT) Working Party on Information Technology has established an Interface Task Force to look at setting standards between laboratory instruments and Blood Establishment computer systems based on HL7 and LIS2 (EC programme promoting the information society in Latin America). The development and implementation of these international standards will take many years and SACIT has long recognised the desirability of developing UK standards for data transfer. The messages defined in this document are well established in the UK and should continue to be used.

This document describes a standard for messages used in communication between Blood Services and their customers. Each message comprises a standard envelope and a message content. The envelope specifies the overall structure of UKBTS messages and identifies the specific message content included inside the envelope. The message content will comply with one of the message protocols defined in this document. Each message protocol defines the content and format of a specific type of data transaction.

The standard does not address the delivery mechanism, or any surrounding envelopes. Thus, it provides a standard which is relevant to delivery mechanisms as diverse as e-mail messages, web page downloads, ftp transfers, or ASCII text files.

At the same time it retains a standard presentation of messages which readily identifies them as belonging to the UKBTS set, and allows a general process to identify the type of message received, the source and the destination.

25.2 Control of message structures

The standard is controlled by SACIT. All messages utilising the UKBTS envelope must comply with an approved message structure.

Proposals for new messages, or amendment to existing messages, should be submitted in the first instance to the Chair of SACIT. These will be reviewed by SACIT and if approved will be incorporated into the standard. While the objective is to obtain standards applied throughout the UK, the two-level structure does allow the flexibility of defining different structures at the message protocol level where essential.

25.3 General protocol

The general protocol defines the general character of the overall message, and elements which are common to both the envelope and the message content. The message uses standard ASCII characters throughout, and lines are terminated with the carriage return (ASCII 13) character. Fields are all fixed width and left-justified. Leading zeros for numeric fields are used only where explicitly indicated.

Please note that this standard does not necessarily conform to any particular operating system standard for specifying a text file. For example, Unix-based operating systems (including Apple Mac OS X) use line feed (ASCII 10) to terminate text lines and Microsoft Windows uses a combination of carriage return and line feed (ASCII 13 and ASCII 10). Apple Mac operating systems prior to OS X used a single carriage return to terminate text lines. Due to these inconsistencies files containing electronic data interchange messages must always be processed character by character and not rely on specific text processing functions.

The following are standard components of every line transmitted:

- The line number: A sequential number defining the line in the file, which is located in character positions 1 to 5 of every line. The header line will always have a line number of 00001.

- The checksum: The checksum immediately precedes the carriage return terminator of each line. The checksum is calculated by taking the sum of the ASCII value of all characters in the line, and then determining the modulus 97 remainder which becomes the checksum.

25.4 Envelope definition

The envelope definition defines the content of the first and last lines of the file/transmission (see Table 25.1).

The first or header line contains an identifier specifying that this is a message complying with a UKBTS specification, the date and time generated, the source and destination of the message, and the protocol number which identifies the relevant protocol to which the message conforms.

Source and destination identifiers for the Blood Establishments will be the ISBT 128 collection facility identification code. It is anticipated that hospital blood banks will use the identifier assigned by their local Blood Establishment.

The terminator line contains a record count indicating the total number of message lines excluding the header and terminator lines, and a standard terminator message.

25.5 Message protocols

Table 25.2 indicates the protocols defined to date.

Table 25.1 Envelope definition

Field	Length	Description	Format	Mandatory?	Notes
Header line					
1	5	Line number	NNNNN	Y	Always 00001 for header
2	10	Fixed text	'UKBTSSTART'	Y	
3	8	Date	YYYYMMDD	Y	
4	4	Time	HHMM	Y	
5	6	Protocol number	NNNNNN	Y	Allocated by UK SACIT
6	6	Source ID	XXXXXX	Y	
7	6	Destination ID	XXXXXX	Y	
8	2	Checksum	NN	Y	
9	1	Terminator	Carriage return	Y	
Footer line					
1	5	Line number	NNNNN	Y	
2	9	Fixed text	'UKBTSSTOP'	Y	
3	5	No. of records	NNNNN	Y	
4	2	Checksum	NN	Y	
5	1	Terminator	Carriage return	Y	

Table 25.2 Message protocol numbers

Protocol number	Title	Description
000001	Blood component dispatch information	Defines the message used to transfer information on blood component issues
000002	Blood derivative dispatch information	Defines the message used to transfer information on blood derivative issues
000003	Reagent dispatch information	Defines the message used to transfer information on reagent issues
000004	Blood component dispatch acknowledgement	Defines the message used to transfer information on blood components received
000005	Blood component fate information	Defines the message used to transfer information on the fate of blood components received

The message protocols contain a range of data defined as either mandatory or optional. The mandatory fields give essential information and must contain valid data. The optional fields give the flexibility to build in a wide range of additional information, but if not required are left as blank (space character) fields.

25.6 Protocol 000001 – blood component dispatch information

Two data line structures are defined within this protocol. The first is a single line containing administrative information (order no., dispatch no.), and the second is a multiple occurrence line with an entry for each item on the dispatch. To distinguish between the two line types, a line type indicator is included as the first field following the line number (see Tables 25.3 to 25.6).

Table 25.3 Message protocol 000001: blood component dispatch information: administration line

Field	Length	Description	Format	Mandatory?	Notes
1	5	Line number	NNNNN	Y	
2	1	Line type	N	Y	='1'
3	12	Order no.	C(12)	Y	
4	12	Dispatch no.	C(12)	Y	
5	8	Date	YYYYMMDD	Y	
6	4	Time	HHMM	N	
7	2	Checksum	NN	Y	
8	1	Terminator	Carriage return	Y	

Table 25.4 Message protocol 000001: blood component dispatch information: dispatch line

Field	Length	Description	Format	Mandatory?	Notes
1	5	Line number	NNNNN	Y	
2	1	Line type	N	Y	='2'
3	15	Unit identifier	C(15)	Y	ISBT 128 donation identification number (data characters with check character, e.g. 'G151797123456L')
4	9	Product code	C(9)	Y	Component code (either a full 9-character Codabar code (including start and stop characters), or an 8-character ISBT 128 product code excluding the data identifier characters)
5	2	Group ABO	C(2)	Y	'A', 'B', 'O' or 'AB'
6	1	Group RhD	C(1)	Y	'+' or '−'
7	8	Date bled	YYYYMMDD	N	
8	8	Date of expiry	YYYYMMDD	Y	
9	4	Time of expiry	HHMM	N	
10	30	Red cell phenotypes	C(30)	N	Position indicates antigen content (see Table 25.5), '+' or '−' for confirmed (tested this time) results, 'P' or 'N' for unconfirmed (historical) results
11	1	HLA flag	C(1)	N	'Y': indicates that HLA information is included either in the comment field or on separate documentation. Space: no information
12	1	CMV	C(1)	N	'+': positive '−': negative Space: unknown
13	1	Irradiated	C(1)	N	'Y': yes 'N' or space: no 'P': info in product code
14	10	Platelet-specific phenotype	C(10)	N	Position indicates antigen, content (see Table 25.6) '+': positive result '−': negative result

Table continues

Table 25.4 continued

Field	Length	Description	Format	Mandatory?	Notes
15	1	IgA	C(1)	N	'Y': indicates that IgA information is included either in the comment field or on separate documentation Space: no information
16	1	High-titre haemolysin	C(1)	N	'Y': present 'N': not present Space: untested
17	1	Neonatal	C(1)	N	'Y': suitable for neonatal use 'N': unsuitable Space: untested 'P': info in product code
18	1	Filtered	C(1)	N	No longer used
19	3	Volume	NNN	N	mL
20	10	Pack lot no.	C(10)	N	
21	1	Methylene blue	C(1)	N	No longer used
22	1	Clinical use	C(1)	Y	'Y': suitable for clinical use 'N': unsuitable for clinical use
23	1	Issue type	C(1)	Y	'R': routine issue 'S': selected, unmatched 'X': crossmatched 'G': autologous
24	10	Cost code/price	C(10)	N	
25	2	Added value code	C(2)	N	
26	30	Comment	Free text	N	
27	2	Checksum	NN	Y	
28	1	Terminator	Carriage return	Y	

Table 25.5 Message protocol 000001: blood component dispatch information. Field 10: red cell phenotype field – antigen codes

Character position in field	Antigen	Character position in field	Antigen
1	C	16	Jk^a
2	c	17	Jk^b
3	E	18	P_1
4	e	19	A_1
5	C^w	20	Lu^a
6	M	21	Lu^b
7	N	22	Kp^a
8	S	23	Kp^b
9	s	24	Unassigned
10	K	25	Unassigned
11	k	26	Unassigned
12	Le^a	27	Unassigned
13	Le^b	28	Unassigned
14	Fy^a	29	Unassigned
15	Fy^b	30	Unassigned

25.7 Protocol 000002 – blood derivative dispatch information

Two data line structures are defined within this protocol. The first is a single line containing administrative information (order no., dispatch no.), and the second is a multiple occurrence line with an entry for each item on the dispatch. To distinguish between the two line types, a line type indicator is included as the first field following the line number (see Tables 25.7 and 25.8).

Table 25.6 Message protocol 000001: blood component dispatch information. Field 14: platelet-specific phenotype

Character position in field	Antigen
1	HPA-1a
2	HPA-1b
3	HPA-3a
4	HPA-3b
5	HPA-5a
6	HPA-5b
7	Unassigned
8	Unassigned
9	Unassigned
10	Unassigned

Table 25.7 Message protocol 000002: blood derivative dispatch information: administration line

Field	Length	Description	Format	Mandatory?	Notes
1	5	Line number	NNNNN	Y	
2	1	Line type	N	Y	='1'
3	12	Order no.	C(12)	Y	
4	12	Dispatch no.	C(12)	Y	
5	8	Date	YYYYMMDD	Y	
6	4	Time	HHMM	N	
7	2	Checksum	NN	Y	
8	1	Terminator	Carriage return	Y	

25.8 Protocol 000003 – reagent dispatch information

Two data line structures are defined within this protocol. The first is a single line containing administrative information (order no., dispatch no.), and the second is a multiple occurrence line with an entry for each item on the dispatch. To distinguish between the two line types, a line type indicator is included as the first field following the line number (see Tables 25.9 and 25.10).

Table 25.8 Message protocol 000002: blood derivative dispatch information: dispatch line

Field	Length	Description	Format	Mandatory?	Notes
1	5	Line number	NNNNN	Y	
2	1	Line type	N	Y	='2'
3	15	Batch number	C(15)	Y	
4	15	Product code	C(15)	Y	Unique pharmaceutical product identification code
5	40	Product description	C(40)	N	Free-format text
6	30	Manufacturer's name	C(30)	N	Free-format text
7	8	Expiry date	YYYYMMDD	Y	
8	4	No. of vials/bottles	N(4)	Y	
9	10	Cost code/price	C(10)	N	
10	5	Actual dosage value	N(5)	N	Decimal values permitted
11	5	Actual dosage units	C(5)	N	Free-format text
12	30	Comment	C(30)	N	Free-format text
13	2	Checksum	NN	Y	
14	1	Terminator	Carriage return	Y	

Table 25.9 Message protocol 000003: reagent dispatch information: administration line

Field	Length	Description	Format	Mandatory?	Notes
1	5	Line number	NNNNN	Y	
2	1	Line type	N	Y	='1'
3	12	Order no.	C(12)	Y	
4	12	Dispatch no.	C(12)	Y	
5	8	Date	YYYYMMDD	Y	
6	4	Time	HHMM	N	
7	2	Checksum	NN	Y	
8	1	Terminator	Carriage return	Y	

Table 25.10 Message protocol 000003: reagent dispatch information: dispatch line

Field	Length	Description	Format	Mandatory?	Notes
1	5	Line number	NNNNN	Y	
2	1	Line type	N	Y	='2'
3	15	Batch number	C(15)	Y	
4	15	Product code	C(15)	Y	Unique reagent identification code
5	40	Product description	C(40)	N	Free-format text
6	30	Manufacturer's name	C(30)	N	Free-format text
7	8	Expiry date	YYYYMMDD	Y	
8	4	No. of vials/bottles	N(4)	Y	
9	10	Cost code/price	C(10)	N	
10	30	Comment	C(30)	N	Free-format text
11	2	Checksum	NN	Y	
12	1	Terminator	Carriage return	Y	

25.9 Protocol 000004 – blood component dispatch acknowledgement

Two data line structures are defined within this protocol. The first is a single line containing administrative information (order no., dispatch no.), and the second is a multiple occurrence line with an entry for each item on the dispatch. To distinguish between the two line types, a line type indicator is included as the first field following the line number (see Tables 25.11 and 25.12).

Table 25.11 Message protocol 000004: blood component dispatch acknowledgement: administration line

Field	Length	Description	Format	Mandatory?	Notes
1	5	Line number	NNNNN	Y	
2	1	Line type	N	Y	='1'
3	12	Order no.	C(12)	N	
4	12	Dispatch no.	C(12)	Y	From associated dispatch information message
5	8	Date of acknowledgement	YYYYMMDD	Y	
6	4	Time of acknowledgement	HHMM	N	
7	2	Checksum	NN	Y	
8	1	Terminator	Carriage return	Y	

Table 25.12 Message protocol 000004: blood component dispatch acknowledgement: dispatch line

Field	Length	Description	Format	Mandatory?	Notes
1	5	Line number	NNNNN	Y	
2	1	Line type	N	Y	='2'
3	15	Unit identifier	C(15)	Y	ISBT 128 donation identification number (data characters with check character, e.g. 'G151797123456L')
4	9	Product code	C(9)	Y	Component code (either a full 9-character Codabar code (including start and stop characters), or an 8-character ISBT 128 product code excluding the data identifier characters)
5	1	Received	C(1)	Y	'Y' or 'N'
6	2	Checksum	NN	Y	
7	1	Terminator	Carriage return	Y	

25.10 Protocol 000005 – blood component fate information

One data line structure is currently defined within this protocol (see Tables 25.13 and 25.14). The data line is a multiple occurrence line with an entry for each item in the message. The data line has a line type indicator in common with the previous protocols to allow for additional line types to be created if required. It is expected that this message will be generated daily and will include information on all units that are:

- free for use

- allocated to a patient (either directly or notionally)

- marked as transfused or wasted in the period from the date the report was last gathered (minus 5 days) up until the present date.

This message will be used for all products with the exception of certain batched products (such as anti-D). Some batched products are excluded as each dose may not be allocated a unique unit number (platelet pools are not excluded).

Table 25.13 Message protocol 000005: blood component fate information: data line

Field	Length	Description	Format	Mandatory?	Notes
1	5	Line number	NNNNN	Y	
2	1	Line type	N	Y	='1'
3	15	Unit number	C(15)	Y	ISBT 128 donation identification number (data characters with check character, e.g. 'G151797123456L')
4	9	Product code	C(9)	Y	Component code (either a full 9-character Codabar code (including start and stop characters), or an 8-character ISBT 128 product code excluding the data identifier characters)
5	2	Group ABO	C(2)	Y	'A', 'B', 'O' or 'AB'
6	1	Group RhD	C(1)	Y	'+' or '–'
7	1	Status	C(1)	Y	F = free A = allocated T = transfused W = wasted C = Confirmed transfusion Note: Confirmed transfusion refers to transfusions that have been positively confirmed by electronic means
8	5	Wasted classification code	C(5)	N	Only used if 'Status' (Field 7) is marked as wasted (W). The wasted classification codes are maintained by the Blood Stocks Management Scheme (see Table 25.14)
9	8	Date used/wasted	YYYYMMDD	N	Only if marked as wasted (W) or transfused (T or C). Presumptive YYYYMMDD should be included if exact date not known
10	4	Time used/wasted	HHMM	N	Only if marked as wasted (W) or transfused (T or C). Optional
11	3	Patient age	NNN	N	Only if marked as transfused (T or C). Optional. Age in number of full years
12	1	Patient gender	C(1)	N	Only if marked as transfused (T or C). Optional. M = male, F = female
13	10	Blank field	C(10)	N	Area reserved for future use
14	2	Checksum	NN	Y	
15	1	Terminator	Carriage return	Y	

Table 25.14 Message protocol 000005: blood component fate information. Field 8: wasted classification code

Product super-group	Code	Full name	Code usage	Date started	Date stopped
RED CELL	TIMEX	Time expiry	The expiry date on the unit has passed	01 Apr 2001	N/A
RED CELL	OTCOL	Out of temperature control outside laboratory	Unit has been left out of temperature range for longer than 30 minutes on the wards, in theatres or in any other non-laboratory location	01 Apr 2001	N/A
RED CELL	OTCIL	Out of temperature control inside laboratory	Unit has been left out of temperature range for longer than 30 minutes in the laboratory	01 Apr 2001	31 Mar 2003
RED CELL	FFAIL	Fridge failure	The unit has been discarded as a direct result of a fridge failure	01 Apr 2003	N/A
RED CELL	MISCN	Miscellaneous	Any other reason the unit is wasted that is not covered by other codes	01 Apr 2001	N/A
PLATELET	MORNU	Medically ordered not used	Platelets ordered for medical procedure but not used	01 Apr 2003	N/A
PLATELET	SORNU	Surgically ordered not used	Platelets ordered for surgical procedure but not used	01 Apr 2003	N/A
PLATELET	STMEX	Stock time expired	If a stock of platelets is held, the expiry date on the unit has passed	01 Apr 2003	N/A
PLATELET	WOSOL	Wasted outside of laboratory	Unit has been left out of temperature range for longer than 30 minutes outside the laboratory	01 Apr 2003	N/A
PLATELET	WIMPT	Wasted import	Unit imported with patient but not used	01 Apr 2003	N/A
PLATELET	MISCN	Miscellaneous	Any other reason the unit is wasted that is not covered by other codes	01 Apr 2003	N/A

Note: These codes are managed by the Blood Stocks Management Scheme. For further information visit www.bloodstocks.co.uk

Chapter 26
Specification for blood pack base labels

26.1 Introduction

This chapter defines the requirements of the UK Blood Transfusion Services for the layout and information content of the blood pack base label affixed to the blood pack by the pack manufacturer.

This specification applies to the base labels provided on all blood component packs either within a blood pack or apheresis assembly or 'stand-alone' (in this context, a blood component is a component as described in Chapter 7). In addition to these labelling requirements, all blood packs must satisfy the validation criteria of Chapter 8.

The base label must be able to accommodate the donation identification number, blood group and blood component overstick labels defined in Chapter 23.

References to linear dimensions in this document are in millimetres.

26.2 Specification

The layout of the blood pack base label is shown in Figure 26.1 and is divided into three areas. Area numbers on the diagram are for reference purposes only and must not be reproduced on the label. Where volumes are to be specified on the base label they must be given in millilitres. Anticoagulant and additive formulations must be in English.

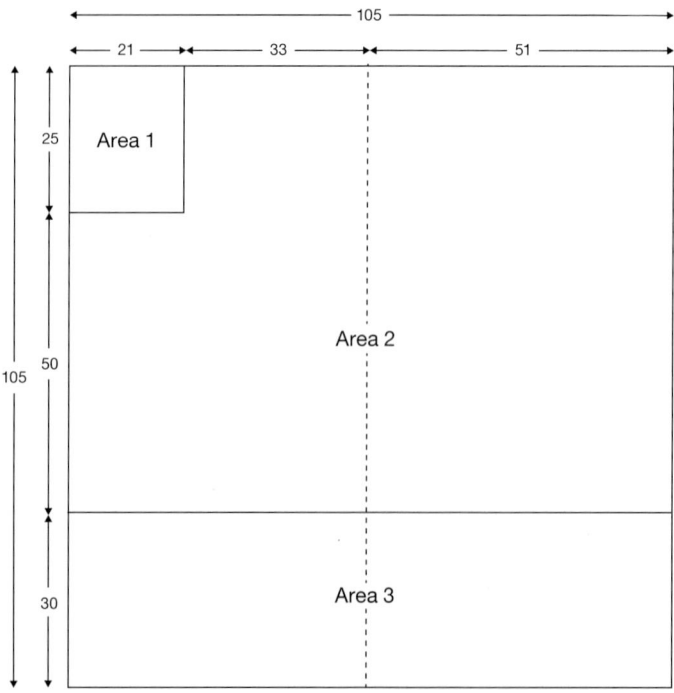

Figure 26.1 Base label layout: dimensions in millimetres for 400 mL to 600 mL pack

The manufacturer's logo may be printed in a colour of their choice. All other printing must be black on white. Labels, adhesive and ink must comply with the requirements of the current version of the International Organization for Standardization Standard ISO 3826-1, Plastics collapsible containers for human blood and blood components – Part 1: Conventional containers.

Area 1 is provided for the manufacturer to print their logo, name and address.

Area 2 is provided for the manufacturer for the following information concerning the medical device. (Note: this area is typically covered after application of Blood Transfusion Service overstick labelling.)

- On all packs the words or approved medical device symbol(s) shown in Figure 26.2:
  - Do not re-use this container
  - Do not vent
  - Contains phthalate e.g. DEHP (if applicable)
  - Sterile
  - Pyrogen free fluid pathway
  - Do not use if damaged/deteriorated
  - Expiry date (see note below)
  - Refer to instructions for use
- On all packs the 'CE' mark and the registration number.
- On primary blood collection packs, the formulation and volume of anticoagulant.
- On additive packs, the formulation and volume of the additive solution.
- The nominal volume of blood/component that is to be collected into the container. (Instructions for use should also give the volume range.)
- Where a pack is specifically intended for the storage of a particular component, the identity of that component, e.g. 'Suitable for the storage of platelets', must be labelled. Alternatively this information can be provided by symbols in the current version of ISO 3826-2 Plastics collapsible containers for human blood and blood components – Part 2: Graphic symbols for use on labels and instruction leaflets.
- Manufacturers should, where appropriate, indicate that the blood pack including its sub-components are latex free. The symbol in Figure 26.2 may be used.

  Note: The expiry date may be expressed as: 'Do not use after DD/MM/YY' where DD is the day number, MM the month number and YY the year. For clarity, the expiry date will be midnight (23:59 hours) on the date shown. It is permissible to use only MM/YY; in this instance the expiry date will be midnight on the last day of the month/year shown.

  The expiry date may alternatively be provided by the manufacturer on the immediate overwrap in which case the following statement must be applied to the base label: 'Use within x days of opening the immediate overwrap', where x is the number of days validated by the manufacturer.

Labelling of the blood pack overwrap and packaging must comply with the current versions of ISO 3826-1 and the EU Medical Devices Directive.

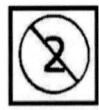 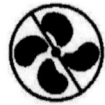 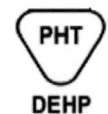 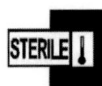

Do not re-use this container | Do not vent | Contains phthalate (DEHP) | Sterile | Pyrogen free fluid pathway

   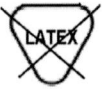

Do not use if damaged/deteriorated | Expiry date | Refer to instructions for use | Latex free

Figure 26.2 Symbols used on blood packs and on critical consumables (ISO 3826-2, ISO 15223-1 and EN 980)

Area 3 is provided for the manufacturer's pack type (list/catalogue) and pack batch or lot number. This information must be printed in both eye-readable and barcoded formats. The UK Blood Transfusion Services are currently in transition from ABC Codabar to ISBT 128 for the provision of this information. Details of both conventions are provided below. The manufacturer's pack type and lot number must remain visible in eye-readable format after application of overstick labels.

Labels must, after sterilisation, conform to the dimensions specified in Table 26.1.

Labelling of the blood pack overwrap and packaging must comply with the current versions of ISO 3826-1 and EU Medical Devices Directive.

Label adhesives applied directly to the plastic film of a blood bag must be tested and approved by manufacturers in accordance with the relevant current versions from the ISO 10993 biocompatibility series of standards (or equivalent national standards). The risk of the adhesive coming into contact with blood or blood components should be established by 'extractables' testing (ISO 10993 – Parts 1, 17 and 18). If testing reveals an unacceptable level of migration, biocompatibility testing should be extended to interaction with blood (ISO 10993 – Part 4) and toxicological testing (ISO 10993 – Parts 3 and 5).

- ISO 10993-1:2009 Biological evaluation of medical devices. Part 1: Evaluation and testing within a risk management process
- ISO 10993-3:2003 Biological evaluation of medical devices. Part 3: Tests for genotoxicity, carcinogenicity and reproductive toxicity
- ISO 10993-4:2002/Amd 1:2006 Biological evaluation of medical devices. Part 4: Selection of tests for interactions with blood
- ISO 10993-5:2009 Biological evaluation of medical devices. Part 5: Tests for in vitro cytotoxicity
- ISO 10993-17:2002 Biological evaluation of medical devices. Part 17: Establishment of allowable limits for leachable substances
- ISO 10993-18:2005 Biological evaluation of medical devices. Part 18: Chemical characterisation of materials.

Table 26.1 Blood bag base label dimensions (width × depth)

100 mL bag	60 × 85 ±5 mm*
250 mL bag	90 × 85 ±5 mm*
400 mL bag	105 × 105 ±5 mm
500 mL bag	105 × 105 ±5 mm
600 mL bag	105 × 105 ±5 mm

* The layout of base labels applied to smaller packs must be controlled within the purchasing specification. Barcode positions are indicated in the ISBT 128 (ICCBBA) product labelling section.

26.3 Manufacturers' blood pack catalogue and lot numbers

Below we describe two data structures for encoding the manufacturer's blood pack catalogue and lot numbers. The structures are fundamentally different but both coding systems use two data structures. For Codabar the manufacturer's code is with the lot number and the catalogue number/pack type is a separate code. For ISBT 128 the catalogue number/pack type is with the manufacturer's code and the lot number is a separate code. For ISBT both the catalogue and lot number are required to uniquely identify a batch of blood bags.

26.3.1 ABC Codabar manufacturer's blood pack catalogue and lot numbers

Currently Blood Services request Codabar barcoded information on each pack. Two classes of data are recorded, namely:

Catalogue number (pack type)

This label defines the type of pack, e.g. whole blood, platelet etc. The code is defined as follows:

$$cppppppk7b$$

Where:

c is the start code

pppppp is the manufacturer's list/catalogue number

k is the modulus 11 check digit

7b is the stop code.

Batch/lot number

This number describes the batch/lot number for each individual pack. The format is:

$$b1XXDDDDDDDC6b$$

Where:

b1 is the start code

XX is the manufacturer's code (see Table 26.2)

DDDDDDD is the batch/lot number

C is a modulus 11 check digit based on XXDDDDDDD

6b is the stop code.

Table 26.2 Manufacturers' Codabar codes

Manufacturer	Code	Manufacturer	Code
Baxter Healthcare	01	ASAHI Medical GmbH	10
TUTA Laboratories	02	Gambro BTC – UK	11
Biotest UK	03	Kawasumi Laboratories Inc	12
Haemonetics	04	Charter Medical	13
NPBI FRESENIUS	05	Baxter Healthcare – La Chatre	14
Terumo	06	Baxter Healthcare – Haina	15
Gambro BTC – US	07	Baxter Healthcare – Mountain Home	16
Maco Pharma	08	Cerus Europe BV	17
PALL	09	Fenwal – La Chatre	18

Note: Not all entries are in current use but are retained for use in look-back situations.

26.3.2 ISBT 128 manufacturers' blood pack catalogue and lot numbers

To achieve ISBT 128 compliance the UK Blood Transfusion Services will adopt the ISBT 128 convention for manufacturers' blood pack catalogue and lot numbers. Details are provided in the current version of ISBT 128 Standard Technical Specification, Data Structures 017 and 018, which is available on ICCBBA's website (www.iccbba.org).

Chapter 27
Specification for labelling consumables used in therapeutic product production

27.1 Introduction

This chapter defines the requirements of the UK Blood Transfusion Services for the labelling by the manufacturer of 'stand-alone' consumable medical devices (critical consumables) used in the production of therapeutic blood components and tissues.

These devices are distinct from blood bags (either individual bags or within a blood pack or apheresis set assembly, including those pre-filled with anticoagulant or preservatives) that are described in Chapter 26 and tissue containers which are described in Chapter 24.

This specification applies to:

- stand-alone intravenous (IV) and other solutions including:
  - preservatives and additives (e.g. platelet additive solution)
  - saline
  - dextrose and dextran
  - anticoagulants
  - pathogen inactivators
- filters (e.g. leucodepletion, prion filtration)
- fluid transfer sets
- injection sites, clamps, one-way valves.

27.2 Specification

All critical consumables used in the manufacture of therapeutic product that either come into contact with the therapeutic or influence its quality or the safety of recipients must be CE-marked medical devices (93/42/EEC).[1]

Where a harmonised European standard exists for such devices this is the preferred route for conformity assessment. A list of 'reference harmonised' EU standards is to be found at the European Commission Enterprise and Industry website.[2]

Labelling of critical consumables and their packaging shall comply with the EU Medical Devices Directive[1] and appropriate harmonised standards.

The critical consumable or, when there is insufficient space, its individual overwrap must bear the following information:

- The 'CE' mark and the registration number.
- The name and address of the manufacturer.
- The manufacturer's catalogue number (product code) and lot or batch number in eye-readable and preferably also barcode format (see below).
- On all products, the words or approved medical device symbol(s) shown in Figure 26.2:
  - Do not re-use this container
  - Sterile
  - Do not use if damaged/deteriorated
  - Expiry date (see note below)
  - Refer to instructions for use.

    Note: The expiry date may be expressed as: 'Do not use after DD/MM/YY' where DD is the day number, MM the month number and YY the year. For clarity, the expiry date will be midnight (23:59 hours) on the date shown. It is permissible to use only MM/YY; in this instance the expiry date will be midnight on the last day of the month/year shown.

    The expiry date may alternatively be provided by the manufacturer on the immediate overwrap in which case the following statement must be applied to the base label: 'Use within x days of opening the immediate overwrap' where x is the number of days validated by the manufacturer.

Containers for intravenous solutions must in addition bear the following information on each container:

- the nominal volume
- the formulation (in English) of the solution
- the words or approved medical device symbol(s) shown in Figure 26.2:
  - Do not vent
  - Contains phthalate (DEHP) (if applicable)
  - Pyrogen free fluid pathway (when applicable)
- Manufacturers should, when appropriate, indicate that the material of the container including its sub-components are latex free. The symbol in Figure 26.2 may be used.

Label adhesives applied directly to the surface of a critical consumable that may come into contact with blood or tissue must be tested and approved by manufacturers in accordance with the relevant current versions from the ISO 10993 biocompatibility series of standards (or equivalent national standards). The risk of the adhesive coming into contact with blood or tissue should be established by 'extractables' testing (ISO 10993 – Parts 1, 17 and 18). If testing reveals an unacceptable level of migration, biocompatibility testing should be extended to interaction with blood (ISO 10993 – Part 4) and toxicological testing (ISO 10993 – Parts 3 and 5).

- ISO 10993-1:2009 Biological evaluation of medical devices. Part 1: Evaluation and testing within a risk management process

- ISO 10993-3:2003 Biological evaluation of medical devices. Part 3: Tests for genotoxicity, carcinogenicity and reproductive toxicity

- ISO 10993-4:2002/Amd 1:2006 Biological evaluation of medical devices. Part 4: Selection of tests for interactions with blood

- ISO 10993-5:2009 Biological evaluation of medical devices. Part 5: Tests for in vitro cytotoxicity

- ISO 10993-17:2002 Biological evaluation of medical devices. Part 17: Establishment of allowable limits for leachable substances

- ISO 10993-18:2005 Biological evaluation of medical devices. Part 18: Chemical characterisation of materials.

27.3 Manufacturers' catalogue and lot numbers

Below we refer to a convention (ISBT 128) for encoding the manufacturer's catalogue and lot numbers. ISBT 128 is recognised by the UK Blood Transfusion Services which are progressing towards full compliance for their therapeutic products and associated critical consumables.

27.3.1 ISBT 128 manufacturers' blood pack catalogue and lot numbers

To achieve ISBT 128 compliance the UK Blood Transfusion Services will adopt the ISBT 128 convention for the manufacturer's catalogue and lot number barcodes on critical consumables. ISBT 128 codes the manufacturer's identity and catalogue number in one barcode and the lot number in a separate barcode. For ISBT, both the catalogue and lot number are required to uniquely identify a batch of critical consumables.

Full details are provided in the current version of ISBT 128 Standard Technical Specification, which is available on the ICCBBA website (www.iccbba.org). The following data structures apply:

- For stand-alone containers of intravenous solution and other critical consumables: Data Structures 021 and 022.

27.4 References

1. Council Directive 93/42/EEC of 14 June 1993 concerning medical devices. *OJ*, L 169, 12.7.1993, pp1–43.

2. References of harmonised standards and of other European standards can be found at http://ec.europa.eu/enterprise/policies/european-standards/index_en.htm

Annex 1
Standards available from the National Institute for Biological Standards and Control

This annex lists some of the various standards and reference materials available from the National Institute for Biological Standards and Control (NISBC) that are relevant to transfusion medicine. Further details of these preparations as well as the complete product catalogue are available on the website www.nibsc.ac.uk.

Table A1.1 Serological, virological and other preparations

	Status	Code
Serological and related preparations		
Anti-Human Platelet Antigen-1a minimum potency reagent	IRR	05/106
Anti-Human Platelet Antigen-5b minimum potency reagent	IRR	99/666
Anti-Human Platelet Antigen-3a minimum potency reagent	IRR	03/190
Anti-Human Platelet Antigen-1a *Intended for quantitation of anti-HPA-1a in International units*	IS	03/152
Anti-Human Neutrophil Antigen-1a minimum potency reagent	IRR	09/284
Anti-A minimum potency for blood grouping reagents	IS	03/188
Anti-B minimum potency for blood grouping reagents	IS	03/164
Anti-D minimum potency for blood grouping reagents *Intended to be used as the reference preparation for minimum acceptable potency of anti-D blood grouping reagents*	IS	99/836
Anti-D (Rho) antibodies, human *Intended to be used in the assay of plasma/serum anti-D levels by automated haemagglutination*	B†	73/515
Anti-c incomplete blood typing serum, human	IS	W1007 (67/160)
Anti-c serum, human *Intended to be used in the assay of plasma/serum anti-c levels by automated haemagglutination*	B†	84/628
Anti-C complete blood typing serum, human	IS	W1004
Anti-E complete blood typing serum, human	IS	W1005
Anti-D for operator proficiency* *Intended to be used to assure the sensitivity of routine antibody screening methods, to assess operator competence in performing and reading antiglobulin tests, to assure the efficacy of red cell washing prior to the addition of an antiglobulin reagent, and as an internal control for antibody titrations*	B	07/304
Anti-human globulin	ICSH/ISBT	96/666
Papain preparation for use with anti-D preparation 91/562*	ICSH/ISBT	92/658
Anti-D for use with papain preparation 92/658* *Intended to check the efficacy of enzyme preparations*	ICSH/ISBT	91/562

	Status	Code
Anti-D immunoglobulin, human *Intended for use in anti-D potency assays of anti-D immunoglobulin products*	IS	01/572
Anti-D immunoglobulin control* *Intended for use as a control in anti-D potency assays of anti-D immunoglobulin products to monitor assay consistency*	NR	99/728
Biotinylated Brad-5 (Bio-Brad-5)* *Intended for use in the competitive enzyme-linked immunoassay of potency of anti-D immunoglobulin products*	NR	99/698
Negative control for FCXM* *For use in flow cytometry cross matching (FCXM) and anti-HLA serology*	B†	09/112
Minimum potency positive control for FCXM* *For use in flow cytometry cross matching (FCXM) and anti-HLA serology*	B†	07/214
Anti-HLA Control *Negative control for Luminex-based anti-HLA serology*	B†	10/142
HLA Class II positive control for anti-HLA serology *Positive control for Luminex-based anti-HLA Class II serology*	B†	08/148
RHD/SRY plasma DNA sensitivity standard *For use in fetal RHD testing using maternal blood*	IRR	07/222
RBC1 gDNA *For blood group genotyping*	IRR	10/232
RBC4 gDNA *For blood group genotyping*	IRR	10/236
RBC5 gDNA *For blood group genotyping*	IRR	10/238
RBC12 gDNA *For blood group genotyping*	IRR	10/234
Blood Group Genotyping Reference Panel *One ampoule of each of 10/232, 10/234, 10/236 and 10/238 above*	IRR	11/214
HLA-A Genotyping Reference Panel *24 samples for use in DNA-based HLA typing*	NR†	05/208-001
HLA-DRB1 Genotyping Reference Panel *39 samples for use in DNA-based HLA typing*	NR†	10/136-001
Virological preparations		
Anti-HAV Immunoglobulin	IS	97/646
Anti-HBc	IS	95/522
Anti-HBs Immunoglobulin	IS	07/164
Anti-measles serum (for use in neutralisation assays only)	IS	97/648
Anti-parvovirus B19 serum (IgG), human	IS	01/602
Anti-VZ Immunoglobulin	IS	W1044
Anti-poliovirus serum, types 1, 2 and 3	IS	82/585
Anti-rubella serum	B†	67/182
Hepatitis B surface antigen (HBsAg) (subtype adw2, genotype A)	IS	00/588
Hepatitis A virus RNA	IS	00/560
Hepatitis C virus RNA	IS	06/100
HCV genotype panel (currently awaiting a replacement)	NR	See NIBSC catalogue

Table continues

Table A1.1 continued

	Status	Code
Hepatitis B virus DNA	IS	97/750
HIV-1 p24 antigen	IRR	90/636
HIV-1 RNA for NAT	IS	10/152
HIV-2 RNA for NAT	IS	08/150
HIV-1 NAT Subtype Reference Panel	IRR	12/244
Anti-HIV-1 British Working Standard (1 in 5 dilution)*	B†	99/710
Low-level control materials for HBsAg and anti-HCV	B†	See NIBSC catalogue for current batches
Anti-HIV-1 British Working Standard*	B†	99/750
Anti-HIV reference panel	IRR	02/210
Anti-HIV-2 Monitor Sample*	NR†	99/674
Anti-HTLV-1 Monitor Sample*	NR†	03/104
Parvovirus B19 DNA Genotype 1	IS	99/802
Parvovirus B19 genotype panel (Genotypes 1, 2 and 3)	IS	09/110
NAT working reagent for HAV RNA*	NR	01/488
NAT working reagent for HBV DNA*	NR†	11/182
NAT working reagent for HCV RNA*	NR†	02/264
NAT working reagent 1 for HIV-1 RNA (medium copy number)*	NR†	99/634
NAT working reagent 2 for HIV-1 RNA (high copy number)*	NR†	99/636
NAT working reagent for B19 DNA*	NR†	11/208
NAT working reagent for multiplex (HCV, HBV, HBV, HIV, B19)*	NR	99/732
Endotoxin	IS	94/580
Tetanus antitoxin	NR	76/589
Anti-HIV 1: Quality Control Serum: Sample 1	QCRHIV1QC1	
Anti-HIV 1: Quality Control Serum: Sample 2	QCRHIV1QC2	
Anti-HIV 1: Quality Control Serum: Sample 3	QCRHIV1QC3	
Anti-HIV 1: Quality Control Serum: Sample 5	QCRHIV1QC5	
HIV1 p24 Antigen : Quality Control Serum: 1	QCRHIV1P24QC1	
HIV1 p24 Antigen : Quality Control Serum: 2	QCRHIV1P24QC2	
Anti-HIV 2: Quality Control Serum: Sample 2	QCRHIV2QC2	
Anti-HIV 2: Quality Control Serum: Sample 3	QCRHIV2QC3	
Anti-CMV Quality Control Serum: Sample 1	QCRCMVQC1	
Anti-VZV Quality Control Serum: Sample 1	QCRVZVQC1	
Anti-Syphilis Quality Control Serum: Sample 1	QCRSYPHQC1	
Anti-Syphilis Quality Control Serum: Sample 2	QCRSYPHQC2	
Anti-Rubella Quality Control Serum: Sample 1	QCRRUBQC1	
Anti-Rubella Quality Control Serum: Sample 2	QCRRUBQC2	
Anti-Rubella IgM Quality Control Serum: Sample 1	QCRRUBIgMQC1	
Anti-Toxoplasma Quality Control Serum: 1	QCRTOXOQC1	
Anti-HSV1 Quality Control Serum: Sample 1	QCRHSV1QC1	
Anti-HSV2 Quality Control Serum: Sample 1	QCRHSV2QC1	
Anti-Malaria Quality Control Serum: Sample 1	QCRMALQC1	

ANNEX 1: STANDARDS AVAILABLE FROM THE NATIONAL INSTITUTE FOR BIOLOGICAL STANDARDS AND CONTROL

	Status	Code
Anti-HCV Quality Control Serum: Sample 1	QCRHCVQC1	
Anti-HBs Quality Control Serum: Sample 1	QCRHBsQC1	
HBsAg Quality Control Serum: Sample 1	QCRHBsGQC1	
HBsAg Quality Control Serum: Sample 2	QCRHBsGQC2	
Anti-HBe Quality Control Serum: Sample 1	QCRHBEQC1	
Total Anti-HBc Quality Control Serum: Sample 1	QCRTHBcQC1	
Total Anti-HBc Quality Control Serum: Sample 2	QCRTHBcQC2	
Total Anti-HAV Quality Control Serum: Sample 1	QCRTHAVQC1	
IgM Anti-HBc Quality Control Serum: Sample 1	QCRHBcIgMQC1	
IgM Anti-HAV Quality Control Serum: Sample 2	QCRHAVIgMQC2	

See the NIBSC website for details of materials currently available.

Key

IRR – International Reference Reagent or Panel

IS – International Standard

ICSH/ISBT – International Committee for Standardization in Hematology/International Society of Blood Transfusion

B – British Standard/Reference Reagent

NR – NIBSC Reagent

* Working Standards supplied as multiples of 5

† CE marked

Table A1.2 Coagulation preparations – WHO International Standards

Factor	Plasma	Concentrate	Purified	Code
ATIII	✓			08/258
ATIII		✓		06/166
Fibrinogen	✓			09/264
Fibrinogen		✓		09/242
II	✓			09/172
II		✓		11/126
IX	✓			09/172
IX		✓		07/182
IXa			✓	97/562
Protein C	✓			02/342
Protein C		✓		04/252
Protein S	✓			03/228
Thrombin			✓	01/580
V	✓			03/116
VII	✓			09/172
VIIa		✓		07/228
VII		✓		10/252
VIII	✓			07/316
VIII		✓		07/350
VWF	✓			07/316
VWF		✓		09/182
X	✓			09/172
X		✓		11/126
XI	✓			04/102
XIII	✓			02/206

Table A1.3 Coagulation preparations – British Standards

Preparation	Code
Blood Coagulation Factor VIII, Concentrate, Human (13th BS)*	10/188
Blood Coagulation Factors II, IX, X, Concentrate, Human (6th BS)*	07/326
FEIBA Concentrate, Human (1st NIBSC Working Reference Standard)*	06/172

* Working Standards supplied as multiples of 5

How to order

NIBSC does not charge for the reference materials themselves; however, there is a handling charge to part-cover administration and storage costs. The current handling charge is GB £70 per ampoule/vial.

Those preparations identified as 'working standards' are supplied as multiples of five with a current handling charge of GB £90 per five ampoules/vials. HLA genotyping panels are £675 each or £900 for both panels; other panels are £140. See the NIBSC website (www.nibsc.ac.uk) for prices of quality control reagents. NIBSC periodically adjusts the handling charge. Any changes to the handling charge are detailed on the website.

This handling charge covers the shipping cost of preparations that can be dispatched by (air) mail.

You can place an order by:

Mail: NIBSC, PO Box 1193, Blanche Lane, South Mimms, Potters Bar, Herts, EN6 3QH, UK
Fax: +44 (0) 1707 641064
E-mail: standards@nibsc.hpa.org.uk
Telephone: +44 (0) 1707 641467

Orders should include the following information:

- your full dispatch address and invoice address (if different)

- your purchase order number

- for EU customers, your VAT number or VAT exemption certificate

- for each item ordered, the NIBSC code number, preparation name and number of ampoules/vials required

- for preparations that are to be sent by courier/air freight, NIBSC must have a contact name along with both contact telephone and fax numbers

- your e-mail address or fax number. NIBSC will acknowledge receipt of your order. NIBSC would prefer to contact you by e-mail.

In addition, orders for infectious materials must be ordered on an NIBSC order form for infectious materials. These forms are available from the website www.nibsc.ac.uk.

Annex 2
ISBT 128 check character calculation

ISBT 128 donation numbers utilise check characters based on the ISO 7064 modulus 37,2 algorithm. This Annex shows how to calculate the check character for a given number. The calculation is based on the donation number string excluding the leading '=' symbol and the flag characters.

The steps in the process are as follows:

1. For each character in the string determine its check value as required by ISO 7064 (see Table A2.1).

2. For each character determine its weighted check value by multiplying the check value from (1) by the nth power of 2 where n is the position of the character from the right-hand end of the string.

3. Sum the weighted check values from (2).

4. Find the modulus 37 value of the sum from (3).

5. Subtract the value obtained in (4) from 38.

6. Find the modulus 37 value of the result of (5). This is the 37,2 checksum.

The calculated checksum is used to generate both the barcode check characters used in the flag positions of the ISBT 128 barcode and the eye-readable check character. The barcode check characters are determined by adding 60 to the checksum. The eye-readable check character is determined by cross-referencing the checksum to Table A2.1.

Table A2.1 Mapping from characters to ISO 7064 check values

Char	0	1	2	3	4	5	6	7	8	9	A	B	C	D
Value	0	1	2	3	4	5	6	7	8	9	10	11	12	13

Char	E	F	G	H	I	J	K	L	M	N	O	P	Q	R
Value	14	15	16	17	18	19	20	21	22	23	24	25	26	27

Char	S	T	U	V	W	X	Y	Z	*
Value	28	29	30	31	32	33	34	35	36

Table A2.2 Example of displayed numbers

Donation number G123 498 654 321				
Position from right (n)	2^n	Character	ISO7064 value (step 1)	Weighted value (step 2)
13	8192	G	16	131072
12	4096	1	1	4096
11	2048	2	2	4096
10	1024	3	3	3072
9	512	4	4	2048
8	256	9	9	2304
7	128	8	8	1024
6	64	6	6	384
5	32	5	5	160
4	16	4	4	64
3	8	3	3	24
2	4	2	2	8
1	2	1	1	2
Step 3	Sum of weighted values			148354
Step 4	Sum mod 37			21
Step 5	Subtract from 38			17
Step 6	Mod 37			17
ISO 37,2 checksum =				17
ISBT128 barcode check characters				77
ISBT128 eye-readable check =				H

Annex 3
Trial components

This section contains information regarding trial components and can only be found on the JPAC website www.transfusionguidelines.org.uk.

Definitions

These definitions are taken from the Blood Safety and Quality Regulations 2005 unless stated otherwise.

Additive solution means a solution specifically formulated to maintain beneficial properties of cellular components during storage.

Allogeneic donation means blood and blood components collected from an individual and intended for transfusion to another individual, for use in medical devices or as starting material or raw material for manufacturing into medicinal products.

Apheresis means a method of obtaining one or more blood components by machine processing of whole blood in which the residual components of the blood are returned to the donor during or at the end of the process.

Autologous donation means blood and blood components collected from an individual and intended solely for subsequent autologous transfusion or other human application to that same individual.

Autologous transfusion means a transfusion in which the donor and the recipient are the same person and in which pre-deposited blood or blood components are used.

Blood means whole human blood collected from a donor and processed either for transfusion or for further manufacturing.

Blood component means a therapeutic constituent of human blood (red cells, white cells, platelets and plasma) that can be prepared by various methods.

Blood component release means a process which enables a blood component to be released from a quarantine status by the use of systems and procedures to ensure that the finished product meets its release specification.

Blood Establishment shall mean any structure or body that is responsible for any aspect of the collection and testing of human blood or blood components, whatever their intended purpose, and their processing, storage, and distribution when intended for transfusion. This does not include hospital blood banks. (EU Directive 2002/98/EC definition).

The four UK Blood Services/Blood Transfusion Services (NHS Blood and Transplant, Scottish National Blood Transfusion Service, Northern Ireland Blood Transfusion Service and the Welsh Blood Service) are Blood Establishments.

Blood product means any therapeutic product derived from human blood or plasma.

Buffy coat means a blood component prepared by centrifugation of a unit of whole blood, and which contains a considerable proportion of the leucocytes and platelets.

Commission means the European Commission.

Cryoprecipitate means a plasma component prepared from plasma, fresh-frozen, by freeze-thaw precipitation of proteins and subsequent concentration and resuspension of the precipitated proteins in a small volume of the plasma.

Cryopreservation means prolongation of the storage life of blood components by freezing.

Deferral means suspension of the eligibility of an individual to donate blood or blood components, such suspension being either permanent or temporary.

Distribution means the act of delivery of blood and blood components to other Blood Establishments, hospital blood banks and manufacturers of blood products, other than the issuing of blood or blood components for transfusion.

Doctor means a registered medical practitioner.

Donor carer means a person who has passed both the written and practical examinations of NHS Blood and Transplant, the Scottish National Blood Transfusion Service, the Northern Ireland Blood Transfusion Service or the Welsh Blood Service in the care of blood donors and who holds a current certificate of competence, awarded by that body, in the care of blood donors.

Emerging infectious disease means a newly recognised, clinically distinct infectious disease, or a known disease whose reported incidence within the past two decades is increasing in a given place or among a specific population (Health Protection Agency definition).

Facilities means hospitals, clinics, manufacturers, and biomedical research institutions to which blood or blood components may be delivered (Commission Directives on haemovigilance/traceability).

Granulocytes, apheresis means a concentrated suspension of granulocytes obtained by apheresis.

Haemovigilance means a set of organised surveillance procedures relating to serious adverse or unexpected events or reactions in donors or recipients, and the epidemiological follow-up of donors.

Health service hospital has the same meaning as in section 128 of the National Health Service Act 1977.

Hospital means a health service hospital or an independent hospital.

Hospital blood bank means any unit within a hospital which stores and distributes, and may perform compatibility tests on, blood and blood components exclusively for use within hospital facilities, including hospital-based transfusion activities.

Imputability means the likelihood that a serious adverse reaction in a recipient can be attributed to the blood or blood component transfused or that a serious adverse reaction in a donor can be attributed to the donation process (Commission Directives on haemovigilance/traceability).

Independent hospital has the same meaning as in Section 2 of the Care Standards Act 2000.

Inspection means formal and objective control to identify problems in accordance with standards adopted to assess compliance with these Regulations.

Inspector means a person appointed by the Secretary of State to carry out inspections pursuant to Regulation 15(10).

Nurse means a registered nurse or registered midwife.

Person responsible for management of a hospital blood bank means:

(a) in the case of a hospital blood bank located in a hospital managed by a health service body, that body, and

(b) in the case of an independent hospital, the registered person.

Plasma means the liquid portion of the blood in which the cells are suspended. Plasma may be separated from the cellular portion of a whole blood collection for therapeutic use as fresh-frozen plasma or further processed to cryoprecipitate and cryoprecipitate-depleted plasma for transfusion. It may be used for the manufacture of medicinal products derived from human blood and human plasma or used in the preparation of pooled platelets, or pooled, leucocyte-depleted platelets. It may also be used for resuspension of red cell preparations for exchange transfusion or perinatal transfusion.

Plasma, cryoprecipitate depleted for transfusion means a plasma component prepared from a unit of plasma, fresh-frozen. It comprises the residual portion after the cryoprecipitate has been removed.

Plasma, fresh-frozen means the supernatant plasma separated from a whole blood donation or plasma collected by apheresis, frozen and stored.

Platelets, apheresis means a concentrated suspension of blood platelets obtained by apheresis.

Platelets, apheresis, leucocyte depleted means a concentrated suspension of blood platelets, obtained by apheresis, and from which leucocytes are removed.

Platelets, recovered, pooled means a concentrated suspension of blood platelets, obtained by processing of whole blood units and pooling the platelets from the units during or after separation.

Platelets, recovered, pooled, leucocyte depleted means a concentrated suspension of blood platelets, obtained by processing of whole blood units and pooling the platelets from the units during or after separation, and from which leucocytes are removed.

Platelets, recovered, single unit means a concentrated suspension of blood platelets, obtained by processing of a single unit of whole blood.

Platelets, recovered, single unit, leucocyte depleted means a concentrated suspension of blood platelets, obtained by processing of a single whole blood unit from which leucocytes are removed.

Qualified health professional means:

(a) a doctor

(b) a nurse or

(c) a donor carer.

Quality assurance means all the activities from blood collection to distribution made with the object of ensuring that blood and blood components are of the quality required for their intended use (Directive 2002/98/EC of the European Parliament and of the Council of 27 January 2003).

Red cells means the red cells from a single whole blood donation, with a large proportion of the plasma from the donation removed.

Red cells, apheresis means the red cells from an apheresis red cell donation.

Red cells, buffy coat removed means the red cells from a single whole blood donation, with a large proportion of the plasma from the donation removed. The buffy coat, containing a large proportion of the platelets and leucocytes in the donated unit, is removed.

Red cells, buffy coat removed, in additive solution means the red cells from a single whole blood donation, with a large proportion of the plasma from the donation removed. The buffy coat, containing a large proportion of the platelets and leucocytes in the donated unit, is removed. A nutrient or preservative solution is added.

Red cells in additive solution means the red cells from a single whole blood donation, with a large proportion of the plasma from the donation removed. A nutrient or preservative solution is added.

Red cells, leucocyte depleted means the red cells from a single whole blood donation, with a large proportion of the plasma from the donation removed, and from which leucocytes are removed.

Red cells, leucocyte depleted, in additive solution means the red cells from a single whole blood donation, with a large proportion of the plasma from the donation removed, and from which leucocytes are removed. A nutrient or preservative solution is added.

Reporting establishment means the Blood Establishment, the hospital blood bank or facilities where the transfusion takes place that reports serious adverse reactions and/or serious adverse events to the Competent Authority (Commission Directives on haemovigilance/traceability).

Reporting year means the period of 12 months ending on 31 March.

Responsible person in relation to a Blood Establishment means the person who has been designated pursuant to Regulation 6 as the responsible person for that Blood Establishment.

Serious adverse event means any untoward occurrence associated with the collection, testing, processing, storage and distribution, of blood or blood components that might lead to death or life-threatening, disabling or incapacitating conditions for patients or which results in, or prolongs, hospitalisation or morbidity.

Serious adverse reaction means an unintended response in a donor or in a patient associated with the collection or transfusion of blood or blood components that is fatal, life-threatening, disabling, or which results in, or prolongs, hospitalisation or morbidity.

Site means any premises at which a Blood Establishment carries out any of the activities listed in Regulation 3(2), but shall not include any premises not owned or managed by the Blood Establishment at which blood is collected, or any mobile blood collection unit.

Statistical process control means a method of quality control of a product or a process that relies on a system of analysis of an adequate sample size without the need to measure every product of the process.

Tissue Establishment means a tissue bank or a unit of a hospital or another body where activities of processing, preservation, storage or distribution of human tissues and cells are undertaken. It may also be responsible for procurement or testing of tissues and cells (Directive 2004/23/EC).

Traceability means the ability to trace each individual unit of blood or blood component derived thereof from the donor to its final destination, whether this is a recipient, a manufacturer of medicinal products or disposal, and vice versa (Commission Directives on haemovigilance/traceability).

Validation means the establishment of documented and objective evidence that the particular requirements for a specific intended use can be consistently fulfilled.

Washed means a process of removing plasma or storage medium from cellular products by centrifugation, decanting of the supernatant liquid from the cells and addition of an isotonic suspension fluid, which in turn is generally removed and replaced following further centrifugation of the suspension. The centrifugation, decanting, replacing process may be repeated several times.

Whole blood means a single blood donation.

Explanation of terms used in the eighth edition

The terms 'Blood Service'/'Blood Transfusion Service'/'Transfusion Service' refer to Blood Establishments. The terms 'Blood Centre'/'Blood Transfusion Centre'/'Transfusion Centre' refer to the sites from which the services of the Blood Establishments are delivered.

The reason for such diversity is that in 2012 the four Blood Establishments in the UK use slightly different titles.

Abbreviations

2,3-DPG	2,3-diphosphoglycerate
Ab	antibody
ADP	adenosine diphosphate
Ag	antigen
AS	additive solution
ASCII	American Standard Code for Information Interchange
ATMP	advanced therapy medicinal product
ATP	adenosine triphosphate
BCSH	British Committee for Standards in Haematology
BS(I)	British Standards (Institution)
BSQR	Blood Safety and Quality Regulations 2005
CD-P-TS	European Committee on Blood Transfusion
cfu	colony-forming unit
CJD	Creutzfeldt-Jakob Disease
CMV	cytomegalovirus
Codabar	American Blood Commission Codabar Barcode
CPA	Clinical Pathology Accreditation
CT	cellular therapy
DAT	direct antiglobulin test
DIN	donation identification number
DMSO	dimethyl sulphoxide
DNA	deoxyribonucleic acid
EC	European Commission
ECV	extra-corporeal volume
EDQM	European Directorate for the Quality of Medicines and Healthcare
EDTA	ethylenediamine tetra-acetic acid
EFI	European Federation for Immunogenetics
ELISA	enzyme-linked immunosorbent assay
EN	European Standard

EU	European Union
F	factor (as in FVIII:C, FXIIa etc.)
FACT	Foundation for the Accreditation of Cellular Therapy
FBC	full blood count
FCXM	flow cytometric crossmatch
G-CSF	granulocyte colony stimulating factor
GMP	good manufacturing practice
Hb	haemoglobin
HBcAb	hepatitis B core antibody
HBsAg	hepatitis B surface antigen
HBV	hepatitis B virus
HCMV	human cytomegalovirus
HCV	hepatitis C virus
HDFN	Haemolytic Disease of the Fetus and Newborn
HIV	human immunodeficiency virus
HLA	human leucocyte antigen
HNA	human neutrophil antigen
HPA	Health Protection Agency OR human platelet antigen (depending on context)
HPC	haematopoietic progenitor cell
HTA	Human Tissue Authority
HTLA	high-titre low-avidity
HTLV	human T cell lymphotropic virus
HTR	haemolytic transfusion reaction
IAT	indirect antiglobulin test
ICCBBA	International Council for Commonality in Blood Banking Automation
ICSH	International Council for Standardization in Hematology
ID	identification
IgG	immunoglobulin G
IgM	immunoglobulin M
IL	interleukin
IMP	investigational medicinal product
ISBT	International Society of Blood Transfusion

ISBT 128	International Society of Blood Transfusion 128 barcode
ISO	International Organization for Standardization
IU	international unit
IUT	intrauterine transfusion
JACIE	Joint Accreditation ICT Europe and EBMT
JPAC	Joint UKBTS/HPA Professional Advisory Committee
LISS	low ionic strength (salt) solution
MCV	mean cell volume
MHRA	Medicines and Healthcare products Regulatory Agency
NAT	nucleic acid amplification techniques
NEQAS	National External Quality Assurance Scheme
NHSBT	National Health Service Blood and Transplant
NIBSC	National Institute for Biological Standards and Control
NIBTS	Northern Ireland Blood Transfusion Service
pCO_2	partial pressure of carbon dioxide
PCR	polymerase chain reaction
Ph Eur	European Pharmacopoeia
pO_2	partial pressure of oxygen
RBC	red blood cell(s)
RCI	Red Cell Immunohaematology
RNA	ribonucleic acid
SaBTO	Advisory Committee on Safety of Blood Tissues and Organs
SAC	Standing Advisory Committee
SACBC	Standing Advisory Committee on Blood Components
SACIT	Standing Advisory Committee on Information Technology
SACTCTP	Standing Advisory Committee on Tissues and Cellular Therapy Products
SAE	serious adverse event
SAGM	saline adenine glucose mannitol additive solution
SAR	serious adverse reaction
SHOT	Serious Hazards of Transfusion scheme
SNBTS	Scottish National Blood Transfusion Service
SOP	standard operating procedure

SSOP	sequence-specific oligonucleotide probe
SSP	sequence-specific primer
TBV	total blood volume
TC	therapeutic cells
TGF-β	transforming growth factor beta
TNF-α	tumour necrosis factor alpha
TRALI	transfusion-related acute lung injury
TTI	transfusion-transmitted infection
UK	United Kingdom
UKBTS	United Kingdom Blood Transfusion Services
vCJD	variant Creutzfeldt-Jakob Disease
vWf	von Willebrand factor
WBC	white blood cell(s)
WHO	World Health Organization
WNV	West Nile Virus

Index

Names of blood components are in **bold** type. Page numbers relating to tabulated information are in *italics*.

ABO grouping
    anomalous 222–3, 224
    antisera 188–96
    of blood 222–3
    of donations 216
    fully automated 222
    indication on dispatch note 68
    indication on labels 316, 317–18
    mismatched transplant testing 226
    molecular genetics 231
    in the presence of autoantibodies 224
    quality control 216
acute coronary syndrome 56
additive solutions 135
advanced therapy medicinal product (ATMP) 293
adverse events/reactions
    EU directives 7, 8, 14
    febrile transfusion reactions 249
    haemolytic transfusion reactions (HTRs) 218
    International Haemovigilance Network categories for 54–6
    recording and reporting 21–2, 42, 51–2
    serious/severe 14, 21, 56, 281
    suspected bacterial contamination of blood components 176
    tissue and organs 281
    TRALI 234, 244, 248–9, 253, 254
    transfusion reactions 176, 178, 218, 249
air embolism 56
air quality 61, 274
alarm systems 44, 144, 296
alert/action levels, processing facilities 175
allergic reactions 55, 56
alloadsorption techniques 223
alloantibodies
    in anomalous ABO grouping 222
    detection in the presence of autoantibodies 224–5
alternative assay testing, definition *161*
ambient temperature 61
amnion donation 266
amotosalen ultraviolet treatment 57
anaphylaxis 56
Anatomy Act 1984 8

anonymity/confidentiality of donors 27, 28, 46, 263, 290
antecubital fossa 48
anti-A 107, 110, 112, 114
    high-titre testing 218
    performance and evaluation testing *191*
    reference preparations 182, 204, *360*
anti-A,B 183, *191*
    high-titre testing 218
anti-A+B 183
anti-A$_1$ *191*
anti-B 110, 112, 114
    high-titre testing 218
    performance and evaluation testing *191*
    reference preparations 182, 204, *360*
antibodies
    clinically important or significant 183
    complex mixtures 223
    detection 202, 203, 252
    extended phenotyping 223, 224
    to hepatitis B *157*
    heterospecific 197
    to HFA 224
    HLA specific 241–4
    HTLA 223–4
    identification 182, 218, 223–4
    irregular 183, 201–2
    to LFA 224
    to malaria 164
    polyclonal 189
    quantification and titration for HDFN 225–6
    screening 182, 217
    to syphilis 163
    titration in ABO mismatched transplant 226
    weak 203, 209
    see also alloantibodies; autoantibodies
Antibody Quantification Quality Assurance Scheme 225
anti-C *191, 192*
    reference preparation *360*
anti-c *192*, 225
    reference preparation *360*
anti-C3c 196
anti-C3d 211

INDEX

anti-C4b 210–11
anti-C4d 197, 211
anti-Ch 223, 224
anti-Co^a 224
anticoagulant
    during apheresis procedures 30, 37, 44
    labelling 357
    weight 60
anticoagulant flow indicator 44, 144
anti-Co^b 224
anti-complement 196, 198, 210
anti-Cs^a 223
anti-C^w *193*
anti-D
    fetal typing 230, 231
    partial 188
    performance and evaluation testing *191*
    in potency testing 208–9, 210
    quantification and titration for HDFN 225
    reference preparations 182, 204, *360, 361*
    weak 188
anti-E *192*
    reference preparation *360*
anti-e *192*
anti-Fy3 224
anti-Fy^a *193*, 210
anti-Fy^b *194*
antigen profile 188
anti-HBc 164–5
anti-HBs 165
anti-HCV 163
anti-HIV 1+2 or HIV 1+2 Ag/Ab combination 162
anti-HLA-Bw4 and anti-HLA-Bw6-specific
    reagents 244, 245
anti-HTLV I/II 163
anti-human globulins
    batch release testing 197–9, 206–12
    manufacturing requirements 196–7
    performance evaluation 197, 206–12
    polyspecific 210–12
    potency testing 197–8
    reference preparations 182, 198, 204, *360*
anti-IgG
    chequerboard titration studies 209–10
    essential component of anti-human globulin
        reagents 196
    potency testing 197–8, 208–9
    reference reagent 209
anti-In^b 224
anti-Jk^a *194*

anti-Jk^b *194*
anti-K *193*, 210
anti-k 224, *193*
anti-Kn^a 223
anti-Kp^b 224
anti-Le^a *196*
anti-Le^b *196*
anti-light chain activity 196
anti-Lu^b 224
anti-M *195*
anti-malaria serum, reference preparation *362*
anti-McC^a 223
anti-measles serum, reference preparation *361*
antimicrobial medication, donors 31
antimicrobial processing, terminal 272, 274, 275–6
anti-N *195*
anti-P$_1$ *195*
anti-parvovirus B19 serum (IgG), reference
    preparation *361, 362*
anti-poliovirus serum, reference preparations *361*
anti-Rg 223, 224
anti-rubella serum, reference preparation *361, 362*
anti-S *194*
anti-s *195*
anti-S1^a 223
anti-*T.cruzi* 164
anti-Toxoplasma serum, reference preparations *362*
anti-U 224
anti-varicella zoster, reference preparation *361, 362*
anti-Vel 224
anti-Yk^a 223
anti-Yt^a 224
anxiety 52
apheresis
    adverse events/reactions 54–6, 289–90
    anticoagulant 30, 37, 44
    blood flow 49
    citrate toxicity 37
    complications 54–6
    donors 25, 246, 290, 292
    equipment 43–4, 144–5, *146*
    frequency of procedures 29
    HPC collection 291, 292
    information leaflets 27
    labelling of donations 42
    mandatory screening tests 156, *156*
    preparation of pack 48
    sample collection 50–1
    serious adverse events/reactions 56
    venepuncture 48, 49

apheresis *continued*
   volume of blood processed per pass 38
   volume collected 29
archiving
   of documents 17
   of results 215, 229
   of samples 179, 187, 268, 296, 299
arm cleansing 48, 168
arterial puncture 54
aseptic processing facilities 274
aseptic techniques, for collection 43, 49
ASII text files 341
aspirin 25, 32
'assumed negative' procedure, not acceptable 215
audit, Blood and Tissue Establishments 21
autoantibodies
   alloantibody detection in the presence of 224–5
   in anomalous ABO grouping 222
   management of patients with 225
autologous donations
   status label 339
   stem cell 161
autologous serum eye drops 173
automated apheresis machines, specifications 43–4
automated microbial detection system 170
automated test systems 216, 220
avidity determination 206

B cell depleted, definition 294
bacterial *see* microbial
barcodes
   on blood group labels 316–17
   Codabar ABC 311–12
   on component labels 323
   converting to ISBT 306
   decodability grade 315
   dimensions 312
   ISBT 128 309–11
   printing requirements 312–13, 329
   quiet zone 315
   reading and interpretation 308–9
   specifications 307, 312–13
base label 307, 326, 327, 330–1
batch identification number label 307
batch numbers, recording 43, 49
batch of reagent, definition 183
batch of tests, definition 183
batch/pool identification number label 326
beds 53
biohazards
   microbiologically reactive 159
   quarantine storage 65
   safe disposal 66
   status label 320, 321–2, 338
   status labelling *337*
   tissue 279
biological variability 71
biotinylated Brad-5 (Bio-Brad-5), reference preparation *361*
blood
   anticoagulation during collection 49
   donation procedure 49–50
   for neonates, antibody screening 217
   rare phenotypes 223, 231
   uniform labelling 306–24
blood bags, evaluation and inspection 43
   see also blood packs
blood collection sets, inspection 43
blood collection teams
   designated clinical lead 39, 41
   evaluation protocol 149, 150, 152
Blood Compliance Report 14
blood components *see* components
blood derivatives, dispatch information (Protocol 000002) *343*, 346, *347*
blood donations *see* donations
Blood Establishments
   consultant with responsibility for donors 25
   guidelines for the use of DNA/PCR techniques 228–9
   message envelope 342
   quality management system 12–13
   regulation 6–8, 9
   standard operating procedures (SOPs) 57
blood filter 144
blood flow 49, 50
blood flow monitor 44, 144
blood group genotyping 223, 231–2
   reference preparations *361*
blood group labels 306, 316–22
blood group molecular typing 230–2
blood group polymorphisms 231, *232*
blood grouping kit, definition 183
blood grouping reagents
   definition 183
   potency test methods 205–6
   potency testing 190, *191–6*
   reference preparations 203–4
blood grouping system, definition 183
blood grouping tests, components 71

blood groups
    classifications *318*
    ISBT 128 label codes 306
blood packs
    evaluation 145–53
    labelling 306, 352–6
    positioning 48
    preparation 48–9
blood pressure measurement 33
blood products, minimum release criteria *217*
Blood Safety and Quality Regulations 2005 7, 13, 46, 154, 221
blood tests, donors 33–5
blood typing antisera 188–96
blood volume 33
    monitoring 50
bone donation 281–2
bone marrow
    collection facilities 291–2
    donors 289, 290–1
    HPCs 286
    mandatory microbiological testing 173
bovine serum albumin, manufacturing requirements 202
bovine spongiform encephalopathy (BSE) 202
    see also Creutzfeldt-Jakob Disease (CJD)
British Bone Marrow Registry 290
British Committee for Standards in Haematology (BCSH) 35, 221
British Standards
    BS 15000 *10*
    BS EN 13612:2002 185, 189, 197
    BS EN 13640:2002 185, 189, 197
    BS EN 13641:2002 185
    BS EN 18113:2011 188
    BS EN 375 183
    BS EN ISO 14971:2012 185
    BS EN ISO 18113:2009 236, 243
    see also European Standards
buffy coat enriched, definition 294
buffy coat layer 213

C3d 196
cadaver donors *see* deceased donors
Caldicott Report (1997) *10*, 226
calibration 18
capacity, for consent 27–8, 265
cardiac disease, donors 35
cardiovascular tissue, retrieval and processing 282–3
Care Quality Commission *10*

cause of death, deceased donors 265
CD34 selected, definition 294
CE mark 57, 144, 155, 224, 239, 357, 358
Chagas' disease *see Trypanosoma cruzi*
change control 16
check character 366–7
checksums 309, 311, 315, 366
chequerboard titration studies 209–10
children, capacity for consent 28
chlorhexidine 283
citrate anticoagulants 37, 44
cleaning/disinfection of processing facilities 176
Clinical Pathology Accreditation (CPA-UK) Standard for Medical Laboratories 221
clinicians, information for 60
clonogenic assays 299
closed system, definition 62–3
Clostridium sp., marker resistant organism 275
CMV (cytomegalovirus) *156, 157,* 165, *298*
    reference preparation *362*
Co(a–) 231
coagulation factors 142, *143*
    standard preparations *364*
    see also factor
Co^b antibody specificity 189
Codabar system 306, 307, 311–12, 355–6
codes
    assigned by SACIT 334
    components 323–4
    status codes *337*
collection facility, identification 319, 332
collection volume preset device 44, 144
colour coding
    labels 314, 316
    reagents 186, *188*
Committee for Medicinal Products for Human Use (CHMP) 5
compensation 52
complaints 20
complement 183, 196, *212*
    see also anti-complement
complement dependent cytotoxicity 241
completion of donation 50, 54
complex antibody mixtures 223
components
    additional tests for donors 34
    allogeneic HLA 234
    apheresis collection 43–4, 50–1
    codes 323–4
    discard limits 58

components *continued*
   discard procedure 66
   dispatch acknowledgement (Protocol 000004) *343*, 348, *349*
   dispatch information (Protocol 000001) *343*, *344–5*
   donation by apheresis 50–1
   evaluation and manufacture 131–53
   fate information (Protocol 000005) *349*, *350*, *351*
   frequency of tests 60
   from high titre group O donors 218
   identification numbers 213
   for intrauterine use, neonates and infants under 1 year 107–30
   investigation of suspected bacterial contamination 176
   irradiated 128–30
   labelling 64, 306–24, 322–4
   leucocyte depletion 70–1
   monitoring tests 58–60
   non-clinical use 67
   non-conforming 65, 66, 67
   novel, evaluation 131–53
   packaging for transit 68
   pathogen inactivation 57
   processing 61–3
   recall 69, 172
   release 66, 67
   returned 65
   shelf life 63–4
   specifications 57–8, 70–130
   storage *see* storage
   traceability 69
   transportation 67–9
   weight:volume ratio 60
   withdrawal criteria 58, 72
computer software
   apheresis equipment 144
   for release of tested components 215
computer-based system, unavailability 66, 215
concatenation requirements for ISBT 128 309–10, 329
confidentiality
   of donor information 27, 28, 46, 263, 290
   of trial data 147
confirmatory testing *159*, 161, 168
confirmed positive samples, definition 171
congenital hypofibrinogenaemia 144
consent
   additional 187
   for bone marrow donation 290
   for cord blood donation 291
   Human Tissue Act 2004 8
   informed 27–8, 30
   for non-clinical use 264
   for tissue donation 263–4
consultant with responsibility for donors 25, 41
continuous flow analyser 225
contracting goods and services 19
control codes, within Codabar 311–12
control samples 155
control sera
   for HNA typing 251
   for HPA antibody detection 255
copper sulphate haemoglobin screen 34
cord blood
   collection 292
   collection facilities 291–2
   definition 288, 293
   donors 291
   HPCs 286, 288, 291, 293
   mandatory microbiological screening 173
   testing 246, *298*, 299
corneal transplantation 284
Coroner, permission to retrieve tissue 264
Council of Europe 3
Creutzfeldt-Jakob Disease (CJD) 32, 270
   see also bovine spongiform encephalopathy
critical consumables, labelling 357–9
cryoprecipitate, leucocyte depleted 100–2
cryoprecipitate, methylene blue treated and removed, leucocyte depleted 104, 122–4
cryoprecipitate, novel, evaluation 142, *143*, 144
cryoprecipitate pooled, leucocyte depleted 102–4
cryopreservation
   cardiovascular tissue 283
   definition 294
   HPCs 296–7
   labelling of products 327
   skeletal tissue 282
   tissue 277
cryosupernatant, novel, evaluation 142, *143*
culture media, for environmental monitoring 175
cytotoxicity
   complement dependent 241
   crossmatch requirements 244
   scores 236

D antigen
   molecular typing to confirm 230
   partial 188, 223

weak 188, 216, 217, 223
D grouping
    anomalous 222–3, 224
    blood 216, 222–3
    fully automated 222
    indication on dispatch note 68
    indication on labels 317–18
    molecular typing 230
    quality control 217
    variants, molecular testing 232
data analysis, processing facilities 39, 175
data identifiers, in ISBT 128 309
Data Protection Act (1998) 226, 261
date bled, printed on label 319, 321, 322
date of manufacture 185–6
death, related to donation 56
deceased donors
    family, duty of care to 267, 268
    medical and behavioural history 265
    neonatal and infant 157, 267
    reconstruction 271
    tissue 267, 271–2
defects, blood packs 43, 48
deferral
    autologous pre-deposit donations 35
    clinical trials 30
    Hb concentration 34
    medications 25, 31–2
    travel history 32
delayed bleeding 54
density enriched, definition 294
deviations, components and tissue 20
dextrose and dextran, labelling 357
direct antiglobulin test (DAT) 220, 222
disability, related to donation 56
'discard', status label 338
discard limits, components 58
discard procedure
    components 66
    HPCs 304
disseminated intravascular coagulation (DIC) 144
distribution
    quality management system 20
    tissues 279
diversion donation 49, 170
dizziness and fainting 27, 33, 52
DNA
    avoidance of contamination 228–9
    preparation 238
DNA-based HLA typing 235, 238–9, 298–9

DNA/PCR techniques 228–9, 231, 238
'do not use after', on labels *317*, 319, 358
Do^a antibody specificity 189
documentation
    accompanying samples in transit 68
    for laboratory test procedures 155
    for look-back investigations 181
    quality management system 17
    transfusion-transmitted infection reports 178
Dombrock typing 230
donation care pathway 51
donation identification number
    barcoded/eye-readable 64, 315, 332–3
    checking 43
    general structure 313–16
    indication on dispatch note 68
    on labels 306, 326
    manual recording 333
    tissue 326, 331–3
    unique 306, 313
donation number *see* donation identification number
donation record
    linked to donor 154, 213
    signing 30
donations
    ABO/D grouping 215–17
    adverse events/reactions 51–2, 56
    allogeneic 46
    antibody screening 217
    apheresis 50
    autologous 35, 46, 268
    bone 281–2
    completion 50, 54
    DAT positive 220
    diversion 49, 170
    frequency 29
    genomic or nucleic acid testing 187
    from high titre group O donors 218
    infectious 178–81
    labelling 42, 213
    microbiological screening 156–69
    non-clinical use 67, 187
    pre-donation sampling 63
    preparation of venepuncture site 48, 49
    records 42
    repeat 291
    testing 187, 213–21
    volume 29–30, *36*
    volume monitoring 50

donation-specific information, on status label 336
donor lymphocyte infusions (DLI) 288
donor samples *see* samples
Donor Selection Guidelines 26, 28, 31, 260, 263
donor transplant coordinator 263
donors
    advice and counselling 54, 267–8, 290
    age limits 28
    anonymity/confidentiality 27, 28, 46, 263, 290
    anxiety 52, 53
    apheresis 25, 246, 290, 292
    arm cleansing 48, 168
    autologous 35, 46, 268, 290
    beds for 53
    blood tests 33–5
    blood volume monitoring 50
    bone marrow 289, 290–1
    care and selection 25–35, 39
    clinical trials 30
    compensation 52
    completion of donation 50, 54
    component 34
    consent 27–8, 30, 187, 263–4, 290, 291
    coping strategies 53
    DAT positive 220
    deceased 157, 267, 271
    deferral 25, 30, 31–2, 34, 35
    DNA-based HLA typing of stem cell donors 246
    duty of care 26
    eligibility 17
    exclusion criteria 32–3, 161
    extra-corporeal volume 25, *36*
    female 249
    first-time 216
    fitness to donate 26
    fluids before donation 52–3
    genetically determined conditions 31
    hazardous occupations/hobbies 26
    health assessment 25, 26, 47, 290
    high titre group O 218
    HLA/HPA testing 245–9
    HNA testing 253
    HPA typing 258
    HPC 289, 290–1
    identification 42, 47, *280*
    illiterate 28
    immune plasma 35
    information to be obtained from 47
    information to be provided to 27, 46–7, 51
    lifestyle exclusions 265
    medical history 27, 30–2, 47, 264–5, 290
    on medications 31–2
    microbiological screening 156–69
    must not be left unattended 41, 49, 53
    opportunity to ask questions 47
    option to change mind 46
    physical examination 33
    points of care 51, 52
    prion-associated disease 32–3
    records 42
    referrals 263
    reinstatement after non-specific screen reactivity *167*, 167–8, *169*
    reporting illness after donation 30
    returning 33
    risks to 27
    screening 53
    seating 53
    selection for tissue banking 263–9
    signature 30, 47
    testing 266–7
    third party information 28
    tissue-specific considerations 266
    transfusion-transmissible infections 32–3, 178–81
    travel history 32
    unpaid volunteers 25
    weight limits 33
double red cell donations, frequency 29
Duffy typing 232
duty of care
    to donors 26
    to family of deceased donors 268

electronic data 42, 226, 341–51
electronic delivery mechanisms 341
electronic signature 226
e-mail 341
emergency use only, label 320, 322
encephalopathies *see* bovine spongiform encephalopathy; Creutzfeldt-Jakob Disease
endotoxin, reference preparation *362*
enucleation 284
envelope 341, 342, *343*
environmental control, of sessional venue 40
environmental monitoring, of processing facilities 174–6
enzyme treatment, control 207
enzyme-treated cells 187, 188
equipment
    log 214

    maintenance 214
    manufacturers' instructions 214
    quality management system 16
    validation 214
errors, minimising risk of 42
Estimation of Fetomaternal Haemorrhage 221
ethical approval 187
ethidium bromide 228
ethnicity 224
ethylenediamine tetra-acetic acid (EDTA) 213
EU Directives
    2001/20/EC 287
    2001/83/EC 7, 287
    2002/98/EC 7
    2003/63/EC 287
    2004/23/EC 8, 260, 286, 290
    2004/33/EC 7
    2005/28/EC 287
    2005/61/EC 7
    2005/62/EC 7, 13
    2006/17/EC 8, 260, 286
    2006/86/EC 8, 260, *280*, 286
    2009/108/EC 185, 189, 197
    93/42/EEC 8
    98/79/EC 7–8, 182, 185, 188, 203
    blood related 5, 6–7
    Good Manufacturing Practice Directive 6
    legally binding 1, 3
    product liability 1
    quality management system 12–13
    tissue and cells 8–9
European Blood Inspection System *11*
European Federation for Immunogenetics (EFI) 234, 238
European Foundation for Quality Management Self-Assessment *10*
European Medicines Agency (EMEA) 5
European Pharmacopoeia 4–5
European Standards
    BS EN 375 183
    harmonized 182, 357
    see also British Standards
European Union 3–5
ex vivo expanded, definition 294
exclusion from donation 32–3, 161
expiry date
    amendment 72
    definition 183
    on labels 317, 319, 327, 339–40
external reports, serious untoward incidents 22–3

extra-corporeal volume (ECV) 25, 29–30, *36*
eye retrieval 284
eye-readable information 154, 213, 222, 312, 315, *316*, 329, 333, 340

FACT-JACIE 173, 286, 299
factor ATIII *364*
factor II *364*
factor II, IX and X concentrate *364*
factor IX *364*
factor IXa *364*
factor V *364*
factor VII *364*
factor VIIa *364*
factor VIII 141, *364*
factor VIII:C 95, 96, 98, 102
factor X *364*
factor XI *364*
factor XIII 100, 102, 122, *143*, *364*
false negative samples, definition 172
false positive samples, definition 171
Family and Law Reform Act 1969 28
fax procedures 226
febrile transfusion reactions 249
FEIBA concentrate *364*
female blood donors, HLA screening 249
fetal amniocytes, HPA typing 258
fetal calf serum, manufacturing requirements 202
fetal typing 230, 231
fetomaternal haemorrhage, testing 221
fibrinogen
    from cryoprecipitate 100, 102
    WHO International Standard *364*
fibronectin, from cryoprecipitate 100, 102
filters, labelling 357
fire exits 40
first-time donors 216
Fisher's notation for Rh genotype 182
'fit for clinical use (Rh D not specified)', status label 337
fitness to donate 26
flooring, non-slip 40
flow cytometric crossmatch (FCXM) 244–5
    reference preparations *361*
flow cytometry 222
fluid transfer sets, labelling 357
fluorescein isothiocyanate (FITC) 245
Food and Drug Administration regulations 187, *188*
'for *in vitro* R&D only', status label 338
freeze-drying 277

freezing 277
fresh frozen plasma, leucocyte depleted 95–7
fresh frozen plasma, methylene blue treated and removed, leucocyte depleted 97–100
fresh frozen plasma, neonatal use, methylene blue treated and removed, leucocyte depleted 119–21
fresh frozen plasma, novel, evaluation 141–2
fresh serum for complement activity, definition 183
ftp transfers 341
full blood count 34

gamma irradiation 276, 282
gene manipulated, definition 294
general practitioner 26, 265
genetic haemochromatosis 31
genetically determined conditions 31
genotyping, blood group 223, 231–2
    reference preparations 361
glaucoma 284
glycerolisation 277
Good Automated Manufacturing Practice (GAMP) 6, 11, 43, 144
Good Manufacturing Practice Directive 6
good manufacturing practice (GMP) 13, 185
goods inward inspection, evaluation protocol 148, 150, 152
gowning 175
grafts see tissue
granulocyte agglutination test 252
granulocyte colony stimulating factor (G-CSF) 290
granulocyte immunofluorescence test 252
granulocyte-bound immunoglobulins, controls for direct tests 254
granulocytes
    cell panel for HNA antibody detection 250
    immunology 250–4
    irradiated 129, 130
    paternal 253
    preparation 250
    transfusions 244
granulocytes, apheresis 92–3
granulocytes, pooled, buffy coat derived, in platelet additive solution and plasma 93–5
Guide to the Preparation, Use and Quality Assurance of Blood Components 13
Guide to Quality and Safety Assurance for Human Tissues and Cells for Patient Treatment 260, 299
Guide for Validation of Automated Systems in Pharmaceutical Manufacture 11
Guidelines for Blood Grouping and Antibody Testing in Pregnancy 221
Guidelines for the Blood Transfusion Services in the United Kingdom 203
Guidelines for Compatibility Procedures in Blood Transfusion Laboratories 221

haematocrit 29, 30, 38, 109, *136*
haematoma 54
haemoglobin
    acceptable lower limits 25, 33
    estimation of concentration 33–4
    screening 47
haemoglobinopathies 31, 219
haemolysis, complication of apheresis 56
haemolysis measurements, red cell components 71
Haemolytic Disease of the Fetus and Newborn (HDFN)
    antibody quantification and titration for 225–6
    fetal typing 230, 231
    scope of donor testing for 221
haemolytic transfusion reactions (HTRs) 218
haemopoietic progenitor cell (HPC) components
    adverse events/reactions 289–90
    clonogenic assays 299
    cryopreservation 296–7
    definitions 293–394
    disposal 304
    HLA typing 298–9
    labelling 299–301, *302–3*
    microbiological testing 297, *298*
    packaging 299
    processing standards 294–5
    records 304–5
    release 301
    sampling 299
    sterility 299
    storage 295–7
    testing 297–9
    transportation 303
haemopoietic progenitor cell (HPC) donors 289, 290–1
haemopoietic progenitor cells (HPC)
    ABO and RhD typing 299
    collection facilities 291–2
    Designated Individual 290, 292, 295
    European Union Directives/guidelines 286–7
    histocompatibility, donor selection and microbiology documents 288
    HPC-A 290–1, 293
    HPC-C 291, 293

HPC-M 290–1, 293
Human Tissue Authority guidelines 288
international standards 286
policy and procedure requirements 289
processing facility 289
reference sources 286–8
terminology 288
thawing and infusion 303
therapeutic cells (TC) 288, 293–4
third party agreements 289
UK legislation 288
hand hygiene 169
hazardous occupations/hobbies 26
Hb *see* haemoglobin
HbS screening 219
HBsAg screening 161, 162
HCMV (human cytomegalovirus) *156, 157,* 165, *298*
reference preparation *362*
Health and Safety at Work Act 19743 40
Health Protection Agency (HPA) syphilis quality control preparation 163
Healthcare Inspectorate Wales 10
healthcare worker, blood injury 270
heart valves and vessels 282
hepatitis A virus, reference preparation *361, 363*
hepatitis B virus (HBV)
core antigen (HBc) 164–5
HBV NAT 166
reference preparations *361, 362, 363*
screening protocols 219, *298*
surface antigen (HBsAg) *157,* 161, 162, 165
hepatitis C virus (HCV) *157,* 165
reference preparations 361, *362, 363*
high frequency antigens (HFA) 224
high titre group O donors 218
high titre low avidity (HTLA) antibodies 223–4
high-efficiency particulate air (HEPA) filters 274
histocompatibility testing, EFI standards 234
HIV
anti-HIV 1+2 or HIV 1+2 Ag/Ab combination 162
HIV NAT 166
mandatory testing *156, 157*
reference preparations *362, 363*
HL7 341
HLA
antibodies 234, 239–44, *242*
antibody characterisation by complement dependent cytotoxicity 241–4
antigens, defined by serological typing 240
DNA typing reagents 238–9
general concepts 234–5
genes and gene products, testing 239
phenotyping 236, 237
reagents 235–9
reference preparations *361*
sensitised patients 244
serological typing reagents 236–7
terminology and nomenclature 235, 239
typing 236
HNA
antibody detection 252
antibody investigation 253
nomenclature 251
sensitised patients 244
typing methods 252
typing reagents 250
hobbies, hazardous 26
'hold' label 320
hospital blood banks
compliance reports 6
computer systems 341
envelope identifiers 342
Good Automated Manufacturing Practice 13
quality management system 14
regulation 6–8
HPA
antibodies 255, 257, 258, 259
nomenclature 256
patient card and information leaflet 259
reference preparations 256
typing 255, 257, 258
HPC, apheresis (HPC-A), definition 293
HPC cord blood (HPC-C), definition 293
see also cord blood
HPC marrow (HPC-M), definition 293
see also bone marrow
human cells, safety precautions 228
human growth factors 292
human leucocyte antigens *see* HLA
human neutrophil antigens *see* HNA
Human Organ Transplants Act 1989 8
human platelet antigens *see* HPA
human source material 187, 243, 250, 255
human T-cell lymphotropic virus (HTLV) I/II *156, 157,* 163, 297
Human Tissue Act 2004 8, 9, 187, 260
Human Tissue Authority (HTA) *11,* 260, 281, 288
Human Tissue Code Database 334
human tissue products *see* tissue

Human Tissue (Quality and Safety for Human Application) Regulations 2007 9, 260
Human Tissue (Scotland) Act 2006 8, 260
hygiene 15, 39, 68, 168–9, 274

icterus 72
identification number, unique 306
identification of donors 42
IgG
    sensitisation 223
    tests for 206
    weak antibody preparations 198, 209
IgM antibodies, detecting 196, 197, 206
immediate container, definition 183
immune plasma 35
immune refractoriness, diagnosis 234
Immuno Polymorphism Database (IPD) 257
immunoglobulin-coated red cells 230
immunohaematology
    donation testing 213–21
    patient testing 221–6
in vitro diagnostic medical devices 7–8, 22
in vitro studies, novel components 135–7, 138, *139*, 141–2, *142*
in vivo studies, novel components 135, 137, 138, 139–40, 143–4
incapacity, related to donation 56
incidents *see* adverse events/reactions
inconclusive sample, definition *161*
indeterminate samples, definition 171
indirect autoglobulin test (IAT) 223, 225
infants
    deceased tissue donors 157
    donor/donation criteria 72, 107
infectious disease, transfusion-transmissible 32–3, 178–81
initial reactive samples, definition *161*, 171
in-line air detector 44, 144
instructions for use
    anti-human globulin reagents 198–9
    DNA typing reagents 238–9
    rabbit complement for use in HLA serology 237
    reagent red cells 200
    reagents 188
    see also manufacturer's instructions
instruments, single-use 270, 284
International Blood Group Reference Laboratory (IBGRL) 223
International Council for Commonality in Blood Banking Automation (ICCBBA) 325, 326, 332, 334

International Council for Standardization in Hematology/International Society of Blood Transfusion (ICSH/ISBT) reference preparations 204
International Granulocyte Immunology Workshops 251
International Haemovigilance Network categories for donor adverse events 54–6
International Society of Blood Transfusion (ISBT) 232, 306
    Working Party on Automation and Data Processing 325
    Working Party on Information Technology 341
international standards
    HPCs 287
    ISO 10993 354–5, 358–9
    ISO 15223-1 *354*
    ISO 17799 *11*
    ISO 3826 62, 353, *354*
    ISO 9000 2000 *12*
    ISO 9001 2008 *12*
    preparations 204
International Standards for Cellular Therapy, Product Collection Processing, and Administration 173
International Standards for Cord Blood Collection, Processing and Release for Administration 173
interpreters 28
intrauterine transfusion
    donor/donation criteria 72, 107
    HbS screening 219
intravenous access 49, 292
intravenous solutions, labelling 357, 358
inventory
    of biohazard samples 66
    control 214, 296
    of storage category/areas 65
    of test procedures 155
investigational medicinal product (IMP), definition 293
iron supplementation 29
irradiation
    components 128–30
    tissue 276, 282
ISBT 128
    barcoding 309–11
    check character calculation 366–7
    labelling of tissue products 325–40
    manufacturers' catalogue and lot numbers 356, 359
    nationally assigned codes 310–11, 329–30
    product codes 325

ISBT 128 *continued*
   Technical Specification 306, 307, 325

Joint Accreditation ICT Europe and EBMT (JACIE) assessment standard 12
Joint UKBTS/HPA Professional Advisory Committee (JPAC) 341
   accountability and structure 1–2
   recommendations from SACBC 131
Js(b–) 231

k– 231

labels/labelling
   alternative 320–2
   barcoded 64 see also barcodes
   biohazards 66
   blood and blood components 307–8
   blood collection sets 43
   blood component packs 352–6
   blood group 316–22
   colour coding *188*, 314, 316
   components 64, 306–24, 322–4
   critical consumables 357–9
   cryoprecipitate, leucocyte depleted 100–1
   cryoprecipitate, methylene blue treated and removed, leucocyte depleted 122–3
   cryoprecipitate pooled, leucocyte depleted 103
   cryopreserved products 327
   deceased donor tissue 271–2
   donation/donor identification 42, 64
   eye-readable 64, 154, 213, 222, *316*, 333, 340
   Food and Drug Administration regulations 187, *188*
   fresh frozen plasma, leucocyte depleted 96
   fresh frozen plasma, methylene blue treated and removed, leucocyte depleted 98–9
   fresh frozen plasma, neonatal use, methylene blue treated and removed, leucocyte depleted 120
   future developments 64
   granulocytes, apheresis 92–3
   granulocytes, pooled, buffy coat derived, in platelet additive solution and plasma 94
   HLA reagents 236
   HPCs 299–301, *302–3*
   irradiated components 129
   layout and information content 352–5
   machine-readable 306
   minimum acceptable height 312
   non-conforming components 67
   physical characteristics 308, 327–8
   plasma, cryoprecipitate depleted, leucocyte depleted 105
   platelets, apheresis, leucocyte depleted 86
   platelets, pooled, buffy coat derived, leucocyte depleted 84
   platelets for intrauterine transfusion, leucocyte depleted 125
   platelets for neonatal use, leucocyte depleted 127
   platelets in additive solution and plasma, leucocyte depleted 88–9
   platelets in additive solution, leucocyte depleted 90–1
   positioning 327, *328*
   pre-printed 64, 314
   printing requirements 312–13, 314–15, 316, 329
   quality management system 19
   rabbit complement for use in HLA serology 237
   reagent red cells 200
   reagents 187, *188*
   red cells for exchange transfusion, leucocyte depleted 112–13
   red cells for intrauterine transfusion, leucocyte depleted 108
   red cells for neonates and infants, leucocyte depleted 115
   red cells in additive solution for neonates and infants, leucocyte depleted 117
   red cells in additive solution, leucocyte depleted 77
   red cells, leucocyte depleted 75
   red cells, thawed and washed, leucocyte depleted 81–2
   red cells, washed, leucocyte depleted 79–80
   separated samples 222
   specifications 306–24
   subsidiary packs 64
   tissue and tissue products 278–9, 325–40
   transit containers 68
   whole blood for exchange transfusion, leucocyte depleted 110
   whole blood, leucocyte depleted 73
laboratories
   Clinical Pathology Accreditation (CPA) accredited 298
   external quality assurance schemes 251, 257, 289
   red cell immunohaematology (RCI) 221
   staff seniority policy 226

legislation, for Blood and Tissue Establishments and hospital blood banks 6–9
leucocyte antibody screening 35
leucocytes
    counting 60
    crossmatching 244–5
    depletion 70–1
lifestyle risks 265
lighting 40
lipaemia 72
liquid nitrogen 277
liver biopsy 143
liver transplant recipients 143
living donors *see* donors
local anaesthesia, for venepuncture 49
location, of sessional venue 40
look-back investigations 180–1, 268
low frequency antigens (LFA) 224
low ionic strength solution (LISS) 203
Lu(b−) 231
lymphocytes, preparation 250
lymphocytotoxic crossmatch 244

malaria testing 164, *298*
mandatory microbiological testing
    archived samples 268
    conformity with 71
    of donors/donations 156–69
manipulated components, definition 293
manual methods, potency testing 205
manual override system 44, 144
manual tests, review 220
Manufacture of Sterile Medicinal Products 175
manufacturer, definition 183
manufacturers' catalogue and lot numbers 356, 359
manufacturers' instructions
    adherence to 213
    apheresis machines 43, 44
    reagents and test kits 155
    SOPs 41
    weighing devices 50
    see also instructions for use
manufacturing processes, quality management system 18–19
Medical Devices Directive 8
medical history
    deceased donors 265
    donors 27, 30–2, 47, 264–5, 290
    patients 222
Medicines and Healthcare products Regulatory Agency (MHRA) 6, 22, 39, 44, 52
Mental Capacity Act 2005 27
mental competence 27–8, 264
message
    content 341
    protocols 341, 342–51
    structures 341–2
methylene blue 57
microbial contamination
    investigation of 176
    platelet components 170
microbial contamination, reagents 186
microbial culture 170
microbial infection, donors 35
microbial processing, terminal 272, 275–6
microbiological testing
    to assess staff hand hygiene 169
    cardiovascular tissue 283
    of donors' arms 169
    for donors/donations 156–69
    environmental monitoring of processing facilities 174–6
    retrospective 180, 187
    standards for 172–4
microplate methods 155, 183, 205–6
mixed-field reactions, unexpected 222–3
mobile donor sessions 39
molecular screening algorithm 159, *159*, *160*
molecular typing, blood groups 230–2
monoclonal antibodies 184, 188, 196, 223, 252
monospecific blood grouping reagent, definition 184
multi-component test systems, HLA reagents 236
'must be sterilized', status label 338
Mycobacterium tuberculosis 283

National Evidence-Based Guidelines for Preventing Healthcare-Associated Infections in NHS Hospitals 168
National External Quality Assessment Scheme 58
National Genetic Reference Laboratory 229
National Institute for Biological Standards and Control (NIBSC) 232
    standards available 360–5
National Patient Safety Agency (NPSA), 22
near misses 22
    see also adverse events/reactions
negative sample, definition *161*
neonates
    antibody screen for blood for 217

deceased tissue donors 157
donor/donation criteria 72, 107
HbS screening for blood for 219
neonatal alloimmune neutropenia (NAIN) 253, 254
neonatal alloimmune thrombocytopenia (NAITP) 259
nerve injury 55
NetCord-FACT 173, 286, 289, 291, 297
NHS Blood and Transplant Authority (NHSBT) 2
   Human Tissue Transport Box 284
   Tissue Retrieval Site Risk Assessment 284
NHS Estates Health Technical Memoranda 270
NHS Litigation Authority risk management assessment programme 12
NHS National Services Scotland 2
NHS Quality Improvement Scotland 10
NHSBT/HPA transfusion-transmitted infection surveillance scheme 180
nitrile gloves 228
Nomenclature for Factors of the HLA System 239
non-reactive samples, definition 161
non-steroidal anti-inflammatory drugs 25
Northern Ireland
   Blood Transfusion Service 2
   devolved government 5
Northern Ireland Department of Health, Social Services and Public Safety 10
Northern Irish Blood Transfusion Centre 180
'not for transfusion' label 320, 321
nucleic acid techniques (NAT)
   HBV NAT 166
   HIV RNA 166
numbers, unusable or missing 314
nurses, training and certification 41

obesity 33
occupations, hazardous 26
ocular tissue, retrieval and storage 284
open system, definition 63
organ transplants, antibody quantification 225
osteochondral allografts 282

package insert *see* instructions for use
packaging
   HPC components 299
   tissue 278–9
painful complications 55
papain, reference preparations 182, 204, *360*
Paroxysmal Cold Haemoglobinuria
   investigations 222

pathogen inactivation, blood components 57
pathogen inactivators, labelling 357
patient samples *see* samples
patient-designated components 71
patients
   anomalous grouping 222–3, 224
   HLA/HPA testing 245–9
   HNA testing 253–4
   HPA typing 258–9
   medical history 222
   multiply transfused 230
   non-Caucasoid 259
   testing 221–6
PCR *see* DNA/PCR techniques
performance evaluation 185, 189–90
pH measurements 72
phenotyping
   additional 218–19, 224
   extended 223, 224
   HLA 236, 237
   rare phenotypes 223, 231
   red cells 218–19
phlebotomy 49–50
phycoerythrin 245
physical examination of donors 33
pipettes, semi-automatic 205
plasma
   citrate levels *37*, 44
   donors 25, 29, 34
   immune 35
   pathogen inactivation 57
   see also fresh frozen plasma
plasma, cryoprecipitate depleted, leucocyte depleted 105–6
plasma and RBC reduced, definition 294
plasma components
   donor/donation criteria 72
   leucocyte count not required 71
   novel, evaluation 141–4
   pathogen inactivation 57
   weight:volume ratio 60
plasma reduced, definition 294
plasmapheresis, frequency of donation 29
Plasmodium sp. *156, 157*
platelet additive solution, labelling 357
platelet components
   donation criteria 71
   microbiological screening 170, *171*
   novel, evaluation for transfusion 137–40
   visual inspection 85, 87, 89, 91, 128

platelet count 25, 34, 71
platelet pheresis, frequency of donation 29
platelets
   cell panel for HPA antibody detection 255
   discard limits *58*
   drugs affecting 32
   immunology 255–9
   irradiated 129, 130
   paternal 259
   refractoriness 234, 247, 259
   weight:volume ratio 60

platelets, apheresis, leucocyte depleted 86–7

platelets, pooled, buffy coat derived, leucocyte depleted 83–5

platelets for intrauterine transfusion, leucocyte depleted 124–6

platelets for neonatal use, leucocyte depleted 126–8

platelets in additive solution and plasma, leucocyte depleted 88–90

platelets in additive solution, leucocyte depleted 90–2

platelet-specific antibodies 234
polyclonal antibodies 189
polymerase chain reaction *see* DNA/PCR techniques
polyspecific anti-human globulin reagent, definition 184
polyspecific blood grouping reagent, definition 184
pool identification number 331–3
pooling, tissues 276
positive diluent control 222
positive reactions, unwanted 197, 198–9, 207
positive sample, definition *161*
post-mortem
   examination 265, 271
   sampling 176, 267
post-result entry verification 220
potency testing
   anti-complement 198
   anti-human globulin 197–8
   blood grouping reagents 190, *191–6*
   manual and microplate blood grouping reagents 205–6
   recommended titration techniques
   tube or microplate methods 190
potency titre 184, 205
power failure 44, 144
pregnancy testing *298*
premises
   component processing 61
   health and safety 40
   hygiene 39
   for preparation of components 39
   quality management system 15
   venue selection 39–40
preservation methods 277
preservative 186
pre-transfusion testing 222–5
PRINCE2 *12*
printing
   eye-readable information 312–13, 329
   on-demand 64, 314–15, 316
prion filters 57
prion-associated disease 32–3, 202, 270
process monitoring tests 58
process simulations 175–6
processing facilities
   aseptic 274
   environmental monitoring 174, 174–6
processing team, evaluation protocol 149, 151, 152
product label, for tissue 326, 334–5
proficiency testing 19
protein C 142
   WHO International Standard *364*
protein S 142
   WHO International Standard *364*
proteolytic enzyme preparations, manufacturing requirements 202
prozone, definition 184
purchased material and services, control 43–4

Quality Assurance Manager 52
quality assurance pack conformance inspection 148, 150, 152
quality control 155, 216, 219
quality management system
   adverse events/reactions 21
   audit 21
   Blood Establishments 13
   change control 16
   collection procedure 17–18
   complaints 20
   documentation 17
   donor eligibility 17
   equipment 16
   good manufacturing practice 13
   hospital blood banks 14
   improvements 20
   labelling 19
   manufacture 18–19

non-conformance 20–1
overview 6
personnel and organisation 14–15
premises 15
proficiency testing 19
recall 21
record keeping 16
release 19
serious untoward incidents 22–3
storage and distribution 19–20
tissue and cell establishments 14
traceability 20
validation 17
in vitro diagnostic medical devices 22
quality monitoring algorithm *59*
quality monitoring, evaluation protocol 148, 150, 153
quarantined material 278
components 65
status labelling 330, 337, 339

rabbit complement 237–8, 241
rare phenotypes 223, 231
RBC reduced, definition 294
reagent control, definition 184
reagent lymphocytes, HLA phenotype 241, 243
reagent red cells
antigens expressed 200–1
identification/screening 200–2
IgG coated 202
immediate container label 200
instructions for use 200
manufacturing guidelines 199–202
specifications and testing 199–200
for use in ABO and RhD grouping 200
for use in antibody screening 200
reagents
dispatch information (Protocol 000003) *343*, *346, 347, 348*
filtering 186
for HLA serology/typing 235–9
instructions for use (package insert) 250
labelling 187, *188*
manufacture 182–212
monoclonal anti-D reagents 223
reference preparations 182
serological testing 205–12
testing by manufacturer 186
real-time quantitative PCR (RQ-PCR) 231
recall procedures 21, 69, 172, 281
reconstruction, deceased donors 271

records
electronic 42
HPC components 304–5
permanent, continuous 65
quality management system 16, 17
'Red Book'
development 1
inclusion of novel components or processes 131
scope 57
red cell components
expiry dates 72
haemolysis measurements 71
irradiated 130
microbiological testing *172*
neonatal 72
novel, evaluation 134–7
validation of preparation processes 71
red cell immunohaematology (RCI) laboratories 221
red cell volume 60
red cells
complement sensitised 210, *212*
discard limits *58*
immunoglobulin-coated 230
immunohaematology
donation testing 213–21
patient testing 221–6
incubation 207
novel, evaluation for transfusion *136*
pathogen inactivation 57
phenotyping 218–19, 223
preparation of suspensions 207
prion filters 57
selection of weak IgG antibody preparations 209
tests with anti-human globulin reagents 209
red cells for exchange transfusion, leucocyte depleted 112–14
red cells for intrauterine transfusion, leucocyte depleted 107–9
red cells for neonates and infants, leucocyte depleted 114–16
red cells in additive solution for neonates and infants, leucocyte depleted 117–19
red cells in additive solution, leucocyte depleted 77–9
red cells, leucocyte depleted 75–7
'red cells not for clinical use', label 320, 321
red cells, thawed and washed, leucocyte depleted 81–3
red cells, washed, leucocyte depleted 79–81

reference preparations
   definition 184
   enzymes 202
   guidelines and recommendations 182
   serological 202, 203–4, 251, 257, *360–3*
   traceability 203
refreshments, provision 40
refrigeration devices 277
   see also storage
regulation, for Blood and Tissue Establishments and hospital blood banks 6–9
Regulation and Quality Improvement Authority (Northern Ireland) *10*
reinstatement of donors, after non-specific screen reactivity *167*, 167–8, *169*
release
   authorised by designated person 65
   concessionary 67
   criteria *217*
   HPC components 301
   inspection of blood bags 43
   quality management system 19
   tested components 66–7, 215
   tissue 269, 278
repeat donations 291
repeat reactive samples, definition *161*
results
   archiving 215, 229
   authorising 226
   recording 154, 155
   reporting 155, 215, 226
resuscitation equipment 39
returned components, status and storage 65
reverse grouping 222
'RhD neg – fit for clinical use', status label 338
'RhD pos – fit for clinical use', status label 337–8
Rh genotype, Fisher's notation 182
Rh grouping
   indication on labels 317–18
   molecular typing 230
   in the presence of autoantibodies 224
RhD *see* D antigen
RHD genes 232
RHD zygosity
   molecular typing 230
RHD/SRY plasma DNA sensitivity standard *361*
riboflavin ultraviolet treatment 57
risk
   assessment 222, 270
   management 9, *12*, 185

road traffic collision, within 24 hours of donation 56
root cause analysis 281
Rules and Guidance for Pharmaceutical Manufacturers and Distributors 2007 39, 61, 185, 274

Safe Management of Healthcare Waste 66
safety-related defects, reporting 48, 52
saline
   labelling 357
   specifications 203
samples/sampling procedures
   acceptance 221
   antibody identification/screening 200–2
   archiving 179, 187, 268, 296, 299
   collection 49
   cryopreservation 296–7
   diversion donation 49, 170
   donor reinstatement 167, *167*, *169*
   environmental monitoring 174–6
   HPCs 299
   identification 154, 213, 215
   investigation of suspected bacterial contamination of blood components 176
   labelling 213, 222
   maternal 267
   post-mortem 176, 267
   pre-donation 63
   for pre-transfusion testing 221–5
   reagents 186–7
   reconciliation 213
   red cell immunohaematology 213–14
   retained and stored 186
   separate 222
   standards for microbiological screening 172–4
   storage and preparation 154, 213
   validation of procedures 60
   visual inspection 213, 221
sclera 284
Scotland, devolved government 5
Scottish National Blood Transfusion Service 2
screening tests
   for donors/donations 53, 155
   for tissue and stem cells *157*
sealing, of blood packs and apheresis harnesses 62
seating 40, 53
'see outer container for product status', status label 339
self inspection 21
sensitivity, definition 184
sequence-specific oligo-nucleotide probes (PCR-

SSOP) 238
sequence-specific primers 238
seroconversion 180
Serious Adverse Blood Reactions & Events
    (SABRE) 21
serious adverse events/reactions 14, 21, 56, 281
    see also adverse events/reactions
Serious Hazards of Transfusion (SHOT) 21–2, 180
serious untoward incidents, reporting 22–3
serological preparations, standard *360–3*
serological reference library 231
serological tests, grading 189
serology screening algorithms 158, *156, 157, 159*
serum albumin 34
service contracts *see* third party agreements
shelf life
    components 63–4
    definition 184
    see also storage
shipping containers, tissue 279
short form unit identifier 307, 310, 329–30, 336
signatures
    on dispatch notes 68–9
    of donors 30, 47
    electronic 226
    separated samples 222
single-test system, platelet components 170
skeletal tissue
    from deceased donors 282
    retrieval and processing 281–2
skill mix 41
skin
    cleansing 168–9
    preparation for venepuncture 48
    retrieval and processing 283
SNBTS National Microbiology Reference Unit 180
Specification and Use of Information Technology (IT)
    Systems in Blood Transfusion Practice 221
specificity, definition 184
specificity testing
    anti-human globulin reagents 197
    blood grouping reagents 190, *191–6*
    HPA typing kits 258
S–s–U– 231
stability testing 185, 189, 197
staff
    consultant grade 226
    hand hygiene 169
    refreshments 40
    seniority policy 226
    training 41
'stand-alone' consumable medical devices,
    labelling 357–9
standard operating procedures (SOPs)
    apheresis process quality monitoring 58
    change control 16
    closed system blood pack assembly 62
    compiling 57
    compliance with 41
    component release 66
    donation testing 213
    evaluation of blood packs 152
    labelling 48–9
    patient testing 221
    pre-donation sampling 63
    tests 215
    tissue banking 260
standards
    for inspection, licensing, accreditation or
        certification *10–12*
    National Institute for Biological Standards and
        Control (NIBSC) *360–4*
Standards for the Medical Laboratory 12
Standing Advisory Committee on Blood
    Components (SACBC) 131, *132, 133, 134*, 324
Standing Advisory Committee on Information
    Technology (SACIT) *132, 134*, 310, 323, 332, 334,
    341, 342
Standing Advisory Committee on Tissues and
    Cellular Therapy Products (SACTCTP) 334
statistical process monitoring methodology, for
    leucocyte depletion 70
status codes *337*
status labels
    tissue 326–7, 335–9
    for use in the 'blood group label' location 320–2
stem cells
    DNA-based HLA typing of donors 246
    donor reinstatement 168, *169*
    samples, testing *157*
    standards for microbiological screening 173
sterilisation, terminal 275–6
sterility assurance level (SAL) 275–6
still births 157
stock
    archive samples 268
    release to 66, 70
    return to 65, 111, 113
    rotation 65
    see also storage

storage
- **cryoprecipitate, leucocyte depleted** 101
- **cryoprecipitate, methylene blue treated and removed, leucocyte depleted** 123
- **cryoprecipitate pooled, leucocyte depleted** 103–4
- **fresh frozen plasma, leucocyte depleted** 96–7
- **fresh frozen plasma, methylene blue treated and removed, leucocyte depleted** 99
- **fresh frozen plasma, neonatal use, methylene blue treated and removed, leucocyte depleted** 120–1
- **granulocytes, apheresis** 93
- **granulocytes, pooled, buffy coat derived, in platelet additive solution and plasma** 95
- HPC components 295–7
- irradiated components 130
- ocular tissue 284
- **plasma, cryoprecipitate depleted, leucocyte depleted** 106
- **platelets, apheresis, leucocyte depleted** 87
- **platelets, pooled, buffy coat derived, leucocyte depleted** 84–5
- **platelets for intrauterine transfusion, leucocyte depleted** 125
- **platelets for neonatal use, leucocyte depleted** 127
- **platelets in additive solution and plasma, leucocyte depleted** 89
- **platelets in additive solution, leucocyte depleted** 91
- procedures 65–6
- quality management system 19–20
- red cells, evaluation during 137
- **red cells for exchange transfusion, leucocyte depleted** 113
- **red cells for intrauterine transfusion, leucocyte depleted** 108–9
- **red cells for neonates and infants, leucocyte depleted** 115–16
- **red cells in additive solution for neonates and infants, leucocyte depleted** 117–18
- **red cells in additive solution, leucocyte depleted** 78
- **red cells, leucocyte depleted** 75–6
- **red cells, thawed and washed, leucocyte depleted** 82
- **red cells, washed, leucocyte depleted** 80
- samples 154
- test kits and reagents 155
- **whole blood for exchange transfusion, leucocyte depleted** 110–11
- **whole blood, leucocyte depleted** 73–4

storage areas 15, 64, 65
storage temperature
- components 63, 64
- permanent, continuous records 65

syphilis antibodies
- mandatory testing 156, *163*
- reference preparations *362*

T cell depleted, definition 294
temperature
- ambient 61
- continuous monitoring and recording 277
- during transportation 67, 68
- *see also* storage temperature

tendon injury 55
teratogens 31
test equipment and procedures
- general specifications 155
- validation and monitoring 214–15

test kits *see* reagents
test monitor 184, *219*
test results *see* results
tested components, release 215
testing
- additional 156, 215, 218–19
- to assess donors' arm cleansing 169
- to assess staff hand hygiene 169
- blood group molecular typing 230–2
- blood grouping reagents 189–96
- categories 215
- confirmatory 161
- **cryoprecipitate, leucocyte depleted** 102
- **cryoprecipitate, methylene blue treated and removed, leucocyte depleted** 123–4
- **cryoprecipitate pooled, leucocyte depleted** 104
- donor reinstatement 167, *167*, *169*
- fetomaternal haemorrhage, 221
- **fresh frozen plasma, leucocyte depleted** 97
- **fresh frozen plasma, methylene blue treated and removed, leucocyte depleted** 99–100
- **fresh frozen plasma, neonatal use, methylene blue treated and removed, leucocyte depleted** 121
- **granulocytes, apheresis** 93
- **granulocytes, pooled, buffy coat derived, in platelet additive solution and plasma** 95

Haemolytic Disease of the Fetus and Newborn (HDFN) 221
HLA typing and serology 234–49
investigation of suspected bacterial contamination of blood components 176
plasma, cryoprecipitate depleted, leucocyte depleted 106
platelet components, microbial screening 170
platelets, apheresis, leucocyte depleted 87
platelets, pooled, buffy coat derived, leucocyte depleted 85
platelets for intrauterine transfusion, leucocyte depleted 125–6
platelets for neonatal use, leucocyte depleted 128
platelets in additive solution and plasma, leucocyte depleted 89
platelets in additive solution, leucocyte depleted 91
reagent red cells 199
red cell components, novel *136*
red cells for exchange transfusion, leucocyte depleted 114
red cells for intrauterine transfusion, leucocyte depleted 109
red cells for neonates and infants, leucocyte depleted 116
red cells in additive solution for neonates and infants, leucocyte depleted 118
red cells in additive solution, leucocyte depleted 78
red cells, leucocyte depleted 76
red cells, thawed and washed, leucocyte depleted 82
red cells, washed, leucocyte depleted 80
resolution of anomalous grouping 222–3, 224
standards for microbiological screening 172–4
whole blood for exchange transfusion, leucocyte depleted 111
whole blood, leucocyte depleted 74
see also mandatory microbiological testing
tetanus antitoxin, standard preparation *362*
thalassaemias 31
thawing, frozen components 96, 97, 100, 121, 303
therapeutic cells (TC) 288, 293–4
third party agreements 266, 270, 284, 289
third party information 28
thrombin, WHO International Standard *364*
thrombophilias 31
thrombophlebitis 55

thrombotic thrombocytopenic purpura 144
tissue
    autologous donation 268
    bacteriostasis and disinfection 272–3
    consent for donation 263–4
    deceased donor 157, 265, 271–2
    discard 264, 268, 270, 278
    distribution 279
    donation identification number 331–3
    donor reinstatement 168, *169*
    EU Directives 8
    labels/labelling 271–2, 325–40, 335–9
    microbiological screening 156, 157–9, *159*
    minimum donor/recipient data to be kept *280*
    notification of serious adverse events and reactions 281
    pool identification number 331–3
    pooling, not permitted 276
    preservation methods 277
    processing 274–84
    processing solutions 277
    recall 281
    release criteria 269, 278
    retrieval 271–2
    samples, testing 266–7
    standards for microbiological screening 172–3
    storage 277–8
    temperature/time relationships *273*
    terminal microbial processing 272, 275–6
    traceability 263, 280
    transportation 272
Tissue Establishments
    audit (self inspection) 21
    audit trail 263
    data protection/confidentiality 261
    Designated Individual 260
    designated medical officer 263
    donor identification *280*
    donor referral policy 263
    donor selection 263–9
    equipment 270
    minimum donor/recipient data set to be kept by *280*
    notification of serious adverse events and reactions 281
    policies and protocols 266
    post-mortem sampling 267
    processing and storage facilities 270
    purchased materials and solutions 270
    reference documents for 260

Tissue Establishments *continued*
    regulatory environment 6, 7–9, 260
    third party agreements 266, 270, 284
toilet facilities 40
total serum protein 34
toxic substances, safe disposal 239
traceability
    biohazards 66
    components 66, 69
    EU Directives 7
    HPCs 304
    quality management system 20
    reagents 155, 187, 214
    reference preparations 203
    tissue 263, 280
transfused patients, molecular typing 230
transfusion reactions
    febrile 249
    haemolytic 218
    suspected bacterial contamination 176, 178
    see also adverse events/reactions
transfusion refractory patients 244
transfusion-related acute lung injury (TRALI) 234, 244, 248–9, 253, 254
transfusion-transmissible infections 32–3, 178–81
transfusion-transmitted infection 32, 178–81
transit containers 67
    see also transportation
transplant physician 295
transportation
    from Blood Establishments to hospital blood banks/users 68–9
    from collection site to processing centre 68
    of components 67–9
    cryoprecipitate, leucocyte depleted 102
    cryoprecipitate, methylene blue treated and removed, leucocyte depleted 124
    cryoprecipitate pooled, leucocyte depleted 104
    fresh frozen plasma, leucocyte depleted 97
    fresh frozen plasma, methylene blue treated and removed, leucocyte depleted 100
    fresh frozen plasma, neonatal use, methylene blue treated and removed, leucocyte depleted 121
    granulocytes, apheresis 93
    granulocytes, pooled, buffy coat derived, in platelet additive solution and plasma 95
    HPCs 303
    ocular tissue 284
    plasma, cryoprecipitate depleted, leucocyte depleted 106
    platelets, apheresis, leucocyte depleted 87
    platelets, pooled, buffy coat derived, leucocyte depleted 85
    platelets for intrauterine transfusion, leucocyte depleted 126
    platelets for neonatal use, leucocyte depleted 128
    platelets in additive solution and plasma, leucocyte depleted 89–90
    platelets in additive solution, leucocyte depleted 91–2
    red cells for exchange transfusion, leucocyte depleted 114
    red cells for intrauterine transfusion, leucocyte depleted 109
    red cells for neonates and infants, leucocyte depleted 116
    red cells in additive solution for neonates and infants, leucocyte depleted 118–19
    red cells in additive solution, leucocyte depleted 78–9
    red cells, leucocyte depleted 76–7
    red cells, thawed and washed, leucocyte depleted 83
    red cells, washed, leucocyte depleted 80
    tissue 271–2
    whole blood for exchange transfusion, leucocyte depleted 111–12
    whole blood, leucocyte depleted 74–5
    written procedures 68
Transposition Guide: How to Implement European Directives Effectively 5
travel history of donors 32
trend analysis, processing facilities 175
trial components 368
Trypanosoma cruzi 156, *157*, 164
tube indirect autoglobulin test (IAT) 223, 225
tumour cell depleted 294
two-test system, platelet components 170
typeface 187

UK Rare Red Cell Exchange 223
ultraviolet treatment 57
undiluted, definition 184
unequivocal reaction, definition 184
United Kingdom
    Blood Services/Blood Transfusion Services 2
    devolved government 2, 5

regulatory environment 1–8
United Kingdom Blood Services Forum 2
United Kingdom Blood Transfusion Services (UKBTS)
   computer systems 341
      labelling requirements 306
      message envelope 341
      standards for electronic data interchange 341–51
unmanipulated components, definition 293
unwanted positive reactions, testing for 197, 198–9, 207
usage limitations, on blood group labels *318*, 319, *320*
UV light, safety precautions 228

validation
   of blood packs 62, 63
   of component preparation process 63
   of component release 66, 155
   of component storage areas/equipment 65
   definition 184
   of HNA typing kits 252
   need for 17
   of prion filters 57
   process simulations 175–6
   of sampling procedures 60
   of storage conditions 65
   of terminal sterilisation 276
   of test equipment and procedures 155, 214–15
variant Creutzfeldt-Jakob Disease (vCJD) 32
   see also bovine spongiform encephalopathy; Creutzfeldt-Jakob Disease
vasovagal episodes 52, 55
Vel− 231
Velindre NHS Trust 2
venepuncture 48, 49, 292
venesection, medical 31
venous access 49, 292
venting, prohibited 62
venue, for donor sessions 39–40
verification, definition 184
visual audible alarm 44, 144
visual inspection
   of platelet components 85, 87, 89, 91, 126, 128
   of reagents 183, 187
   of samples 213, 221
volume
   apheresis 44
   blood processed per pass *38*
   of donations 29–30, *36*
   see also blood volume; extra-corporeal volume; weight:volume ratio

von Willebrand factor 100, 102, 122, 141, 142
   WHO International Standard *364*
V^w antibody specificity 189

waiting area 53
Wales, devolved government 5
washing facilities, for staff 41
waste disposal areas 15, 41
water quality 203
web page downloads 341
weight:volume ratio, components 60
Welsh Blood Service 2
Welsh Bone Marrow Donor Registry (WBMDR) 290
West Nile Virus (WNV) *156*, *157*, 166
whole blood
   frequency of donation 29
   weight:volume ratio 60
whole blood for exchange transfusion, leucocyte depleted 109–12
whole blood, leucocyte depleted 73–5
workflow 40
working standards 360–4
   anti-HBc 164
   anti-HCV 163
   anti-HIV 162
   HBsAg 162
World Health Organization
   Expert Committee on Biological Standardization 39
   guidelines and recommendations 2–3
   international reference reagents 182, 251, *364*
   Nomenclature Committee for Factors of the HLA System Report 235, 239
   Nomenclature for Factors of the HLA System 235, 239
World Marrow Donor Association Accreditation Programme *11*
Wr^a 189

Xg^a 189

Yt^a 189, 231

Notes